SOFTWARE QUALITY ASSURANCE

A Guide for Developers and Auditors

Howard T. Garston Smith

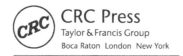

CRC Press
Taylor & Francis Group
Boca Raton London New York

CRC Press is an imprint of the
Taylor & Francis Group, an **informa** business

Contents

Part 2: The Process

Part 4: Appendices

For Faith

*After 25 years of happily
married life, our joy to-
gether deepens with each
passing day.*

1 John 4:9

About the Author

Howard Garston Smith graduated with a BSc in Chemistry at Queen Mary College, London, in 1968 and joined Upjohn Ltd as an analytical chemist. After graduating with an MSc in Pharmaceutical Chemistry from London University in 1971 and spending two years in analytical research and Quality Review at Glaxo Laboratories, Greenford, he joined Pfizer Ltd, Sandwich, rising to become Chief Analyst, Quality Control, in 1982.

During the following years he gained extensive experience in BASIC and FORTRAN programming, writing nearly 100,000 lines of code associated with laboratory automation and information management systems. He was an early practitioner of software quality assurance and computer-related systems validation in the regulated pharmaceutical environment. He has since been appointed Software Quality Assurance Auditor for the European region of Corporate Information Technology within Pfizer, responsible for the evaluation of the engineering quality of all business, commercial and technical software prior to purchase and installation. He has wide experience in auditing and advising software vendors throughout the United Kingdom, the United States, Canada and continental Europe.

He is a Chartered Chemist, Fellow of the Royal Society of Chemistry and Qualified Person under European Union Directives'

Medicines Regulations. He has lectured at Interphex and is a member of the United Kingdom Good Automated Manufacturing Practices (GAMP) Forum under the auspices of the International Society for Pharmaceutical Engineering.

Previously, he published "Automation in HPLC Analysis" in *Manufacturing Chemist* (Volume 53, No. 11—November 1982).

Acknowledgments

The author would like to express his gratitude to

- **Mr. Jonathan Cronk**, formerly Director of Corporate Information Technology (CIT), European Region of Pfizer and **Mr. Steve Woodcock**, presently Business Manager, CIT Europe, for their kind permission to write about the experiences gained in the course of his employment by Pfizer Limited as a Software Quality Assurance Auditor.

- **Dr. Robert Thomas** of Pfizer Ltd for advice on aspects of company law mentioned in chapter 3.

- **The British Standards Institution** of 389 Chiswick High Road, London, W4 4AL, UK, for kind permission to reproduce figure 5.9 and associated extracts from version 3.0 of *The TickIT Guide*, and to quote from the ISO standards 8402 and 9000-3 in the introduction and in chapter 6, respectively. Complete editions of *The TickIT Guide* and ISO standards can be obtained from the above address.

- **Knight Features**, the UK agents of United Feature Syndicate Inc., for permission to reproduce one of the Dilbert cartoons (figure I.3).

- **The Massachusetts Institute of Technology** on behalf of the **W. Edwards Deming Institute** for kind permission to reproduce figure 1.2 and extracts from *Out of the Crisis* by W. Edwards Deming in chapter 1. *Out of the Crisis* is published by MIT, Center for Advanced Educational Services, Cambridge, MA 02139, and is copyright 1986 by the W. Edwards Deming Institute.

- **Mr. Joseph Richardson,** Customer Services Director of S & S International, producers of the *Dr. Solomon's Anti-Virus Toolkit* suite of software, and **Mr. Russell Hobby** of Second Sight UK Limited, suppliers of the *InVircible* antivirus product, for technical assistance in drafting chapter 13.

- **Mr. Ian Whalley** of Virus Bulletin Limited for kind permission to reproduce the Virus Prevalence Table.

- **The Controller of Her Majesty's Stationery Office** for permission to quote or reproduce from the following Crown Copyright documents:

    1. *Software Quality Standards: the Costs and Benefits—A Review for the Department of Trade and Industry,* a report produced by Price Waterhouse

    2. *Software—A Vital Key to UK Competitiveness,* a report by the Advisory Council for Applied Research and Development

    3. *The STARTS Guide,* a National Computing Centre publication

- **Mr. John Riley** of Reed Publishing Publishing, The Quadrant, Sutton, Surrey, SM2 5AS for kind permission to include sundry quotations from *Computer Weekly.*

- To **John Wiley and Sons of Chichester, England** for permission to reproduce the V model as figure 1.8 and to quote briefly from *Stategies for Software Engineering* by Martin V. Ould, copyright 1990, in chapter 3.

- To **Mr. John Foxton of AT&T** for permission to quote the essential structure of the Personal Performance Guide originally published by AT&T.

- To **Addison Wesley Longman Ltd** of Harlow, UK for permission to reproduce figure 5.7 from *Software Inspection* by Tom Gilb and Dorothy Graham (1993).

- To **Intel Corporation (UK) Limited, Pipers Way, Swindon, UK** for performance data on the Intel family of processors (the MIPS speed for the Pentium Pro® processor is not published but for comparative purposes an estimate has been given).

- To **John Murray (Publishers) Ltd 50 Albermarle Street, London W1X 4BD** for permission to adapt John Piper's illustration included in *Church Poems* by John Betjeman © 1981, for use as figure 11.3.

- To **Helicon Publishing Limited**, publishers of the Hutchinson Multimedia Encyclopedia, for permission to reproduce therefrom the cuckoo illustration as figure 3.1.

- To **Random House UK Limited** 20 Vauxhall Bridge Road, London and the **Curtis Brown Group** of London and New York for permission to quote in the Epilogue from *Future Shock* by Alvin Toffler, published in 1970 by The Bodley Head.

- To the Standards Department of the **Institute of Electrical and Electronic Engineers** at Piscataway, NJ, USA, for permission to quote from ANSI/IEEE standard 610.12-1990 in the Glossary of Terms. The ANSI/IEEE standard 610.12-1990 "IEEE Standard Glossary of Software Engineering Terminology" is Copyright © 1990 by the Institute of Electrical and Electronic Engineers Inc. The IEEE disclaims any responsibility from placement or use in the described manner.

- Finally to the many companies it has been his pleasure to visit and from whom he has learned so much of the practical realities of producing quality software in today's frenetic and competitive marketplace.

Preface

Modern science is simply wonderful—it would take
50 people 20 years to make the same mistake a computer
with faulty software can make in a millisecond.

Anon

Information Technology (IT) today affects almost every household and occupation in the civilised world. Computer systems are now at the heart of national defence and government, of every commercial company, manufacturing enterprise and financial institution, becoming the foundation upon which much of life from the international level down to the personal is conducted. Every developed economy is now totally dependant on IT. Linking them all together is a web of wireless-based communications that is steadily integrating business and commerce across geographical and political boundaries. At the heart of IT and of every single computer system lies software—the essential execution steps which give the computer's hardware its ability to perform its intended function. World demand for software is now estimated to be well in excess of $100 billion annually. Software, therefore, is critical to the world's economy and fundamental to life as we now know it.

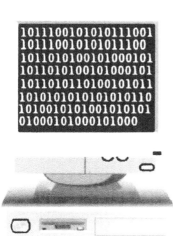

However, herein lies a difficulty. Software, being just a binary pattern of 0's and 1's in a computer's memory, is intangible. It is "soft"—it can neither be seen nor touched. Its ethereal nature makes it hard for people to understand what it is. When it works as intended, it is easy to accept it complacently. But when it fails, both the causes of the failure and the solutions to the ensuing problems seem infinitely remote and far beyond the comprehension of ordinary people.

For the first 20 years or so of the computer revolution, purchasers of software found themselves in a sellers' market and hostage to the computer manufacturers on whom they had come to depend. The defects which accompanied software, over whose functionality users had very little control, were endured with stoical fortitude as an unavoidable inherent characteristic, much like the spots of the leopard.

But times are changing fast. Although world demand for software continues to soar, users of software are tumbling to the realisation that they should not be obliged to accept software that does not do what they require and that is riddled with errors. They are beginning to be as intolerant of these as they are of defects in any of a host of other kinds of consumable merchandise. They are cottoning on to the fact that defects are put into software and that in many application areas they are beginning to have a choice. They are demanding software that does exactly what they want and that has a vanishingly small level of errors, and they want it TODAY! For software developers who have been accustomed to contemptuously treating their customers as a captive market, the game is up. Software quality is becoming to software vendors a burning issue of competitive advantage and ultimately of commercial survival itself.

In industrial terms, the development of software is a new activity. It is labour intensive and still largely carried out by craft level methods. Most programmers have not been professionally trained and do not have an in-depth mathematical background or training in logical thinking. They pick up their skills by experience. This weakness is ironically being exacerbated by the emergence of the

graphical Windows™ environment and the availability of sophisticated development tools. These can be used even by a relative
novice programmer to cobble together an application extremely
quickly. Software houses need to mature from a craft-based labour-
intensive operation to the adoption of a capital-intensive engineering process from which all chance has been eliminated. The scarcity
of niche markets is accentuating competition from which only the
successful will emerge.

*It is to the practical everyday needs of software vendors to
improve the quality of their products, their productivity, profitability and prospects of survival that this book is directed.* The
principles of good software engineering practice, aimed at predictably delivering software of the right quality, on time and within
budget have been established as standards for some years. The
problem for vendors, and especially the small ones of fewer than
20 employees, is to find simple, cost effective, nonbureaucratic
practices that can enable them to quickly achieve substantial compliance with the standards and reap the financial and business benefits that such compliance is demonstrably capable of bringing.

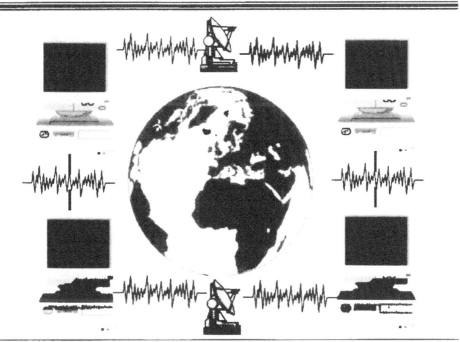

Computers Surrounding a Changing World

Since 1994, I have been a software quality assurance auditor for one of the world's largest multinational pharmaceutical companies. As a major purchaser of software, the company has recognised that the purchase of software involves the obligatory incorporation of the vendor's development process into the company's operations; in other words, that this is unavoidable. Therefore, it aspires to confine its software purchases to those products that can demonstrate a sound pedigree of engineering integrity upon which the business can safely rely. The growth of the software industry over the last few years and the extent of competition between its members has now made this a realistic expectation. Indeed, in the particular realm of its manufacturing operations, now extensively computerised in a variety of ways, the confinement of software to that produced by a quality-assured process is now a legal requirement on which its manufacturing licence depends, and which, therefore, cannot be circumvented.

The fact is, regrettably, that many of the smaller vendors in the software industry worldwide have yet to understand how to develop quality software cost-effectively. They need practical help, not just through a one-off licence purchase, but guidance on improving their software development process towards reaping the financial and business benefits inherent in a quality assured methodology. The role of the auditor is, therefore, not only to assess the vendor's current level of maturity but also to powerfully assist the programming team by recommending down-to-earth practical improvement actions that will lead in this direction.

The use of the word *audit* to describe my visits to vendors is probably too well entrenched to be changed. This is rather unfortunate since it conveys overtones of a negative connotation focusing only on shortcomings, caricatured perhaps with the sinister implications of a police raid! In practice, 90 percent of the time spent during an audit visit is actually *consultancy,* positive practical advice given in the spirit of working as a team with the vendor to raise standards, quality, productivity and profitability. This is the bedrock on which long-term business relationships can be securely founded between purchaser and supplier, to the mutual benefit of both.

I have now conducted over 40 audits of software vendors of all shapes and sizes, in a variety of application areas, and at every level of capability. Twenty years as an analytical chemist in quality control in the pharmaceutical industry has bred into me a familiarity with the disciplines of good manufacturing practice, documentation and control which have extensive parallels with the established principles of good software engineering. The need for specific computer software, unavailable commercially, in an expanding laboratory led me to spend nearly 10 years writing almost 100,000 lines of FORTRAN code to process analytical data on pharmaceutical products. Through hard practical personal experience, I discovered the consequences to which good (and not-so-good!) software engineering practices inexorably lead.

The layout of the book reflects the perspective of the audit/consultancy process, tracing the team's examination of the successive stages of the development life cycle from conception through to maintenance. I share what I have found to be cost-effective and practical activities directed at compliance with standards. When implemented through the documentation of the process in written (either on paper or electronically) procedures these enable a company to quickly assemble a quality management system capable of introducing the benefits of lower support costs and a higher quality product with a reduced level of residual defects. Each element of practical guidance given in this book is presented on the assumption that the software developer reader will relate the recommendations given here to the situation in his or her own company. The layout of the presentation is as follows:

Keep It
Simple

Practical Guidance

(The actual guidance appears here.)

The guidance provided is designed to repeatedly emphasise and reinforce two cardinal principles which I regard as axiomatic for the company's successful migration to a quality culture:

1. Each procedure must represent as far as is possible the best of the existing practice within the concern, so that the quality assurance arrangements are accepted and owned by everyone. Procedures foreign to the organisation and imposed from outside should be kept to the very minimum, since they are likely to be resisted, certainly in the early days.

2. Each procedure should be kept as simple as is humanly possible, directed at preventing a recognisable danger. In this way the cost of the quality assurance arrangements (they do not come free!) will be minimised while their

effectiveness will be maximised, and thus the greater the likelihood of compliance and the greater the benefit to the operation. The "Keep It Simple" logo is intended to be a constant reminder of this.

The emphasis is on practical measures aimed at avoiding the evils of bureaucracy, guidance which has been shown in one company after another to promote a predictable engineered software development process and consequent commercial success. However, it is only guidance, not a prescription. There are many different ways of achieving quality in software engineering, although the recommendations given here represent what I believe to be the irreducible minimum set of procedures that ought to be featured in any quality management system.

In the course of addressing every other major activity in the operations of a software house, this book has grown out of my practical experience both of quality control and quality assurance, the discipline of programming in submission to the remorseless logic of the digital computer, and the emergent consensus of good software engineering practice expressed in the ISO 9000-3 TickIT standards. My sole aim throughout the book is to address the practical needs of today's software vendor to adopt sound development practices, in order not just to survive, but supremely to prosper, in a frenetically changing world.

Finally, I should emphasise at the outset of this work that the views and opinions expressed herein are entirely my own. These views and opinions are not necessarily endorsed in whole or in part by the Pfizer Group of Companies, nor may they necessarily be so endorsed in the future.

Howard T. Garston Smith
Margate, UK
May 1997

Part 1

The Company and the Culture

Introduction

Computers will never replace human beings.
Someone has to complain about the errors.

Anon

In the last 30 years of the 20th century, the world has undergone one of the most profound transformations in human history. Dubbed as the second industrial revolution, this extraordinary change is not only as fundamental as the first revolution of the 19th century, but is taking place at a much faster pace. The transformation has two principal foci. One is the extraordinary processing power and miniaturization of the silicon microprocessor, born[1] in the fervor of the space missions of the 1970s. The other is the transition from fixed location, wired telegraphy to mobile, wireless communications, a closely related evolution also stemming from the fruits of research in space technology. Its effect is to release the potential of the computer from fixed location processing of a discrete task to global shared processing of information independent of geographical or political boundaries. The impact on every aspect of human life, business, commerce, politics, the home and the foundational presuppositions on which much of everyday life is based is proving to be nothing short of phenomenal.

While the potential and pace of this revolution is exciting and largely of great benefit to mankind, it brings in its wake huge social problems. Despite the fact that computerization is generating far more jobs than it is destroying, social dislocation and human suffering are arising from the displacement of thousands of workers from their source of livelihood through the automation of traditional processes. The mystery which surrounds the computer, which contrary to popular myth is still very difficult to learn, breeds in many a sense of exclusion and alienation. Many, especially the elderly, feel left behind in a world whose basic technological tools seem to be understood with ease by younger folk, even the very young. Furthermore, the great advantages that well managed and successful computerization can bring are counterbalanced by a steady stream of disasters, where a lack of understanding of the challenges presented by the new technology has tarnished its image and caused severe financial losses.

This is especially true in the area of software, to which subject this book is devoted. Software is that mysterious commodity which makes computers work and which so few really understand. This lack of understanding spans the entire age range and all levels in business, being especially acute among the captains and decision makers in industry, business and commerce. It lies at the heart of much of the waste and incompetence that mars the application of this powerful new force. The cheap availability of programming tools exacerbates the problem, making it possible for small software companies, with almost no understanding of how to produce software predictably that can be guaranteed to be fit for its intended purpose, to spring up everywhere.

With the amazing possibilities that computers offer for wealth creation in any business being so apparent, how can purchasers of software discriminate between products which possess adequate inherent quality and those that do not? Again, can responsible software houses be helped to understand how to develop and maintain a robust, defect-free product that meets the market's needs in a cost-effective and profitable manner? It is to these issues that this book is devoted.

HISTORICAL REVIEW OF DATA PROCESSING

It is during the last 15 years that the real revolution has occurred in the world of computing and data processing, driven principally by the advent of the now ubiquitous personal computer and the standard platform it has established. Although initially viewed by many in corporate data processing departments as something of a toy, with little relevance to the real world of computing, it quickly became apparent that its effect on the *status quo* would be cataclysmic.

This revolution has by no means been confined to the realm of hardware, although such a misconception is still extremely common. The wide availability of cheap computing power presented software programmers with the opportunity to distribute the fruits of their creativity to a wide audience at a small fraction of the price of existing software. Previously, software had been confined for its usefulness to costly proprietary mainframes affordable only by larger commercial enterprises. It was generally developed to serve the needs of a single, specific function reflecting entrenched organizational boundaries within the enterprise. Financial applications[2] such as general ledger and bookkeeping were common.

It is instructive to reflect on the culture that surrounded software development in those days. Programmers focussed their thinking heavily on becoming the recognized technical experts in the applications for which they wrote their software, and on the products that represented the crowning glory of their individual creativity. Their principal concerns centered on technical accuracy, bound up with the intimate details of the hardware and its relationship to their work. Users were involved only as far as was absolutely necessary; the software being seen as shaping the business activity to a considerable degree rather than vice versa, and users being treated, even if ever so politely, on a take-it-or-leave-it basis. The delivery and commissioning of the software into use was regarded as the culminating event of all their highly skilled efforts. Their main fear tended to be that of technical inaccuracy or other undiscovered defects in the program. To the objection that such a description is a gross caricature, it need only be pointed out that enough of this culture remains throughout the software industry today to demonstrate the truth of it!

THE CENTRALITY OF THE CUSTOMER

The new generation of software, designed to exploit the potential of the relatively inexpensive new standard platforms, transformed the place that computing occupies in the business and commercial world. The explosive rate at which this transformation has occurred has left many breathless and has given rise to a yearning for technological stability which continues to be elusive. Indeed, the rate of change seems geometric rather than arithmetic, perspicaciously predicted by Frank Fraser Darling in his BBC Reith Lectures in the early 1960s in relation to the then emerging science of ecology, and beautifully expressed by his term *the technological exponential*. In the course of just 15 years, the bulk of generic business and office processes, together with much of their associated communications, have become based on the technology of the personal computer and its local and wide area networks. The vision adumbrated in 1975 by Bill Gates and Paul Allen, the founders of Microsoft, of *one per desk—one computer on every desk in every school, office and home*—which seemed fanciful at the time, has now become a reality. Perhaps the most significant milestone in the realization of this dream was the launch of the Windows™ graphical user interface program as version 3.0 in 1990. Based on a concept originally developed by Apple computers for the Macintosh (so named, incidentally, after a variety of North American apple), it transformed the use of the computer from an experience constrained within a command-based dialogue (where command syntax had to be learnt) into one of a visual and intuitive character based on point-and-click activities. This has released the computer from its confinement within an eclectic group of enthusiastic, professional users to a mass audience, with no previous technical training or experience, and which has since penetrated every area of business.

This has borne with it profound implications for the software development process itself, since software and its quality is now so business critical. These issues, of which relatively so few people in general appreciate the importance, form the focus of much of the material in this book. At their heart lies the centrality of the customer or user, no longer the hapless captive of the programmer's conception of the job, but the central player in the business process. This metamorphosis of the user's or customer's role is exemplified to perfection by the Ford Motor Company. Henry Ford's attitude to the customer, summed up in his immortal phrase *"You can have any color so long as it's black!"*[3] has been supplanted by the firm's current advertising slogan *"Everything we do is driven by you"*, an inspired epithet illustrated in figure I.1 and perfectly encapsulating the centrality of the customer in Ford's strategic vision of its own business. The link between this and Ford's outstanding commercial success is no coincidence.

The Centrality of the Customer

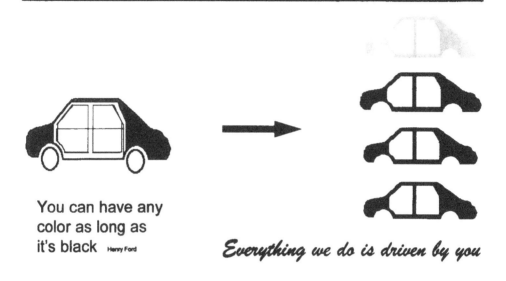

You can have any
color as long as
it's black Henry Ford

Everything we do is driven by you

Figure I.1. The Customer Focus of the Ford Motor Company

For the software developer in a customer- or business-focussed environment, the new frame of thinking becomes centered on the satisfaction of the user, for which technical accuracy is just one (albeit a crucial one) of a number of dimensions. The software product becomes not just an entity in itself, but part of an overall *service* to the customer; the details of hardware and software must be integrated into a larger concern for the whole business process involving hardware, software, liveware (people) and processes. Human relationships and the ability to get alongside users, bringing technical expertise to bear as the servant rather than as the dictator of the application, assume preeminent importance. Hence the user or *application expert*[4] becomes the key player at every stage in the process and to whom the programmer is a service provider. The developer's fear of technical inaccuracy gives way to a fear that the software product will either not be used as intended and, therefore, deliver the intended business benefit, or not be used at all. The failure of the command and control system project for the London (UK) Ambulance Service is just one well publicized example of the results of attempting to introduce a complex system against the will of its staff.

THE RELATIVE IMMATURITY OF SOFTWARE

Why is there still so much concern over software? A superficial comparison between the comparative evolution of hardware versus software over the last decade illustrates how far software is lagging behind hardware in reliability and performance. Most of us continue to be amazed at the engineering marvels achieved almost daily by hardware manufacturers. The growth in processing power and the decreasing price of the silicon chip have become a vast engine driving the relentless expansion of global IT (figure I.2). This is largely due to the maturity and extremely high standard of the electronic design techniques employed, aided to a large degree by formal methodologies used throughout the manufacture of high technology hardware. When the spotlight is then switched to the software industry, the contrast could not be more stark. Here the advances have been far less dramatic; to a large extent, the industry today still retains the appearance of a fragmented cottage industry dominated by labor-intensive craft methods and approaches. The meteoric rise in hardware power is demanding larger, more sophisticated programs; as their complexity increases, so does their level of residual defects. Software now lags far behind hardware both in quality and capability, a fact to which the instability of today's personal computer testifies (a subject to be addressed again in a moment). This gap has become an enormous problem.

THE EFFECTS OF POOR QUALITY SOFTWARE

Even as late as mid-1996, scarcely a month passes without the media reporting some kind of failure in a major computer project. Here are just a few examples gleaned over the past few years (see also figure I.3):

> *The London Ambulance Service lost four emergency calls
> . . . the details were eventually found and an ambulance
> dispatched but the patient later died.*[5]

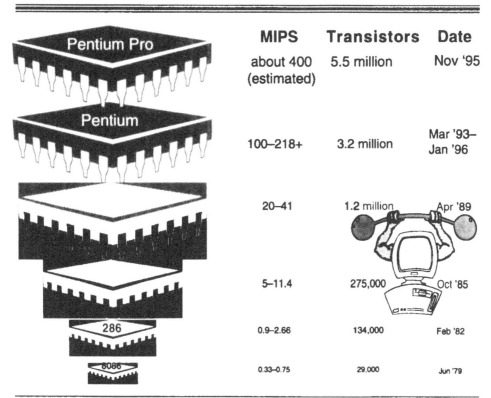

	MIPS	Transistors	Date
Pentium Pro	about 400 (estimated)	5.5 million	Nov '95
Pentium	100–218+	3.2 million	Mar '93–Jan '96
	20–41	1.2 million	Apr '89
	5–11.4	275,000	Oct '85
286	0.9–2.66	134,000	Feb '82
8086	0.33–0.75	29,000	Jun '79

Figure I.2. The Meteoric Rise in Hardware Power

On July 1st there was a six hour telephone system outage affecting over one million customers in the Pittsburgh area . . . had been attributed to a hitherto undetected but reproducible software fault.[6]

Some 400,000 Internet users in the US were left without a service for 13 hours last week when the country's largest provider suffered a software fault.[7]

A UK bank has accidentally transferred £2 billion to UK and US companies because a software design flaw allowed payment instructions to be duplicated.[8]

Flawed software supplied by the Further Education Funding Council to colleges for their £3.5 billion Individual Student Record Scheme ran into problems . . . software hitches made it difficult to reconcile student data with exam results . . . problems with the system led to funding

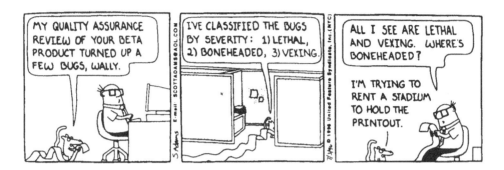

Figure I.3. Software Defects Are Everyone's Business
(DILBERT: ©1996 United Features Syndicate Inc. Reproduced by
permission.)

*estimates ranging from £300,000 to as high as £2 million
. . . the software . . . was initially unable to cope with the
complex task it had to fulfill.[9]*

*The UK's biggest banking network, which handles transac-
tions worth £5 million a second was brought down for almost an entire banking day because of a software bug . . .
which held up bank transfers of more than £100 billion including payments for everything from shares and foreign
exchange to . . . funds from people buying houses . . . all
money transfers in and out of the Clearing House Automated Payments System (CHAPS) were blocked for about
six hours . . . CHAPS is absolutely fundamental to the way
the UK economy works . . .[10]*

These are only a few recent examples of the problems that have
beset the computer industry for decades. As far back as 1962, the
year of Sputnik, a missing hyphen in its software was responsible
for the $18 million U.S. *Mariner* satellite going off course instead of
to Venus. Still in the aerospace arena, the *Columbia* spacecraft had
to abort its planned landing in 1983 due to computer faults, and almost unbelievably, both the first and second backups also failed.
Fortunately for the crew, the third backup worked! Much closer to
home and much more worryingly for all of us the near meltdown at
the Three Mile Island nuclear power station in 1979 was believed to
have involved computer defects.

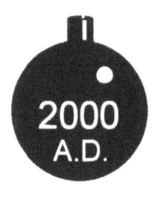

On a more topical note and of great concern worldwide at the present time is the so-called *millennium bomb,* perhaps the most devastating defect ever to afflict the world's business computers. Caused by programmers (many of whom are now in senior executive positions) who, in an effort to conserve scarce memory and expensive storage, or minimise data entry time, abbreviated the year in the date to a two-digit shorthand; this defect is present in tens of millions of lines of code across the world.[11] On 1 January 2000, computers that control banks, government services, public transport ticket machines, traffic lights and office entry systems, to name just a few, will shudder to a catastrophic halt unless they are corrected beforehand. Most will treat the date as 1900 by default, while many personal computers will revert to 1980. Some of the ramifications are extremely bizarre, such as the possibility of hospital admission systems directing geriatric patients to paediatric wards! Ian Taylor, UK Minister for Technology, has warned that the fault could lead to thousands of pensions remaining unpaid, legal actions being deleted, 100 years of credit interest being added to credit card balances, and perhaps even weapon systems and safety-critical software in nuclear power plants failing. The systems of Marks and Spencer, one of the UK's most prestigious retailers, have just been reported[12] as rejecting a tin of corned beef with a sell-by date of 2000 for being 96 years old! Martyn Thomas, the charismatic chairman of Praxis plc, a leading UK software house, has alluded to the implications for fly-by-wire aircraft and air traffic control systems:

> *Not many safety-critical software experts are keen to fly as the millennium changes—there are too many lines of code that someone may have forgotten to change.*[13]

Although the millennium defect can often be repaired quickly in any one program, the simplicity of the problem is leading organizations to grossly underestimate the scale of the action required. The Gartner Group (a highly respected U.S. consultancy house which comments on IT issues) has estimated that a medium sized company running about 8,000 programs will need to spend between $3.6 and

$4.2 million to repair date-defective software.[14] It is likely that should such action be delayed beyond 1997 it may be too late in many cases, since experts will by then be overwhelmed by demands for help and insufficient time will remain for the adequate testing of repairs. The problem is not just confined to disc-based software, since the millenium defect can just as easily be incorporated into code burned onto programmable read-only memory chips. These are commonly to be found embedded within process control systems, so the possible ramifications span a wide spectrum of devices, ranging in size and importance from video recorders, through passenger elevators to electricity distribution systems. The crisis is a perfect example of the widespread lack of understanding among commercial management at large of the full implications of IT, a subject discussed in more detail in chapter 6. According to a survey published by *Viasoft* in August 1996, over a quarter of the users at more than 300 sites were unaware of the issues or simply dismissed them.[15]

Millennium compliance has begun to underline the increasing intolerance on the part of software purchasers of defects in purchased software. It is now widely believed within the legal profession that an avalanche of legal disputes between users and suppliers will be precipitated over who carries responsibility for the estimated £5 billion cost of repairing defective software. The IBM Computer Users Association has drawn up a legal document that software suppliers will be asked to sign as part of their contract with purchasers that their code is year 2000 compliant. Suppliers unwilling to provide this guarantee may be blacklisted.[16] This development flies in the face of the limited warranty disclaimers in software licences from most software suppliers. These limit their liability for loss or damage arising from defects in delivered software to the cost of the software itself, to which the magnitude of the damage may bear no relation whatsoever. Software, being intellectual property, is usually warranted to perform only *substantially in accordance with documentation* (whatever that means); in contrast, hardware is usually warranted to be free from defects in materials or workmanship under normal use and service for a set period. The following example is typical of the wording of software liability disclaimers:

> **Suspect Software** *is a copyrighted, proprietary program offered as is without any warranty of merchantability or fitness for a particular purpose, performance, or otherwise;*

all warranties are expressly disclaimed. By using **Suspect Software,** *you agree that the author will not be liable for any use of (or inability to use), or performance of this product, or for any damages whatsoever.*

There are other straws in the wind that suggest that the days of disclaiming legal liability may be numbered. In a recent British court case,[17] the court declared that if the purchaser has bought or leased the medium (disc, CD-ROM, etc.) on which the software is delivered, then the latter becomes part of the goods. (The significance of this is that goods in the UK are subject to the Sale of Goods Act 1979, which imposes on the supplier an obligation of fitness for purpose, and freedom of the product from defects). In this instance, the judgment declared that this remained the case even if the supplier contract specifically excluded liability, since fitness for purpose was inherent in the contract. While defect-free software is almost never achievable, a legal category defining exactly what is meant by *acceptable* in the context of software quality may well emerge in the foreseeable future, as there are several further cases (involving totally different parties from those in the case already mentioned) pending in the British Courts which are likely to hinge on the fitness of software for its intended use. It is quite possible that, over the next few years, the fear of litigation may assume greater prominence as a driving force in the improvement of software development practice as the containment of cost, or the perceived satisfaction of the user.[18]

THE COSTS OF POOR QUALITY SOFTWARE

Concern over the additional costs incurred both by users and by software suppliers from poor quality software is by no means a recent phenomenon either. As far back as the mid 1980s the U.S. Department of Defense had become so concerned over the quality of military software that it had launched a number of initiatives on improving software reliability. These included the Ada program and another known as STARS. It also founded the Software Engineering Institute at Carnegie Mellon University in Pittsburgh to establish standards for excellence in software development and to promulgate good methodologies. At the same time, on the other side of the Atlantic, there was a widespread feeling that if UK suppliers were to survive, let alone prosper in the increasingly competitive international software market, they had to remain at the forefront of trends toward higher quality software. Sensitive to this, the UK's Department of Trade and Industry commissioned a report from Price Waterhouse to review the costs and benefits of quality management systems in software development. This report (Price Waterhouse 1988) proved to be a landmark in the development of standards and certification schemes and formed a critical link in the formation and launch of the TickIT Accreditation Scheme, founded on international standard ISO 9000-3.

The report set out to identify the origins of the costs of poor quality in software and attempted to quantify them. It went on to show how an effective quality management system could not only avoid these costs but also deliver benefits that far outweighed the overhead cost of the quality system itself. These costs were those spent on the resources deployed to prevent defects creeping into the software in the first place.

Four principal areas of software failure cost were identified:

1. Costs of correcting defects, both before and after delivery to the customer

2. Overruns against time and budget

3. Unnecessarily high maintenance costs

4. Indirect costs which users incur due to residual defects in delivered software

Their research led them to conclude that for software produced by UK suppliers and sold to UK users, the costs resulting directly from poor quality software was at that time £500 million annually, equivalent to one-half of the magnitude of the software market as it then was. This estimate was deliberately conservative! Of this total, 40 percent was borne by suppliers, although almost all of this was eventually passed on to users. But the situation seen in its totality was reckoned to be far worse, as no account had been taken of imported software. No evidence was found to discriminate between the quality of UK software and that produced abroad, and on this basis the total costs of failure were estimated at twice the figure quoted, that is, equivalent to the entire value of the software market in the UK (figure I.4).

In the intervening years, we have seen the establishment of the very successful TickIT certification scheme in the UK. Indeed, this

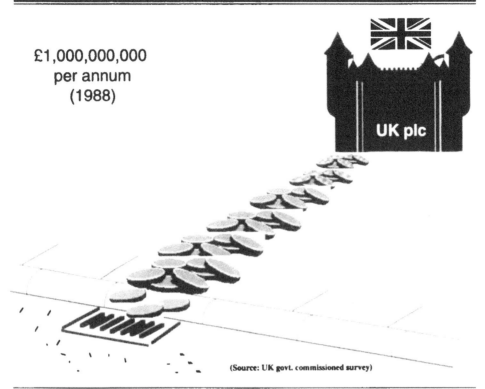

£1,000,000,000
per annum
(1988)

UK plc

(Source: UK govt. commissioned survey)

Figure I.4. Costs of Lack of Quality on Faulty and Unsuccessful IT Projects

has been taken as a model for a number of similar initiatives abroad. Over 1,000 organizations had obtained certificates under the rules of the scheme by late 1995. However, it must be remembered that this constitutes but a small proportion of the total software industry, much of which is composed of small companies. In the experience of the author, it is in these firms that the greatest need for improvement in software quality resides, confirming the impression of the Price Waterhouse investigators.

Businesses are now far more dependent on software than was the case at the time of the Price Waterhouse report, and the need for improvements correspondingly more urgent. Just recently, the prevalence of major IT project disasters has driven the UK government to launch guidelines[19] on the management issues that senior executives in software houses or organisations with in-house software development groups must focus on in order to keep projects on track, together with a list of telltale warning signs indicating when things are beginning to go wrong. These *BuyIT Guidelines*, backed by the Confederation of British Industry, the Computer Software Services Association and the UK National Computing Centre, reflect the fact that two thirds of UK firms have suffered at least one IT project failing to deliver business benefits, with 20 percent suffering financial loss. Across the Atlantic, one third of an estimated 250,000 projects in the United States were canceled in 1995, at a combined loss of $80 billion.

There is, therefore, gigantic scope for cost savings both for the supplier and for the user. We still have a long long way to go.

COMPUTER–RELATED SYSTEMS VALIDATION

The awareness of the need in recent years for software of adequate quality has not been confined to government and the software industry itself. A number of user industries have developed standards for suppliers in response to regulatory pressures, and foremost among these has been the pharmaceutical industry. In the early 1980s, it became apparent that the increasing use of computers in manufacturing and laboratory operations could not be separated from the principles of good manufacturing practice, which by then had long since conditioned the way in which medicinal products were manufactured, tested, stored and distributed. These principles rest on the foundations of statistical process control developed by Deming, Shewart and others, which will be discussed in more detail in chapter 1. What they clearly demonstrate is that the quality of any finished product is a direct result of the process that produced it. Regulation in the pharmaceutical industry grew as a result of a series of spectacular process failures, leading to a realization that to ensure satisfactory products, the process which produced them had to be *validated*. It was recognized that very strong parallels existed between the process-focussed principles of good manufacturing practice on the one hand, and the development of quality software on the other. The disciplines of documentation, building quality into the product within the process (rather than vainly attempting to test it in at the end), which had long since been meat and drink in the established world of good manufacturing practice, applied with equal validity in the newly emerging world of software development.

Process validation was defined by the U.S. Food and Drug Administration (FDA) as follows:

> *Establishing documented evidence which provides a high*
> *degree of assurance that a specific process will consis-*
> *tently produce a product meeting its pre-determined speci-*
> *fications and quality attributes (FDA 1987).*

The now generally accepted definition of *computer-related systems validation*, given originally by the validation committee of the Pharmaceutical Manufacturers' Association (PMA) in the United States in 1986, is as follows:

> *The establishment of evidence that a computer system*
> *does what it purports to do and will continue to do so in*
> *the future (PMACSVA 1986).*

Both of these definitions bear a remarkable resemblance to the ISO standard for quality published in ISO 8402:1994:

> *The totality of characteristics of a product or process that*
> *bear on its ability to satisfy stated and implied needs.*

As computers forced their way into the manufacturing areas and testing laboratories of pharmaceutical companies it was realized that although they were just another kind of equipment and, therefore, needed to be validated in just the same way, in another respect they were quite different. They critically depended on a new, unfamiliar, rather mystical and generally invisible commodity called *software*, which only a very few esoteric individuals knew anything about. Poor or unknown quality in software was recognized as a loose cannon on deck that ill fitted an environment in which every margin for error had to be ruthlessly excluded. This unease was exacerbated by the intimidating nature of the technology, understood only by programming experts reluctant to share their expertise with lay people and seldom regarding themselves as an integral part of the manufacturing team. However, at the same time many users of computerized systems were discovering the benefits of their use in terms of the improved quality and productivity of the processes into which they were introduced. The analytical laboratories of the time furnish an instructive example. The evolution of high pressure liquid chromatography as a specific analytical technique was beginning to deluge chemists with an avalanche of raw data that made computer-aided data processing and reduction an urgent necessity. Microprocessors were beginning to appear in manufacturing machines and analytical instruments. The regulatory insistence on the *validation* of computer-related systems was, therefore, timely and inevitable.

A full summary of the history of validation is beyond the scope of this work, but has been ably documented by Chapman (1991a; 1991b) and others (PMACSVC 1993a; Trill 1993a; Trill 1993b; PMACSVC 1993b) in a number of articles, which are highly recommended to the reader. The wide consensus of agreement that has now been reached on all of the key issues in this area is evident from the conformity in the regulatory requirements for computer-related systems validation in the United States (the FDA), the European Union and Australia (ISPE 1996). The recent guideline published by the U.S. Parenteral Drug Association (PDA 1995) is one of the most succinct summaries of current "good computer-related system validation practices" yet published. These standards have also been accepted in many related areas such as that of clinical research (Korteweg 1993).

REGULATED AND NONREGULATED SYSTEMS

Because of the regulatory involvement under medicines legislation, the need to validate computer-related systems has now long since ceased to be a matter of debate; the same cannot be said for business systems. Why, it is objected, should departments, such as finance and accounting, which are not directly related to the manufacture of medicines be saddled with the overhead of validation? From a superficial standpoint it is easy to understand this point of view. However, it arises fundamentally from a *compliance mentality* which must be grown out of in much the same way as childhood and adolescence. In the early days of regulation, the principal driving force behind the implementation of improvements was the regulatory sanction, from whose obligations and expense there was no escape if manufacturing licences were to be retained. Gradually, even those temperamentally averse to compliance came to realize that, far from being inimical to the firm's best interests, compliance was *entirely compatible* with it. Management had actually as much need to be convinced of the integrity and security of manufacturing and testing procedures as did regulators. Indeed, it has long since been taken for granted that by providing evidence to satisfy the legitimate concerns of *management* that the manufacture is under control regulators will, **by the same token**, also be satisfied.

THE COMPLIANCE MENTALITY

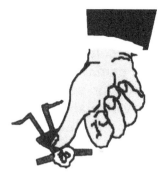 The same principle is slowly at work in the business and commercial systems arena, though decades behind it. There is still a widespread belief even within the pharmaceutical industry (to quote one example) that software assessment is a process that only has value in relation to regulation. It is a requirement imposed as part of computer-related systems validation by a demanding regulatory agency on a reluctant industry struggling to remain competitive in a rapidly changing healthcare environment. It really has nothing to do with the core business activities of making drugs and selling them.

Even the most cursory examination of this attitude will reveal how distorted a view of the industry's vital interests this is. Knowing the importance of quality-assured validated software in the manufacturing areas, suppose a financial director hears the following:

> *We aren't going to bother to carry out any quality assurance checks on the new software for the accounts department, so you won't mind if it's of poor quality and contains quite a lot of residual defects, will you? We don't think we need to ensure the adequacy of software quality in non regulated application areas because there aren't any regulations to comply with. Is that OK?*

The reader will be left to imagine the likely response. Would any responsible business manager willingly acquiesce to such a suggestion? Not only is quality-assured software that *does what it purports to do* and *does not do what it purports not to do* essential in the manufacturing area because of regulations, it is vital in every other area for the well-being and prosperity of the business. In fact, the well-being of the business should be the prime motivation **even in regulated areas**. If we can satisfy ourselves on our level of control of our systems for the sake of our business, we will also, *in so doing*, satisfy the requirements of regulators. We need to shed our compliance way of thinking as a snake sloughs its worn-out skin, adopt a mature business mentality and in so doing, avoid the associated hypocrisy of double standards.

It would seem, then, that when the chips are down, the business sees no dichotomy between regulated systems and nonregulated systems as far as quality requirements are concerned. The business needs sound validatable systems in both arenas. It has been argued that some relaxation of the formality of some of the controls required in computer-related systems validation would be appropriate for business systems, but as far as the quality of the software is concerned, there can be no distinction. Both must be engineered in accordance with a QA system either to ensure mitigation of business risk and supportability of users (business area) or validatability (regulated area). But how do today's systems match up for the average computer user?

TODAY'S UNSTABLE DESKTOP

The principal motives for auditing software are user-focussed—reliability, supportability, maintainability. There is an additional factor, however, in a client/server environment: to reduce, and hopefully eliminate, the interference with other processes simultaneously executing on the network. Although the major server operating systems such as Windows™ NT and OS/2™ are now extremely robust, the Windows™ 3.x desktop operating systems are much less so. All users in this environment have to accommodate themselves to the chronic instability of this environment where the desktop is liable to lock up and lose data at any time for reasons that are rarely adequately understood or explained and are certainly beyond their control. Many users with previous experience of the rock solid traditional proprietary operating systems of the 1970s and 1980s find the acclimatization to this risky way of life hard to tolerate, let alone accept, in contrast to the stoical acceptance of these weaknesses by other users, who have never known anything better. At the heart of the problem lies the management of memory, fundamental to the success of any operating system. This is especially critical for Windows™, where the complexity of the memory scheme inherited from DOS, the widespread misunderstanding both of the various memory areas and the principles of memory mapping, coupled with the huge range of configuration options involved, has turned the subject into something resembling a complicated puzzle, a minefield for all but the expert. The all too frequent Unrecoverable Application Error (Windows™ 3.0) or General Protection Fault (Windows™ 3.1) can often be traced to a failure on the part of an individual program to manage its memory usage strictly in accordance with standards. The process of writing this book for example, has been plagued with software defects of various kinds, despite the fact that the hardware and local area networks on which the work was done are managed by staff of the highest calibre whose commitment and professionalism are exemplary. Of all the categories of software, printer drivers and video drivers are by far the worst offenders in this respect. In fairness also to Microsoft, the principal vendor in the desktop arena, it should be pointed out that these standards are available on CD-ROM, although the complaint that they are extremely extensive, and quite laborious to work through, is often expressed. Regrettably, human nature being what it is, many programmers have been unwilling to make the effort to explore them thoroughly; the temptation to take a shortcut and make assumptions has frequently proven irresistible. Once a program attempts to address a region of memory to which it is refused access, a General Protection Fault will usually result, frequently corrupting the data of other active programs resident there and rendering the Windows™ environment unstable. To add insult to injury, the subsequent failure banner message will often attribute the disaster to the innocent application rather than to the guilty party. Once instability has set in, other applications may subsequently trigger the same error, despite themselves also being above reproach.[20]

Other design weaknesses within Windows™ are another burden. It is widely known that Windows™ 3.1 suffers from the well-known limitation imposed by its 64K graphics device interface and USER 16-bit memory heaps used to store graphics or memory object information, occupancy of which is usually indicated as available free space from the HELP "About . . . " menu option. Once reduced below a certain minimum value consequential on the calls of programs to the Windows™ API, the system will report itself *out of memory* despite a huge amount of free memory still being otherwise available! Since this is a defect in Windows™ itself, even the most prestigious programs are just as vulnerable to failure as are less well-known programs if several are active simultaneously. This infuriating cause of instability has been ameliorated to some extent in Windows 95® as many data structures formerly stored on these heaps have been moved to 32-bit heaps; however, considerable instability remains to haunt the user.

The huge variety of Windows™-based software now in circulation and the gargantuan number of possible mixes in an environment where standards are not rigidly followed will ensure instability remains a persistent problem for some time to come. The greater robustness of the Windows 95® desktop operating system, through increased system resources and improved memory management, has been a step in the right direction. However, the need to accommodate legacy 16-bit applications has necessitated retaining the scope for programmers to circumvent rigid discipline in program design. Windows™ NT is an example of an operating system designed in a far more integrated manner (rather like the proprietary predecessors of yesteryear mentioned earlier), and for this reason is much more stable, making it likely to be favored as one of the operating systems of choice for the client-server commercial world. However, its design necessarily limits the range of 16-bit applications that it will run successfully to those that comply with its strict standards. It is believed that Windows™ NT is likely to be enhanced[21] to accommodate a wider spectrum of 16-bit applications without sacrificing its stability. Clearly, this will thereby lead to the automatic exclusion of many legacy 16-bit applications which usually run successfully under Windows™ 3.x or Windows 95® but are not completely compliant with the NT standards. Such a transition would begin to weed out some of the worst software currently in widespread use and be a welcome development. In the meantime and because of this, auditing of software destined for server installation is an especially important preventive strategy. Confinement of software of suspect provenance to stand-alone workstations can reap the business benefits of such software while at the same time mitigating the risks inherent in its use.

THE QUALITY ASSURANCE AUDIT

By purchasing a piece of software and using it, a customer is incorporating within his or her business the strengths and weaknesses of the engineering processes of the supplier, whether this is realized or not. By so doing, in total ignorance of the supplier's methods and practices, the purchaser is taking a risk of unknown magnitude; to a certain extent the purchaser is abrogating a measure of control of the business that would have been retained had other means of fulfilling that part of the business process been adopted by, for example, conventional paper-based manual methods. The use of a supplier's software implies a greater intimacy of business partnership and a measure of dependency, even if the customer fails to appreciate this. Many software purchasers only become aware of this dependency in the event of a major software failure, a fact reflected in the liability disclaimers that, as we have seen, have become part and parcel of most software licence agreements.

The fact must be faced that many of the most senior managers and chief executives in the businesses of today have not kept abreast of technical changes that computerization has imposed on all of us. To some extent this is understandable. The rate of change has been unprecedented and has overwhelmed everyone. Despite slick advertisements, personal computers are highly complex pieces of equipment difficult to learn and use, prone to failure from unstable operating systems, and require high levels of expertise not only to resolve their frequent failures but also to modify and upgrade them.

There is, however, a much more important issue. Managers today, in general, have not yet understood the implications of incorporating this mysterious commodity called software into their business. In yesterday's world, business processes operated within the medium of pen and paper within the intellectual grasp of everyone. But software is intangible. When seen in its raw state as source code, it is totally baffling to all but the elite high priestly caste of programmers. Managers are subconsciously aware of their total ignorance and lack of control of an area that is becoming vital to the success of their business. This is uncomfortable, even threatening. The intuitive defensive reaction tends to be:

> *I have great responsibility and understand everything that*
> *is important in my business. But I have no understand-*
> *ing of software, and therefore software just cannot be*
> *important.*

The thought that one may not understand something of vital importance, and thus need education about its implications, dare not be entertained, since it would betray ignorance, undermine credibility and reputation and be too injurious to personal pride. So ignorance is tolerated, risk ignored and software procured with no action to assess innate quality, in the blind optimism that functionality is all that matters, and nothing will ever go wrong. In a few years' time this widespread attitude will be seen in retrospect for what it is— breathtakingly irresponsible. In the meantime, the most prudent software purchasers are seeking to mitigate the risk of software acquisition by implementing a software quality procurement policy, of which the QA assessment is the tangible expression.

This development is far less innovative and revolutionary than it sounds. The partnership approach between the supplier and the consumer is exactly analogous to the practices adopted in many other industries committed to a quality culture over many decades. The revolution in Japanese industry after the Second World War was based on just this approach. The leading companies in quality-regulated industries, such as the pharmaceutical industry, have also been highly successful commercially. A quality philosophy focussed on the centrality of customers and their needs, regarding the supplier as part of the overall quality-oriented product delivery process, has produced a consistent pattern of success for its proponents around the globe.

The QA audit, along the lines described in ISO 10011-1:1990 and in concept only in British Standard 4778, is intended to promote and strengthen this supplier-customer partnership. It is designed to help suppliers improve their own processes, to reduce costs and improve quality, to ensure their survival in today's cut-throat competitive environment. It is also aimed at ensuring an adequate level of structural integrity of software acquired for any part of the business, whether subject to regulation or not, and to provide reassurance that future versions and releases will possess no less a level, and ideally a superior level, of quality than existed at the time of the audit. Furthermore, the containment of the number of different suppliers and the standardization of packages for specific business functions such as word processing, text retrieval, document management, financial accounting and the like minimizes a purchaser's internal support costs and IT overheads. Although the benefits of the QA audit to the supplier can become apparent very quickly, those to the purchaser are not immediately quantifiable, since the return on the investment of the cost of the audit is medium to long term. Although the audit can never ensure with certainty the absence of critical defects in purchased software, it can greatly decrease their likelihood. By screening out software produced without a recognizable life cycle methodology or without other evidence of in-built quality, the firm can avoid those sources of business interruption and loss whose prevention and cure has proved be the most difficult and intractable.

THE QUALITY ASSURANCE AUDITOR/CONSULTANT

How can a purchaser firm protect its interests and ensure that the acquisition of new technology is going to be a boon rather than a bane? The first essential is to recognize that the software is the heart and essence of any system. Hardware is simply the environment and the tool by which to execute the software, to incorporate its functionality into the business in order to derive benefit from it. It is also generally manufactured to a very high level of quality. But in contrast software is intangible and utterly beyond the understanding of the layman. Glossy brochures extol the functionality, but what lies beneath it? If it is indeed the Achilles heel of the system, what can go wrong? Does Murphy's Law[22] always apply?

The mission of the software QA auditor/consultant is to act on the purchaser's behalf to address these issues. His or her mission is to measure whether the software that the business intends to acquire is indeed fit for its intended purpose. This book will describe the features of a software engineering approach capable of producing software with an extremely low level of defects that will meet the purchaser's needs at minimal risk. The perspective taken will be that of the examination made by the auditor, working in a team partnership with the supplier's own programming staff, of the way that the software has been constructed. As a necessary preliminary to exploring the nuts and bolts of the process, we first need to review the essential characteristics of organizations capable of producing software that is fit for its intended purpose. It is to this that we will devote our attention in the next chapter.

Notes

1. The silicon chip microprocessor was invented by Dr. Marcian (Ted) Hoff and first announced to the world by Intel in November 1971. The 4004, as it was known, was a 4 bit chip that ran at 0.1 MHz, possessed what then seemed an astonishing 2,300 transistors and cost $299. It was claimed to have the same computing power as the Eniac computer, then worth $0.5 million and run by the U.S. Army, which had 17,468 valves, 70,000 resistors, 10,000 capacitors, 1,500 relays and 6,000 switches.

2. Throughout this book, the word *application* is used as a synonym for *a task or process within the enterprise*.

3. To be totally fair to Henry Ford, the lack of choice over the color of the Model T in the years 1914–1926 was actually a manufacturing necessity. It took just an hour and a half to assemble a vehicle, and Japan black was the only paint then available which would dry within this time.

4. A term coined by K.G. Chapman in the context of validation teams for computer-related systems validation in the pharmaceutical and medical device industries.

5. News item in *Computing,* 20 February 1992.

6. Risks Forum, ACM Software Engineering Notes, July 1991.

7. News item in *Computer Weekl,y* 27 June 1996.

8. News item in *Computer Weekly,* 19 October 1989.

9. "Slow, bug-ridden software hinders college funding", news item in *Computer Weekly,* 13 June, page 14.

10. "Software Crash hits UK Banking System", news item in *Computer Weekly,* 22 August 1996.

11. Printing out 10 million lines of code produces 25 *miles* of listing. A scary thought, don't you think?!

12. News item in *Computing,* 12 September 1996.

13. News item in *Computer Weekly,* 4 July 1996.

14. The total cost of dealing with the millenium bomb have been variously estimated. The Gartner Group reckoned in 1995 that the sum would lie between $400 billion and $600 billion worldwide. The U.S. consultancy Software Productivity Research, on the other hand, has put the cost even higher at $1000 billion.

15. News item in *Computer Weekly,* 3 September 1996.

16. News item in *Computer Weekly,* 13 June 1996.

17. Appeal Court Case *ICL v. St. Albans District Council.* The court decided that the sale of package software is a "goods" contract subject to the Sale of Goods Act 1979. As such, it had to be fit for its intended purpose, a feature implied, the court ruled, by the specification the client had issued for the software. The court awarded the Council £700,000 against ICL for financial loss arising from the effect of a software defect.

18. The journal *IT Law Today,* published by Monitor Press (57-61 Mortimer St., London, W1N 8JX, UK) addresses all of the legal issues surrounding IT, not just in the United Kingdom, but also in Europe and in the United States, from the perspective of both supplier and purchaser alike. Edited by Susan Singleton, with an editorial board including some of the United Kingdom's leading computer lawyers, it provides expert and authoritative comment and practical advice. Subscription information available from the above address; by telephone (+44 1787 467 232); or by fax (+44 1787 880 201).

19. *Now there's no excuse,* article in *Computer Weekly* June 13, 1996, page 20.

20. It would be disingenuous, and unfair, to suggest that careless programming is the only cause of General Protection Faults (GPFs) in Windows™. Faulty desktop configuration is frequently to blame. For example, suppose a network card, using the memory block defined by the address range D800h-DFFFh has been installed. Unless Windows™ is configured to exclude this block from the pool of available memory, Windows™ may subsequently attempt to allocate this block to a running program, leading to a GPF. It so happens that such a reservation can be secured

by means of a particular usage of the expanded memory manager program EMM386.EXE, involked in the CONFIG.SYS file, with syntax such as

DEVICE = C:\DOS\EMM386.EXE NOEMS X=D800-DFFF

The fact that Windows™ itself does not use expanded memory (memmory mapped by software onto the system's upper memory area of 640K to 1,024K) illustrates the subtle and complex nature of memory management under this operating system!

21. At the time of writing (9/96), it appears to be Microsoft's intention to introduce a version (possibly numbered 5.0) of NT incorporating many of the features of Windows 95® sometime in 1997. It is thought to be codenamed Cairo. One of these features, the user interface, has now been brought forward into NT version 4.0, already released.

22. "Nothing is as easy as it looks; everything takes longer than you expect; and if anything can go wrong it will, at the worst possible moment!"

1

The Software Development Process

*A foolish man built his house upon the sand; and the rain
fell and floods came and the winds blew and beat against
the house and it fell; and great was the fall of it.*

Matthew 26: 26–27

THE NEED TO IMPROVE THE PROCESS

In the early days of IT, the arrival of computers promised immediate
benefits to many industries and commercial concerns in the automation of repetitive tasks. These operations had been difficult and
expensive in the years prior to the advent of computers, requiring
large numbers of people with high levels of numeracy and concentration performing essentially routine tasks. The banking industry is
one obvious example among many where the introduction of com-
puterisation brought an enormous reduction in the level of mistakes, the abolition of many labor-intensive activities and the
consequent release of people to more fulfilling spheres of activity in
an era of low unemployment.

From the standpoint of business as a whole, though, the permeation of computerization was very limited. The vast majority of systems had been created from a strictly limited functional view of one part of a business, rather than on an enterprise wide view. As a consequence, a major computer failure had the potential to affect only one area of the business, albeit a central or vital one; most parts of the operation would be able to continue, at least for a time. There are many such legacy systems, which remain important assets, still in successful use today. As software tends to improve with time, with defects being brought to light and corrected, operators become extremely familiar with the system's idiosyncrasies, and so both reliability and financial payback improve with each passing year.

On the other hand, such systems have an indirect disadvantage. Many of them are confined only to the high volume repetitive tasks in the business, where the user's involvement in the design and construction of the software had been regarded as of only minor importance. Quality was an issue which rarely arose since the algorithms on which the software design had been based were relatively straightforward, generally being simple, well-defined and well-understood financial or statistical calculations. The impression is created in the minds of many that today's enterprise wide systems can be developed in the same way as these legacy systems, with the same likelihood of successful and cost-effective implementation, the same life expectancy and return on investment.

The instances of computer failures cited in the introduction underline the folly of such delusions. This is serious because IT is now no longer seen in this limited way. It is regarded as holding the key to competitive advantage as the lifeblood, or perhaps (to use a more appropriate medical metaphor) the central nervous system of the entire organization. As this perception has altered, the commercial pressures to which the IT group is subjected have increased. Customers (computer users) are becoming increasingly discriminating and perceptive where IT costs are concerned. The need for an internal IT organization to demonstrate competitiveness with external service providers would have been unthinkable just a few years ago. Outsourcing (the transfer of service provision to an independent, external company) has now become commonplace, especially among UK government departments. These factors have made it essential to transform the manner in which systems are developed into a more predictable, quality-engineered event. The evolution of life cycle methodologies coupled with the capabilities of CASE (computer-aided software engineering) have combined to make this possible. The sophistication of customers is expressing itself in demands for greater usability, reliability and functionality in the product, and that it be delivered on time and on budget. As a result, software developers are being subjected to a huge cultural transformation from technical specialists into providers of *business solutions*. What is needed is not simply a change in the way that developers practise their skills, but the way in which they *see themselves*.

If developers need to undergo cultural change, the need for management to do so is even greater. Corporate business plans average five to eight years in scope, whereas many IT plans span no more than three years, reflecting the limitations that technological evolution at breakneck speed imposes on mental horizons. The dichotomy between the two views of the business leads to friction at the heart of an organization, and a consequential failure to reap the full benefit of IT investment. The situation is exacerbated by the brief spell which many IT managers spend in one post—the average stay now being only three years. IT investment must be made under a *profit center approach* (underlining IT's critical role in business competitiveness and the generation of revenue) rather than under a traditional *cost center approach* (portraying IT as just another unavoidable overhead cost to be reluctantly borne with stoic fortitude as a necessary evil).

These factors combine to demand a faster and more predictable system solutions delivery line. Moreover, modern systems must be amenable to adaptation to the changing needs of the business in a cost-effective and secure manner, ideally without wholesale redevelopment. This would enable the IT plans of an enterprise to be made on a scale more closely approximating those of the business as a whole.

THE HALLMARKS OF QUALITY–ASSURED SOFTWARE

The Price Waterhouse report (1988) has already been mentioned in the introduction; it categorized the attributes of good quality software under five headings which abide, despite the huge changes in technology that have occurred since then. Therefore, they will be restated here without apology.

Cost

A quality process delivers the required software product within the allocated budget. This means that the product is financially viable, assuming the presuppositions on which the original market forecasts were made were realistic. Changes in the market's needs and the vagaries of competition were always a hazard and remain so, despite the shorter development times made possible by the tools of the object-oriented graphical programming environment. To some extent, this trend drives software development in the direction of being less labour intensive and more capital intensive. However, the process today remains largely labour intensive; therefore, the profitability of the company is likely to be critically dependent on the productivity of the development team.

Standardization delivered both by a quality-assured process methodology, and by the accumulation of a library of reusable program modules or objects, obtained either by internal development (preferable) or purchase (nowadays ubiquitous), greatly reduces the extent to which the wheel must be reinvented. The use of programming standards (a theme to be probed in depth in chapter 8) enables programmers other than the author to maintain code safely and without the incorporation of further adventitious errors. The utilization of staff, therefore, improves.

A formal project life cycle methodology ensures that everyone knows what they are supposed to be doing and when, and what they are supposed to deliver. This avoids unrealistic assumptions and expectations arising, with the waste of time and money this implies. A configuration management system (described in chapter 5) ensures that each change to any item that forms part of the process of developing the product is recorded and documented. For example, as each new build of the software is made during development (perhaps under a rapid application development or rapid prototyping life cycle), it is certain beyond doubt which version of each individual source code file or dynamically linked library has been used to construct the final executable on which tests will be conducted.

Perhaps the overwhelming cost benefit of a quality process is the avoidance of incorporated errors that are so difficult and expensive to remove and live with. Building quality into software means ensuring that errors are not created in the first place. Many to whom these concepts are quite new are astounded when confronted by the fact that most errors are already present in the requirements or design before a line of code is ever written. It is a supreme irony that programmers are obliged to endure a reputation of being responsible for coding errors into software, when all they do is faithfully implement into the product the errors that are *already present in the design they are given*. If the inclusion of errors into software can be systematically weeded out, the scale and expense of subsequent testing can be radically reduced.

Timeliness

Almost every single vendor visited in the course of software quality audits has complained of the difficulty of delivering software to the market on time. In some cases, the competition has beaten them by a whisker, with disastrous marketing results for the original vendor. Of course this can always happen, but if project overruns can be eliminated and market intelligence is at least reasonably good the hazard and risk of becoming an expensive "Johnny Come Lately" can be minimised.

The project life cycle methodology should include the creation of a project plan, which should spawn individual plans for each of the players. The use of GANTT charts is increasingly common suggesting that the message of timeliness is getting through, a fact confirmed by the recent publication of the *BuyIT Guidelines* in the UK also mentioned in the introduction.

Getting the requirements right still remains the most serious cause of overruns. It is extremely difficult to get users to involve themselves in the documentation of requirements to an extent necessary to ensure that these are free of serious errors. This reflects to a large degree the inability of lay people to subject their thinking to the remorseless, logical disciplines to which all computers, being dumb and unimaginative, are subject. Whilst programmers are trained to submit themselves to thinking in this way, ordinary mortals find it irksome, irritating and frustrating. The most serious, intractable and expensive flaws in delivered computer systems can still be traced to inadequate, ambiguous or otherwise defective requirements. Prototyping in today's graphical environment is helping to alleviate this a little, but it remains one of the most serious causes of project delays.

The measurement and recording of how long it takes to complete the stages of a project can hone the skills of managers so that the quality of estimation can continue to improve. If no records are kept, nothing much will be learnt from mistakes and no improvements to the process itself will result. How can tenders be drawn up except on the basis of solid (and maybe bitter) experience? Project post mortems are invaluable in this regard[1] and are discussed in chapter 3.

Reliability

Avoiding putting defects into software (and incidentally paying people to do so!) is the best way of improving reliability. The reason why testing (and the people who carry out this activity are usually paid too!) is such a blunt instrument for removing them will be explained fully in chapter 5. The technique of configuration management that aims to ensure that the user receives the same version of the software that the vendor intends to deliver, and is planning on supporting, will also be explained. Furthermore, the effectiveness of software inspection for the affluent company, and code walkthrough to a lesser extent for the humbler concern, both of which seek to remove nascent errors and are intended to deliver software with a defect level approaching zero, will also be covered. Chapter 7 will describe the main elements of the functional requirements and design specification phases of the life cycle, where inspection can be used to such devastating effect.

But there is no intention to convey the impression that testing has no place in a quality-assured process. No vendor has yet reached the state of celestial perfection where the defect removal process has matured to such an extent as to render retrospective testing redundant. Testing provides valuable confirmatory evidence on a sampling basis of the effectiveness of the precursor life cycle stages. It is a powerful indicator of success or failure and will always have its place, though it should not be as prominent and as expensive a stage in the life cycle that it generally is today.

If the estimating discipline is poor, it may impair reliability. As anyone who has ever worked in a QC role in any process-related industry will testify, quality control are always at the end of the line. Delays earlier in the process lead to product being delivered to quality control late (since they are by necessity the last link in the chain), and giving rise to the loudly trumpeted half truth that *the product is in quality control and the product is late (again)!* (an implied causal relationship that QC personnel the world over bitterly resent). Tremendous pressure is then exerted to attenuate the testing and get the product out (it *must* be all right, mustn't it?). As a result, a product with a high residual defect level gets released.

Functionality

The defects in requirements alluded to above, to whose removal inspection is directed, are often in the nature of incorrect or inadequate behaviour. The program did not do what it was supposed to do, or what the users thought they had expressed, or what they thought they had meant when they said whatever they did say! Failure to be precise, unambiguous and comprehensive underlies a large proportion of the waste and rework in modern IT project development. It is to this fact that the examples quoted in the introduction testify (and had the author been feeling particularly uncharitable, he could have wearied the reader with many pages of them).

Change in the course of software development is a fact of life. To imagine that the vagaries of change can be kept at bay, and that requirements will not be revised as development continues, is quite unrealistic. In the real world, what is needed is a tight change control discipline to keep track of every change in requirements and to thoroughly explore all of its implications. These will bear both on the project life cycle (when will we *now* get it finished and what will it *now* cost?) and on the software development life cycle (what else needs to be changed now because of this?). In this regard, the quality management elements both of design review described in chapter 7, and of structured test plans described in chapter 9, are crucial.

Maintainability

There is evidence (Lientz and Swanson 1980) to suggest that about half the total life cycle effort is devoted to the support and maintenance of software. Getting functional requirements right, weeding out the errors through inspection, and controlling changes securely and cost-effectively all reap a major reduction in support costs. It is amazing that so few firms ever view support costs critically. They are accepted as a fact of life. When it is suggested that every help desk call, that would have been forestalled had the process been better, is itself a measure of nonquality, that such calls account for about three-quarters of all help desk activity in most cases, and that this is part of the measure of the inadequacy of today's modus operandi, vendors often feel wounded and hurt. It is in this sphere, and that of retained business that would otherwise be lost that the pay back of the quality management system principally, though not exclusively, occurs. It is much cheaper to retain a current customer than to find a new one!

What then are the changes that organizations need to make to improve the quality of delivered software? In order to answer this question, a development group needs a *measure* of where they are now and of where they aspire to be. The indispensability of measurement in the pursuit of knowledge was immortalized in the famous quotation attributed to Lord Kelvin:

> *When you can measure what you are speaking about and express it in numbers, you know something about it; but when you cannot express it in numbers, your knowledge is of a meager and unsatisfactory kind; it may be the beginning of knowledge, but you have scarcely in your thoughts advanced to the stage of science.*

We could sum up his lordship's dictum with the following epithet:

> *If you cannot measure it, you cannot manage it.*

Since we have already recognized that software development is a process requires *measurement* as a first step to control it, we have unwittingly entered the world of **statistical process control.**

THE LESSONS FROM
STATISTICAL PROCESS CONTROL

The ideas and principles of statistical process control are not new. They were originally conceived back in the 1920s by Walter Shewart at Western Electric Company, a manufacturing subsidiary of AT&T in the United States. His theory was that a process could be continually improved if subjected to his continuous Shewart cycle, shown in figure 1.1. The cycle comprises four essential steps:

1. **Plan**—decide what you are going to do

2. **Do**—carry it out

3. **Check**—measure how successful it was and thereby identify where it can be improved.

4. **Act**—make the improvement, and then **Plan** etc.

Bringing a process under statistical control involves documenting and describing every element in the process to **control** it, thus removing every source of indeterminate error (i.e., every error of *unknown* cause). Once a process has been brought under statistical

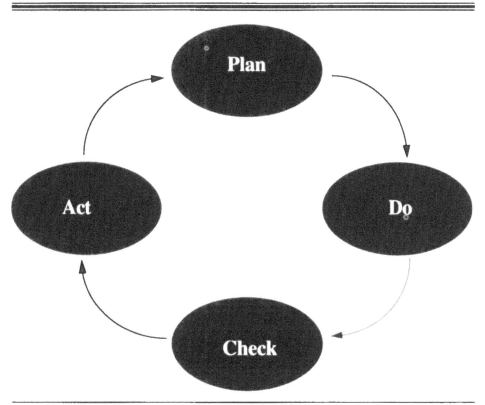

Figure 1.1. The Shewart Cycle

process control, a consistently better result can only be achieved by improving the process itself. Indeed, the absolutely vital corollary of this principle is that while the process remains in an uncontrolled state, sustained and predictable progress is quite impossible. It has been shown on a much broader canvas that *those who have no knowledge of history are condemned to repeat it.* The first task therefore in statistical process control is to gain that knowledge of the process that will lift the sentence of endlessly repeating past mistakes that ignorance has imposed.

These ideas were further developed by two of Shewart's assistants, W. Edwards Deming and J. M. Juran, in the years up to the Second World War.[2] After the war, Deming tried unsuccessfully to engage the interest of American industry in the benefits of a process under statistical quality control, capable of producing goods of the required quality within the expected limits of cost and at the expected time. Rebuffed and disappointed, but nevertheless undeterred, Deming took his ideas to Japan, in 1950 a devastated country of negative net worth, lacking in most natural resources, even wood, but whose stricken and exhausted industry embraced and enacted his philosophy wholeheartedly simply to export to feed its people. Whereas hitherto Japanese goods had had a reputation for being shoddy and "tinny", Western markets were suddenly horrified, and shaken to their foundations, by a flood of hi-fi separates, cameras, watches, automobiles and a host of other goods of a quality far superior to those of western manufacture, while at the same time being no more expensive and sometimes even actually cheaper! Deming later wrote the book *Out of the Crisis* (1986) which became a classic of its time, and for which he is now chiefly remembered.

To illustrate the fact that most faults arise from the *system* rather than from special attributable causes, Deming (1986, p. 7) describes a plant production line known by its supervisor to be in trouble. The supervisor concluded that the 24-worker team made a lot of mistakes and that if they pulled their socks up there would not be any mistakes at all. The first step was to get hold of the inspection data and plot the fraction defective day to day over the previous six weeks. This is the run chart illustrated on the left in figure 1.2.

It showed a stable random variation above and below the mean of 11 percent. So the level of mistakes was predictable and, therefore, it indicates that here we have a stable system for *the production of defective items*! The stability is indicative of the fact that the errors are a property of the system itself. It follows then that it is absolutely no use whatsoever for the management cajoling, berating or pleading with the workers to improve their performance. They are quite incapable of reducing the level of errors any further by working either harder or more conscientiously. The only way to decrease the level of defectives is to improve the system, which is the *responsibility of the management.*

So what were the management to do? It turned out on close examination that the people on the job and the inspector were not completely clear as to what kind of work was acceptable and what was not. Once the manager and two supervisors accepted the truth of this, they set to work to write clear, operational definitions of what constituted a failure, with examples of good and defective items, published for everyone to understand. (This activity is an example of what we now describe as documentation of the process). Within 7 weeks, the rate of defectives had fallen to 5 percent, less than half the previous rate, at no cost whatsoever, with the same

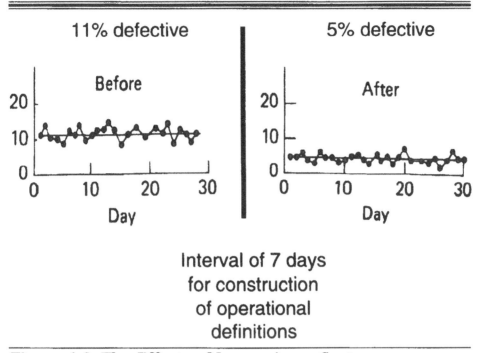

Figure 1.2. The Effects of Improving a System

work force working under the same pressures, and no new plant. Quality up, production of good product up 6 percent, capacity up 6 percent, lower cost per unit, improved bottom line, customers happier, everybody happier! As Deming concludes, this is an example of a gain in productivity accomplished by a change in the system, in this case an improvement in documentation (definitions as it happened) effected by the management, enabling people *not to work harder but to work smarter.*

But why stop there? Since the line was now stable at 5 percent defectives, further gains would have to come, once again, from *action on the system.* They might look at incoming materials that were difficult to work with, or at machines that did not work properly, or attempt to further tighten up the documented definitions, and so it could go on.

Deming's principles apply with equal force to the process of software engineering. In fact, it was in the age of the rapid growth of mainframe systems and the complexity of large software projects in the 1970s that the parallels between statistical process control and software engineering began to be spotted. One of the areas of most acute concern at that time was that of military software and the need to improve it. It was in response to this that the U.S. Department of Defense started a number of projects to try to improve software quality, as was mentioned in the introduction and which led to the foundation of the Software Engineering Institute at Carnegie Mellon University. It was from this institution that Watts S. Humphrey published (1988) one of the clearest categorizations of the various possible states in which a software development group can find itself. This model, known as the Capability Maturity Model, has passed into software folklore, becoming one of the most helpful models assisting software development groups of all sizes everywhere to measure where they are now and where they aspire to be in the future.

THE CAPABILITY MATURITY MODEL

The model, based on an earlier software process maturity grid published by Crosby (1979), is presented diagramatically in figure 1.3. The five levels were chosen because they reflect fairly closely the stages that most software development organizations actually go through as they improve. Each level can be clearly distinguished from those adjacent to it by objective criteria which clarify the measures that must be taken to reach the intermediate improvement goal. Once it becomes clear where an organization presently lies on the model, both managerial and technical staff can see the changes that are the most important. The international standardization program known as SPICE (Dorling 1993) (Software Process Improvement and Capability determination), which is the embryo for what is expected to become a new ISO standard, is defining a framework in which these models can be used to compare one organization with another, and to drive internal improvement programs forward.

So what does each level mean in terms of how an organization functions? Each level is briefly discussed below.

Initial Level

Many, many software development groups are still at the initial level which can be euphemistically described as creative chaos. There are no formal procedures and no more than the most rudimentary of cost estimates (written, perhaps, in the vernacular of the British

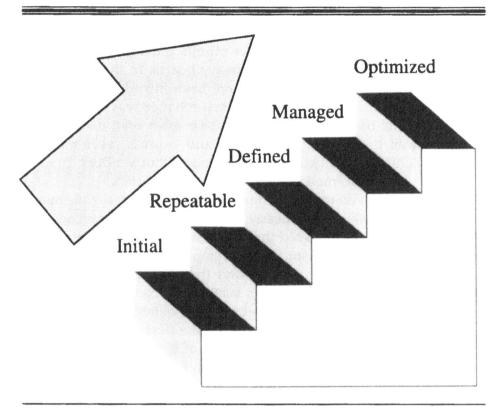

Figure 1.3. The Capability Maturity Model

working man, *on the back of a fag packet!*). There is little or no control exercised over change, both in the project process itself or in software. As a result, projects can never be guaranteed to run on time or at the expected cost, nor is there any certainty over exactly what will be produced in the end. Problems tend to be swept under the carpet, or rather passed on to unfortunate users. If procedures have ever been written, they are not used when it really matters—in a crisis. Just like individuals, organizations reveal their true characters under pressure. In the heat of a crisis, the group will behave in accordance with what it really believes. Any formal procedures are jettisoned with the cry "for heaven's sake, do something", and the disease that one wit has described as the *frantic fumble syndrome* sets in. The *quick fix* that results often creates as many defects as it purportedly resolves.

Even as late as the early 1980s some large, well-known scientific instrument suppliers were delivering software of this kind to the endless frustration of users. Defects seemed to be everywhere, with page after page of known problem reports and suggested workarounds appearing month after month. Each new release was greeted with trepidation and with heavy hearts, in the certain expectation that new defects would have been introduced in the efforts to rectify older errors, and minimal reliance was to be placed on the veracity of the documentation. Year after year, user groups would bewail the quality of software and express resentment at their involuntary use as so-called *beta testers*, but vendors, though anxious to please, seemed at a loss to improve matters.

Why on earth do organizations still behave like this? One might say contemptuously and tactlessly that it is because they know no better; the fact must be faced that there is much truth here, and it hurts. The underlying reason is that companies at this level do not realize what creative chaos is costing the organization, believing that the creativity of programmers is all that is required to develop software. There is always time and money available to put matters right, it seems, but none to do it right in the first place. But the total cost of quality is composed of the cost of trying to find, through testing, the defects that staff have been paid (!) to put into the product already, plus the cost of correcting them before delivery, plus the cost of dealing with defects discovered in the field, plus the cost of loss of business from one dissatisfied current customer, plus the cost of loss of business from other potential customers frightened off by a poor product quality reputation. Is this not sheer lunacy—employing a team of firefighters to extinguish blazes set alight by the squad of arsonists on the same payroll?

Programmers are frequently blamed for the presence of defects that are the fault of the system under which they work, which is the *management's responsibility*. Deming (1986, p. 315) proposed to ask the man in the street why a car manufacturer had recalled a certain model for essential safety repairs. Most respondents would pinpoint careless workmanship on the assembly line as the cause. But they would be wrong, absolutely wrong! The problem lies somewhere in the design of the car or of the assembly line, or management's failure to take cognizance of test results. How well many of us remember the British cars of the 1960s rushed to market to beat the competition but riddled with faults! We used to imagine the fundamental cause as being the cantankerous strike-happy production line workers, incited by communist-inspired rabble-rousers who noisily invaded our television screens night after night, but we were wrong! While such people may have earned Britain the unenviable reputation during that period of a strike-prone banana republic, stricken with what became known by the pejorative expression *The British Disease,* the root cause was actually defects in the manufacturing system. No amount of dedication, care and skill in the workers (and these qualities were present among many, despite the media images) could ever have overcome fundamental flaws in the system. Premature body shell corrosion was just one deficient quality feature. Many cars of that era were notorious rust buckets, attributed quite wrongly at the time to carelessness in body spraying. But motor body shells perforate from corrosion emanating from the *inside out,* not from the *outside in.* No amount of care in vehicle finishing affected this to the slightest degree. The problem was eventually solved in the motor industry by electrostatic deposition of paint inside body shell sections supplemented by wax injection, and the removal through design of the *causes* of internal water entrapment. The moral of the story is that an accurate understanding of the *causes of defects* in effecting their removal is equally as important in software engineering as it is in automotive engineering.

Another analogy of the need for a quality-assured process is provided by the question of what is required to get from A to B in the shortest possible time. Some would say nothing more than a fast car. But there is a fundamental difference between speed and progress. A fast car (creative programmers) is certainly indispensable, but what is also needed is a *map* (the quality management system).

Repeatable Level

At the repeatable level, a company has begun to introduce basic controls so that at least there is a some chance that the same thing can be done twice in the same way. This, of course, presupposes that there is a correct way of doing it. The first and most essential control is that of the time and effort of everyone employed in the business. Management has defined everyone's job at least in general terms by creating a *job description.*

Next, it has begun to manage the project process by producing a *project plan.* This is designed to set out what the project is intended to create, who is responsible for what, the resources needed, and how long it is expected to take. Senior management is now required to endorse all projects to demonstrate responsibility and commitment—the first and most vital step in changing the culture.

It might have also issued a *mission statement* or *quality policy* concerned with performance and quality (an example of the latter is provided in chapter 5).

The second step, almost as critical as the first, has been the creation of a QA post or group. Instead of being seen as free-wheeling passengers who live off the backs of those who do the *real work,* quality assurance ensure that things are done in the approved manner. To do this successfully, it is vital that they be independent of the developers and report directly at a very senior level of management. Again, such an appointment has a powerful effect in changing the culture, since permanent staff means money and money is the authentic indicator of commitment (we spend our money on those things we really value). It also reinforces the message that to do it right the first time is smarter than having to put it right retrospectively.

The third and final step has been the institution of some control over changes, both in the project process and in the software and its documentation. Projects thrive on stability but wilt in the face of uncontrolled change. Change, however, is a fact of life. It cannot be ignored, avoided or imperiously be commanded to retreat out of sight, like King Canute against the incoming tide. Its deleterious effects must be mitigated through strict control. Without change control, an ordered life cycle sequence of design, coding and testing stages cannot be achieved, and any quality plan will be ineffective.

The vast majority of software enterprises in business today are at this level. In most cases, they sincerely believe that they have solved the critical problems of successful software engineering, because the improvement over the state of affairs which appertained at the initial level has been so profound. This is undeniable, but serious problems remain. Nothing much is documented—most things are communicated by word of mouth. The process and its success still critically depend on each individual and his or her experience. Each will operate processes in a repeatable manner (because programmers, generally speaking, are very professional, dedicated, enthusiastic and skilled), although there is no certainty that anyone will execute a given process in exactly the same way as a colleague. While the group remains very small and staff turnover is limited or nonexistent, the weaknesses of the company can, to a large extent, remain masked.

Once a key person leaves and a new recruit joins, however, things begin to fall apart. How on earth is the new recruit to learn the ropes? Who will tell him or her how things are done? Since there are no official company standards, is there even an answer to the question of how things are done? Will they remember to tell the recruit everything? How long will it take them? Can they be released to spend time with the recruit? And in any case, will he or she understand? Experience shows that this is one of the most common sources of breakdown of control and a rise in defect rates in organizations at this level, the importance of which will be emphasized in chapter 5.

Other events soon reveal the vulnerability of such organizations. Technology is changing rapidly. What happens when new languages or tools change the process, or what happens when the firm needs to develop a new kind of product? Any event outside the experience of the group has the potential of being highly disruptive and may even threaten the very existence of the company.

Defined Level

For the first time, a member or a group within the organization has been allocated to spend some time examining and documenting the processes by which software is developed.[3] Until the process is documented, it cannot be brought under control, which is an indispensable prerequisite for ever improving it. In days of intense competition and short product lives, improvement of the process in terms of speeding the time to market of a better quality product, with fewer defects, at a lower and better controlled cost, has frequently become a matter of survival. Larger companies usually do this by a small interdisciplinary group, whereas smaller ones may need the temporary help of external consultants for a while.

Such documentation must include a basic description of the underlying process methodology or life cycle that the organization has used or will use. This description will include the documents that the methodology will naturally deliver, the procedures to be followed to make the process work, quality controls which measure success, and the quality standards that must be met.

It should be stressed that the words *written* and *documentation* no longer imply the necessary use of paper, although carefully designed paper systems can still be efficient and nonbureaucratic. The imaginative use of groupware products, such as Lotus Notes®, can deliver huge efficiency savings in having one master document available to a wide audience, and in providing a medium for documented discussions. Many software houses operate well-documented life cycle methodologies, managed through the effective use of this medium in the modern electronic office suite, and its use will be explored further in chapter 10.

The organization now has a defined software methodology. It will include a document management and control system to control the revision and issue of documents. It will include standard procedures for the review, approval and sign-off of documents (easily achievable in Notes®). It will include procedures and standards for assembling functional requirements and design documents. It will include measures to ensure traceability between them. It will include references to any formal design methods and the use of CASE tools that the organization has selected. It will also describe the use, intention and limitations of any prototyping approaches, now an especially popular approach in today's graphical user environments.

Organizations at this stage have all the ingredients to comply with the International Organization of Standards (ISO) 9000 suite of standards, in particular, the ISO 9000-3 standard for software development, known in the United Kingdom as the TickIT standard, with its pithy slogan of *making a better job of software*. This standard is the application of the general, two-party contractual standard, ISO 9001, to the special needs of the software engineering discipline. In the overwhelming majority of cases, organizations that have achieved TickIT certification have also been commercially successful, a fact that is no accident. The disciplines that lie at the heart of ISO 9000-3 imply control of the project process, the economic removal of defects at the earliest possible moment in the development process, and the avoidance of the huge costs inherent in their retrospective removal from product already in the marketplace.

Managed Level

Now that the process has been brought under effective control and thoroughly defined, how effective is it? We are now able not only to ask this question from an informed standpoint but also to take action with measurements or metrics toward actually improving the process itself. This is the approach most likely to deliver a consistent reduction in the level of residual defects in the product and to form the basis of major reductions in expenditure in hitherto exhaustive product testing.

The organization has now examined its defined process and es-tablished measurements of both the cost of quality measures such as error detection procedures, and the measurable benefits, such as logs of defects identified and removed, that they are delivering. As process improvements are tried, their effect on productivity can be impartially measured. The quality of each delivered product can be measured, and departure from quality targets identified quickly and explored. Quality assurance control points and metrics are identify-ing strengths and weaknesses in project control disciplines. Assur-ance of product delivery on time, within budget and with minimal defects, is becoming increasingly reliable in an engineered and pre-dictable process.

Since quality can now be systematically built into the product to an ever-increasing extent, costly efforts to prove this once the prod-uct has been built may be scaled down accordingly. So also can many of the overheads hitherto necessary to manage the *absence* of quality, such as exhaustive testing and large help desk operations. (A minimal help desk operation should always be in place, not least as a channel for enhancement requests, even if the thrust of process improvement is to deprive the goodly souls employed therein of much of their job content!) What defect reports do arise may be used in process improvements actions, thus completing the virtuous circle of continuous improvement (known as *kaizen* by the Japanese) and making possible the Shewart cycle *plan-do-check-act* on a sys-tematic and regular basis.

Managers now understand just where help is needed in the process and how to support and channel the creativity of program-mers. They, in turn, can communicate with each other in structured, unambiguous and quantitative terms which avoid misunderstand-ings and reinventions of the proverbial wheel. They are also able to understand how to be productive as well as creative and avoid in-corporating defects into the code. Very few organizations have achieved this level of maturity.

Optimized Level

At the optimized level, the process has been improved to such a de-gree that the law of diminishing returns has begun to operate. There is little scope for effective improvement in the process, and the cost of effecting incremental improvements outweighs the benefits of those improvements. The risk in the process is now virtually nil, and a state of optimal stability has been reached.

If few organizations reach the managed level, practically none reach the optimized level. This is not because it is fundamentally impossible to achieve. It is largely because the rate of change of technology in the present era makes it extremely difficult to optimize any software development process, since the underlying technology is not stable long enough for this to happen.

RISK AND STRUCTURAL INTEGRITY

Software development is a risky business, not only for the software developer but also for the purchaser. Modern business is built on software, the medium through which most of its core business processes execute. Every new piece of software added to the computer networks of an enterprise poses a risk, both in terms of other processes executing within the same environment, and to the success of the business process for which the software was intended. As the developer's software capability maturity increases, there is an increasing level of structural integrity in the software product produced—a consistency of internal order and design reducing the scope for defects, ensuring a high level of probability that the software will do what it purports to do and will **not** do what it purports **not to do**. The risk to the purchaser firm and those dependent on it is thereby reduced. This factor is of special importance in certain industries, such as those of pharmaceuticals, nuclear power, aeronautical engineering and others, where human life or well-being is directly or indirectly dependent on software quality.

Maturity also reduces the risk to the developer. As capability maturity improves, there is a marked decrease in the total cost of producing software and in the time to delivery as figure 1.4 illustrates. Total costs include all those costs appertaining to nonquality which have already been mentioned. Boehm (1981) has estimated that as much as two thirds of maintenance costs arise directly from faulty design. De Marco (1982) has calculated that about half the costs of maintaining a software product are incurred during the first 15 percent of its life. Most of these costs are due to errors which only crop up when the system is passed into the hands of users, and many of these turn out to reflect *requirements that were either not specified at all or specified incompletely, ambiguously or otherwise erroneously*. In this regard, Boar (1984) has reported that about half to three quarters of subsequent system faults are in this

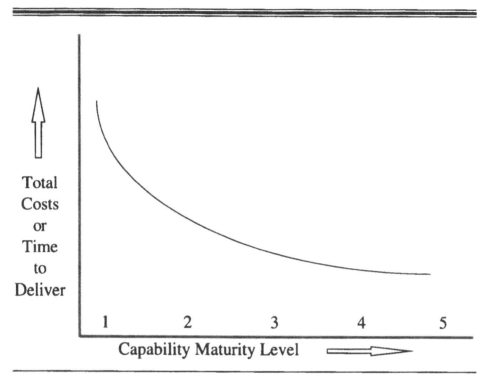

Figure 1.4. Total Costs and Time to Deliver Versus Capability Maturity

category! The reduction in testing and help desk costs, together with the unknown and unknowable costs associated with the loss of repeat business from existing customers, and loss of business from potential customers had the software been of better quality, vastly outweigh the additional costs involved early in the process to remove defects (e.g., to get the requirements right) and to ensure the incorporation of quality and structural integrity. The improvements in the project management process from a defined and managed project life cycle methodology and its associated disciplines ensure a more predictable process. As figure 1.5 shows, there is a marked decrease in the variability of delivery time for comparable stages between projects, and also an increasing correspondence between the time of actual appearance of deliverables in projects and their expected arrival time. An overall reduction in the length of time from product conception to delivery into the field always accompanies such improvements, all other things being equal. Both of these

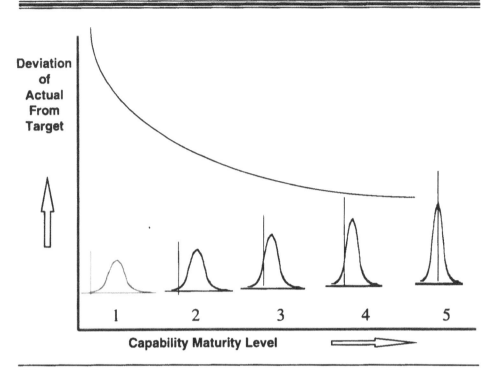

Figure 1.5. Project Management Performance Versus Capability Maturity

factors markedly reduce the risk to the developer inherent in any new software project and improve the likelihood of the developer remaining in business to continue to support product in partnership with customers.[4]

The ensuing chapters will describe the scope of the team's assessment in detail and refer extensively to the applicable standards defining best practice that have emerged in recent years. Comments will be made on practices that have been found by experience to be conducive to the cost-effective creation of sound software, especially as appropriate to the small software house, where cost control is particularly critical and pressure to take the shortcut to quick profit the most irresistible.

SOFTWARE DEVELOPMENT:
AN ENGINEERING PROCESS

In the course of establishing contacts with a large number of software vendors, particularly very small firms, it is extraordinary how frequently the concept of a process approach to software development is either quite novel or only a recent acquaintance. But such an approach is by no means new. One of the first descriptions of a stagewise method of creating software appeared is attributed to Benington (1956, pp. 15–27) and many have followed since. All of them are characterized by certain common elements, which are as follows:

- Documenting the user's requirements (what the system is supposed to do)

- Describing the system technically (how it will fulfil the requirements)

- Building the system

- Testing the system

- Delivering the system, supporting it and enhancing it

These stages taken together share many of the characteristics of engineering processes in general leading to the term *software engineering*, originally coined as the title of a 1968 conference organized by the Science Committee of the North Atlanatic Treaty Organization. This type of approach to software development is in stark contrast to the widely held delusion that software development requires nothing more than the flair and creativity of clever programmers. However, it has long become apparent (Dijkstra 1976) that without the discipline inherent in a process-orientated view, there is very little chance of a software development project delivering a system that will do what it is supposed to do (and will **not** do what it is **not** supposed to do!) within budget and on time. This view has been endorsed more recently through a fresh emphasis on a disciplined approach to software engineering from no less a figure than the legendary Watts Humphrey (1994; 1995). These are the business-critical issues of survival in the highly competitive commercial environment of the 1990s and beyond. The engineering approach is nowadays described as a *system development life cycle*. The term *life cycle* is pregnant with meaning, since it implies an *iterative* process (i.e., a rerun of the process from the beginning). One example of this iterative characteristic is the enhancement element introduced into the basic life cycle in some of the later expressions of the basic model. Enhancement has assumed great importance of late as the rate of technological change has shortened product life-times drastically, enforcing a much more frequent redevelopment of systems to match accelerating changes in user requirements. A detailed description of life cycle models is beyond the scope of this book, but three will be briefly mentioned.

The Waterfall Model

The Waterfall model is the oldest and perhaps the most common model in use, particularly in the many vendors who are scarcely aware that they have any development methodology at all! The model, first recognized by Royce (1970) who originally gave this model its name, is shown in Figure 1.6. It portrays the basic

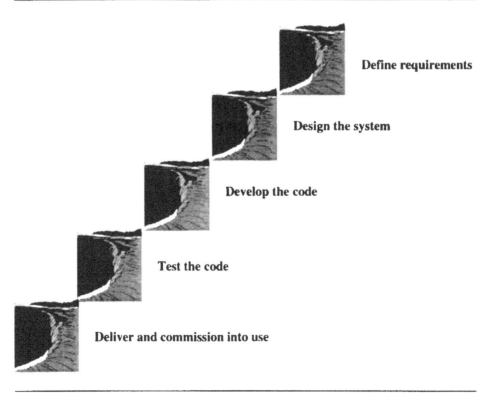

Define requirements

Design the system

Develop the code

Test the code

Deliver and commission into use

Figure 1.6. The Classic Waterfall Model in an Ideal World

skeleton of stages, though these are frequently amplified into greater detail, for example, by exploding the "define requirements" stage into three by adding "analyze requirements" and "specify system". The model implies a smooth progression of activities from inception through definition through production into implementation. Unfortunately, it shares one of the characteristics of the ideal gases of classical physics expressed by the laws of Charles and Boyle: that the real world is never as simple as the model predicts. Though a useful conceptual tool, most projects of any complexity are bedeviled by concurrent changes in requirements and technology which threaten the quality and traceability implicit in the model. Thus, a real world model might bear regressive arrows to indicate iterative repetition of stages, as shown in figure 1.7. This recycling from one phase back to its predecessor may be inevitable, but must,

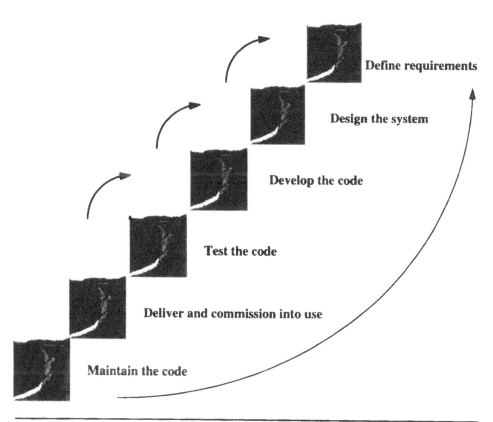

Define requirements

Design the system

Develop the code

Test the code

Deliver and commission into use

Maintain the code

Figure 1.7. The Real World Waterfall Model

nevertheless, be controlled so that the output from each phase constitutes a credible and stable baseline. All reiterations of the previous stage's work must be completed in that stage and not carried forward. Without this care, the cost of subsequent recycling becomes catastrophically expensive extremely quickly. The model also carries an additional stage—maintenance—which applies to most (though by no means all) products, and shows that when enhancements are envisaged, the entire process recommences from the beginning.

The V Process Model

The V process model marks a considerable improvement on the Waterfall model, in that it demonstrates the relationships between activities that precede coding to those following coding, thus reinforcing the key principle of traceability.

A simple diagram of the model appears in figure 1.8. Each specification created prior to building the software is used to develop the test plans on which the subsequent testing of the software is based. In this way, traceability is preserved, and testing becomes a systematic exploration of all of the major pathways and features incorporated into the design. Described another way, the left-hand down-going process creates each specification from the previous document in a decomposition or explosion process, transforming the user's ill-considered, vague and probably ambiguous expressions of requirements into a strict, logical and definitive statement of functionality in technical terminology fit for use as a basis for coding. The right-hand up-going arm describes the testing (delivering test reports) that demonstrate the achievement of the corresponding specifications on the left. Thus, the final delivered system based on acceptance testing is an accurate and complete expression of the original requirements.

The V Model in Regulated Environments

A version of the V model suitable for the regulated pharmaceutical environment is featured in the GAMP guide (1996). Here the model is applied not to the software engineering process but to the validation of a computer-related system. The purpose of introducing this concept lies in the importance of software vendors who supply systems to users subject to regulation, understanding their role in contributing to the user's compliance in a fundamental way. The two

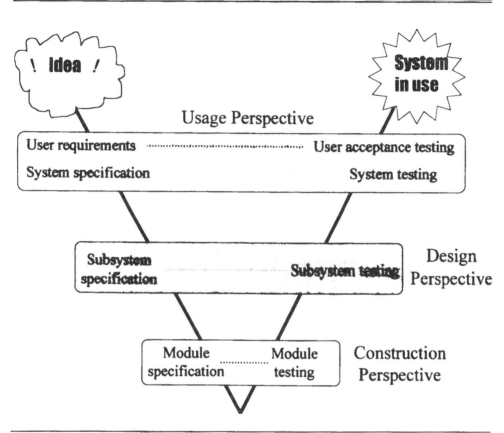

Figure 1.8. The V Model (adapted from an original illustration by Ould (1990, p. 39)

processes are closely linked since the assessment of the quality of the software to measure its validatability is an activity subsumed within a computer-related systems validation plan. The two processes, though quite distinct, have much in common. The model is accordingly couched in the terms that have now become accepted in the realm of computer-related systems validation.

These requirements, now part of good manufacturing practice and good laboratory practice around the world, require the presentation of documentary evidence that a computer system does what it purports to do. The emphasis is, therefore, on *delivered documents*. All life cycle models echo this emphasis, since they seek to formalize and control the two-way flow of information on which all successful software development depends. These flows are as follows:

- Forward: each phase delivering the document constituting the foundation for the subsequent phase

- Reverse: a much smaller flow of problem and feedback reports

The objective of every life cycle methodology is to root out the use of informal, undocumented information. The V model shown in figure 1.9 introduces some new terms referring to user activities. The full list of definitions is as follows:

- **User Requirements Specification:** Documentation created by the *vendor* in close association with the user describing what a system is supposed to do, and linking to performance qualification which tests these requirements.

- **Performance Qualification:** Documentation created by the *user* demonstrating that when operated within set

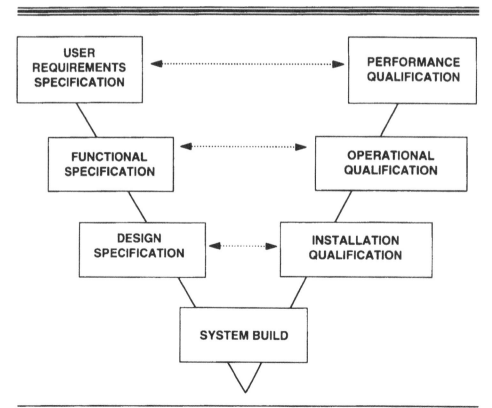

Figure 1.9. The GAMP Version of the V Model

parameters, the process (in this case the automated system) will consistently produce product meeting its predetermined specification. In practice, when a system is running correctly, it produces acceptable quality product and that *sufficient documentary evidence exists to demonstrate this*.

- **Functional Specification:** Documentation describing the detailed functions of the system, and linking to operational qualification which tests all functions.

- **Operational Qualification:** Documentation demonstrating that the equipment or system operates as intended throughout representative or anticipated operating ranges. In practice, the installed system works as specified and *sufficient documentary evidence exists to demonstrate this*.

- **Design Specification:** A complete definition of the system created by the *vendor* in sufficient detail to enable it to be built, and links to installation qualification which checks that the correct system is supplied to the required standards and that it is installed correctly.

- **Installation Qualification:** Documentation created by the *user* that the equipment design and configuration is as intended; that instrumentation has adequate accuracy, precision and range for the intended use, and that services (such as power supplies) are of adequate quality. In practice, the system has been installed as specified and *sufficient documentary evidence exists to demonstrate this*.

The formal exercise of computer-related systems validation only applies in areas subject to regulation. In this context the principal responsibility of the software QA auditor is to seek out whether a system development life cycle methodology exists *at all*, and, if so, the nature of the documentary evidence demonstrating the presence of quality controls within it. By evaluating this evidence, the extent to which quality has been incorporated into the software, and hence the level of innate structural integrity, can be measured. This is closely related to the probable level of remaining unknown defects and, therefore, to the fitness of the software for its intended purpose. From a computer-related system validation standpoint, this effectively is a measure of its validatability. Conversely, of course, in the absence of a quality-assured development methodology, a software product is *unvalidatable* regardless of how exhaustive or comprehensive the user testing program deployed to validate it has been, a lesson that some pharmaceutical companies have had to learn very painfully.

The Spiral Model

The last model we will examine is of particular importance to to-day's object-oriented environment and is known as the spiral model of software development. It was originally attributed to Boehm and introduced by him at a conference held near Los Angeles back in 1985. Illustrated in figure 1.10, its interesting feature is that it is

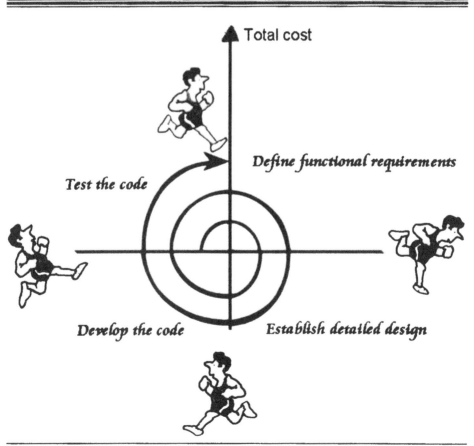

Figure 1.10. The Spiral Model

conceptually endless, with each twist of the spiral retracing the steps of its predecessor. Each twist proceeds clockwise, starting in the upper right-hand corner with defining (or redefining on the second and later iterations) functional requirements, proceeding to firming up the design in the lower right-hand quadrant, and finally building and testing the system. Thus, the two preceding models can be considered as special cases of this more general model, representing a single twist only. The relevance of the spiral model today is that much development of software for the Windows™ graphical user interface environment is based on the approach of *rapid prototyping*, sometimes called *rapid application development*.

Each *prototype* is constructed through one twist and evaluated for conformity to requirements as part of the testing. This would take the form of a critical review by users for the purpose of clarifying and elucidating the functional requirements. The next twist would then be driven by the degree of departure of the prototype from the final intended system. As each iteration proceeds, the spiral deviates further from the center indicating the increasing cost, measured by an imaginary radius. However, as the product more closely approximates (hopefully) to what is required, the risk diminishes. In fact it was the concern with risk which inspired this model in the first place.

Object-Oriented Programming

Very much the vogue today, the object-oriented approach to software development arises from the prevalence of libraries of common screen objects used in Windows™ programs of all kinds. These are used to assemble the user interface or front end of an application very quickly, with little or no original code from the developer. In this sense, development comes to resemble the construction we associate with a child's Lego® kit. At a conceptual level, object-oriented programming differs fundamentally from the traditional life cycle which represents a top-down approach (requirements, analysis, design, development). In contrast object-oriented programming is a bottom-up approach, where code creation is the first activity. Because of this, object-oriented programming can lead to problems when attempting to incorporate it into a top-down life cycle. These difficulties usually relate to the failure to think clearly enough and early enough about the role, limitations and planned deficiencies of prototypes.

Disposable Prototypes Versus Incremental Development

In object-oriented programming, the prototype is little different from the application itself. It is not just an empty shell for demonstration purposes, as might have been the case with a prototype constructed in a third generation language. It is in every respect a working product component, though it may lack other essential functionality, such as a database engine or other critical modules behind it. This extraordinarily powerful aspect of object-oriented programming has a profound effect on third generation language programmers, who positively drool over the ease with which working code can now be constructed, remembering the rigid discipline and the remorseless gargantuan effort needed to make corresponding progress in the past. While the rapidity of object-oriented programming is beyond doubt an incredible *strength*, it is also, at the same time, a *weakness*, in that it places an overwhelming temptation in the path of developers to misunderstand the purpose of a prototype and skip the discipline of documenting functional requirements. Instead, developers can jump straight into development with both feet, throw together (yes, that is often just how it happens!) the front end and take it straight back to users who are instantly taken with the speed at which "the product" is progressing. Euphoria, enthusiasm and impatience then conspire to eclipse sober judgement, in that the rest of the development is pursued with a dismissive disregard for what are instinctively regarded as the unglamorous and prosaic life cycle QC disciplines (another loaded word) that hamper "real progress".

What then are the advantages of prototypes? First, they contribute strongly to a mitigation of *risk*. The emergence of a working model of what developers believe users require can be produced earlier and more cheaply, thus exposing dichotomies of view between users and developers before a great deal of investment has been made, and reducing the risk of developing something no one will eventually buy. Second, a working prototype can be used as a *training aid*, especially since a customer representative intimately familiar with the application will often have assisted in producing it. The prototype can help clarify the requirements which, as we shall see again in chapter 7, continue to be a major source of misunderstanding, ambiguity and defects. Finally, the prototype can assist in system testing, since it defines how the final system should behave. Thus, by comparing outputs from the system against that of the prototype using an output file comparison, errors can be identified earlier, with less effort and in greater depth.

With such a glowing set of attributes, can prototypes have pitfalls? We have already alluded to the temptation to take the shortcut. Indeed, prototyping can only be successful if it is subjected to the same degree of management control and quality assurance as the rest of the life cycle. Unless there is a strong degree of control, the activity can become endless; the project manager must know constantly how the prototype is progressing and what it is costing. To counter the tendency to confuse the prototype and the product, it is essential that if prototyping is anticipated as part of the project, then the prototype's purpose, planned limitations and expected deficiencies should all be elaborated in advance in the project plan. For example, in the interests of speed and economy, the prototype may be permitted to be riddled with defects yet still be useful. In this case, the quality controls to be applied, and the resources which are **not** to be exceeded, should also be defined.

It is critically important for everyone to understand which process model—disposable or incremental—is being followed. There must be no confusion as to whether the prototype is *disposable*, purely intended to elucidate functional requirements (in which case it operates strictly within one discrete phase of the life cycle, and is to be discarded prior to the formal commencement of development), or whether the *incremental development model* is in use (the prototype forms the basis of development and straddles most of the phases of the life cycle). In the former, prototyping is an excellent means of validating the requirements (making sure that what is intended to be produced matches what is actually required). In these circumstances, the deficiencies of the prototype should be outlined clearly, emphasizing its limited value. In the latter case, the cyclic nature of the (spiral) model must be firmly gripped, imposed and reinforced, the sequence *requirement-design-develop-test* with appropriate documentation at each stage being rigorously observed; however, many twists of the cycle are finally made. The alluring temptation to jump across the radius or make other shortcuts in the supposed interests of economy must be fiercely resisted. In any event, prototyping should not commence (or, at worst, not continue past a very early, and strictly limited, stage), unless and until any fundamental architectural decisions have been made and elucidated. If followed, this rule will ensure that the prototype can be kept within its predefined conceptual and practical boundaries.

Finally the old adage still applies: *No job is finished until the paperwork is complete.* When the prototype is agreed to be complete, its functionality and design must be documented. The capabilities of rapid application development reinforce, rather than diminish, the importance of the control disciplines that this book, and the standards which undergird it, are striving to advocate. The interests of both developers and purchasers are most powerfully served if the potential of rapid application development tools is brought to bear in *assisting* the elucidation and documentation of the user's requirements, rather than in seeking to *usurp or avoid them.*

Having reviewed, therefore, the principles by which software that is demonstrably fit for its intended purpose must be engineered, other questions immediately arise. To which types of software does the need to establish this conformity most pressingly apply, and what practical means are now available to a purchasing organization to do this? It is to provide answers to these that the next chapter is devoted.

Notes

1. A regrettable metaphor perhaps—we hope that neither the project nor the firm has terminally succumbed to whatever went wrong!

2. A fuller and fascinating historical review may be found in the *AT&T Technical Journal,* March/April 1986.

3. A case study describing the experience of inaugurating a Software Engineering Process Group (SEPG) in a Japanese electronics manufacturer, producing microprocessor embedded systems including ATMs, POS terminals and railway ticketing machines, has been described by Sakamoto et al. (Sakamoto 1996). The corporation, self-assessed as being at level 1, was involved in producing embedded software of considerable complexity with hundreds of input/output data items managing numerous complex hardware devices and running to more than a million lines of code. The paper describes the results of the SEPG's efforts, their improvement activities, the lessons learned and how the Capability Maturity Model guidelines were accordingly modified after a successful technology transfer.

4. The frequency with which software houses cease trading as going concerns, either through insolvency or through takeover, has become painfully apparent recently from the author's enquiries regarding the millenium compliance of software products.

2

Audit Approaches

An auditor's pat on the back, though only a few vertebrae removed from a kick in the pants, produces inestimably better results.

Anon

CATEGORIES OF SOFTWARE

In our discussions so far of the IT revolution, now in full swing, we have treated software as if it were a single entity. The term, however, embraces a broad spectrum of program types which vary widely in functionality, complexity and market penetration. This of itself implies a differing level of risk exposure for the software purchaser; it follows, therefore, that the need for a quality assessment is by no means uniform. It is important to understand the distinctions between the various classes so that efforts to ensure quality in procurement may be wisely directed. One of the most helpful categorizations of software so far published has been that included in the GAMP guide (1996) which, although written primarily for systems used in pharmaceutical manufacturing actually applies to software of all kinds. The guide groups software into five classes.

Operating Systems

No convincing case can be made in normal circumstances for attempting to assess established, commercially available operating systems. These systems are installed in tens of thousands of computers around the world. Consequently, their logical pathways are being exercised every time any application program installed on them is executed. Therefore, it is highly likely that any significant flaw will emerge quite quickly after release. The clear implication from this, on the other hand, is that a new release should be most carefully reviewed in terms of the impact that new, amended or removed features included in it might have on existing application software developed on an earlier version. A formal retesting of each application should be instituted and the results recorded, with actions being taken and recorded for any deviations from normal behavior. Such deviations will deepen the understanding of the changes effected in the new release and their implications, not just for other existing programs but also for the ongoing projects for new applications, thus avoiding the unintentional incorporation of subtle defects with all their attendant costs. Test records of these checks should be retained as part of the application's documentation. The use of automated testing techniques can be especially cost-effective in these circumstances.

Instrument Firmware

There is a huge variety of instrumentation in use today throughout industry, especially in such fields as manufacturing and chemical analysis, that is driven by software encoded onto programmable chips. Such code, possessing characteristics both of hardware (in that it resides in a chip) and software (in that it can be readily changed) is known as *firmware*. The disciplines used to develop this code are as fundamental to the successful operation of the instrument as are those used to develop conventional software. Therefore, it is perfectly appropriate and just as beneficial for firmware to be audited in the same way as application software.

Standard Software Packages

Standard Software Packages are often known as canned or configurable off-the-shelf (COTS) packages; examples of this genre are Microsoft Access® and Lotus 1-2-3®. The most successful of these packages share some of the characteristics of operating systems in terms of their ubiquity. Once a release has become established in the market, a review may be carried out of their market history. Success in the marketplace implies at least a minimum level of structural integrity in the product although, of course, it does not prove it. This being so, a user company may issue an *implied structural integrity certificate*, described in more detail below, thereby publicly confirming the acceptance of the product in a particular version as being acceptable for purchase on the basis of the implied level of structural integrity, without attempting to carry out a formal assessment.

On the other hand, the use of these products invariably involves the creation of application scripts and tables. It is quite easy to produce an application with a high level of defects, despite the integrity of the COTS platform itself, where there is a lack of strict life cycle disciplines and formal controls. This is frequently overlooked and even deliberately ignored, a fact all the more serious when it is remembered that key financial decisions in an organization are often based on spreadsheet applications with virtually no in-built quality assurance. Accordingly, an audit of this activity and all its attendant documentation is, therefore, just as beneficial to the business as the assessment of applications written in native code.

Configurable Software Packages

Often called custom configurable packages in the United States, examples of this type of software are Laboratory Information Management Systems, Supervisory Control and Data Acquisition packages, Chromatography Data Systems and Material and Resource Planning systems. These systems allow users to develop their own applications by *filling in the blanks* (i.e., by configuring the modules of which the package is composed so as to tailor its specific behaviour exactly to the user's need within the overall constraints of the application in general). This configuration effects no change whatsoever in the executable code of the package.

In these cases, an audit of the application to assess the level of in-built structural integrity is as essential as that for any other software written in native code. But that is not all. Since the functional requirements of the package will be to some extent general, it will also be necessary to audit the quality of the configuration work built on top of the package (the contents of the blanks). Both audits taken together can yield a reliable assessment of the level of structural integrity of the application as a whole and also ensure regulatory compliance where applicable.

Bespoke[1] or Custom-Built Systems

The category of bespoke or custom-built systems is one where the need for thoroughness of the audit process is greatest. Since the system is unique, there are unlikely to be more than a few copies in use anywhere. Thus, the scope for the discovery of defects in the field is extremely limited, and deprived of this, the need to avoid the inclusion of defects in the first place is greatest. Since the development costs must be borne on such a narrow base, there is a strong trend away from such software in all but the most esoteric applications; any case put forward today for the development of such software ought to be subjected to the most thorough and critical examination.

IMPLIED STRUCTURAL INTEGRITY CERTIFICATE

The Implied Structural Integrity Certificate (see appendix 6) is a document that publicizes the results of an assessment of the probable level of in-built quality of a commercial software product and summarizes the available evidence. Such evidence centers around the number of licences that have been sold, and thus by implication, the approximate number of individual users who may be reckoned to be exercising, and in a real sense, *testing* the product. Once this figure reaches the tens of thousands, the probability of serious structural weaknesses or other major operational errors remaining undiscovered becomes quite small, as does the likelihood of such errors appearing for the first time.

If reliable information of this nature can be gleaned from the vendor, a certificate summarizing the market history can be issued. This certificate is intended to give confidence to other prospective purchasers of the product within the organization. It also assists in confining software for generic tasks, such as word processing and spreadsheets, to one or two standard products, thus reaping the benefit of lower support costs.

It is vital, however, to disabuse readers of the certificate of the impression that the assessment is capable of affording the same degree of quality assurance as that delivered by a formal audit. In addition, certificate holders must be warned that new versions of well-tried software cannot be assumed necessarily to possess the same quality pedigree as their predecessors, since the rigor of change control and other essential software life cycle disciplines has not been evaluated. New versions must be treated with the same caution as that appropriate for any other new product.

It is disappointing to relate that some major international vendors are still unwilling to release this kind of information, citing grounds of commercial confidentiality as the reason for the refusal. It is difficult to understand how such reticence can be justified or how the release of such information on a retrospective basis could be commercially damaging. The suspicion lingers that underneath it all the vendor may fear the data incapable of substantiating a favourable conclusion in this respect, and reinforces the impression that software quality remains a very sensitive issue, even among blue chip suppliers.

INITIATION OF THE AUDIT REQUEST

A successful audit program can only survive in a purchasing organization with a clear quality policy that extends to the procurement of IT resources, of which software is a major component. The policy should be expressed and implemented in a family of procedures describing the business processes. The most progressive commercial and industrial organisations, those whose IT groups are reinforcing their commitment to a customer-focused ethos in the most tangible ways, are beginning to formalise these relationships in *service level agreements* or in the publication of catalogues of *service offerings* that internal customers can procure from an advertised catalogue, along similar lines to that of any mail order or retail supplier. Each service, which includes, behind the scenes, the documented procedures on which service delivery depends, must bear a quality metric in one form or another in whose terms the standard offering or specific customer agreement is framed. This kind of approach can be elegantly implemented using a groupware vehicle such as Lotus Notes® and is one of the most effective ways by which internal IT groups can demonstrate their commercial competitiveness and resist any pressure to become outsourced.[2] The software quality assurance audit service is just one example of a service that might feature in such a catalogue. It is worth noting that the management and control of service provision exhibits many parallels with the disciplines of good software engineering, and forms the subject of a separate ISO standard, ISO 9004-2:1991.

Ideally, the request for an audit assessment should immediately precede the decision to purchase, following the purchaser's review of the software's functionality and his or her perception of its suitability to meet a particular business need. Should events not proceed in this order, the request should always precede the decision to install the software, as a final safeguard.

THE QUALITY REVIEW

There are, however, a number of instances where a *quality review* is more appropriate than an audit. This exercise is far less expensive than a full-blown assessment visit but only delivers a shallow insight into the level of innate software quality. As always, you get what you pay for. It may take a number of forms. If a number of competing products are being evaluated and a quality assessment is included as part of the sifting process, it will usually not be cost-effective to audit each one. A *vendor screening* has been found to be useful and can be carried out with the aid of a bald questionnaire, an example of which appears in appendix 2. This is a rather blunt tool for differentiating between vendors and is only capable of identifying the most glaring contrasts, such as distinguishing a vendor who at least has a quality management system of some sort, from a vendor who has no procedures whatsoever! It cannot and must not be pressed into service in an attempt to resolve finer discriminations between vendors, since the bland answers to its *closed* questions (those that call for nothing more than a yes or no answer) conceal so much. Although telephone enquiries are capable of illuminating such responses, they can only do so to a limited degree.

A more in-depth questionnaire designed to elicit much fuller information and phrased to avoid closed questions can be used where the inclination toward a particular vendor is crystallizing. An example of such a *vendor quality assurance/life cycle enquiry* appears in appendix 10. Clearly, this requires much more work on the vendor's part to respond to the enquiries on the document than the simpler questionnaire, and many vendors would be unwilling to cooperate in completing it without a fairly firm prospect of some business eventually materializing. Successful use of this document has been made in certain circumstances, where for one reason or another an audit could not be carried out, but a decision on software had to be made quickly for business reasons.

Another case where the expense of an audit can often be avoided is that of standard software packages, especially where an Implied Structural Integrity Certificate has been issued. There is seldom any new native code in such applications which might present a hazard to other coexecuting software if installed on a network server. A good example of this is database applications written entirely in Microsoft Access® and with no other native code. In these cases, the auditor's concern focusses on the supportability of the product and especially the documentation that has been generated as part of the development life cycle. Summaries of such documentation, which should cover the main phases of the life cycle, can be requested and give a sufficient degree of quality assurance without incurring the expense of an audit assessment. In some cases, the developer has visited the purchasing company prior to commencing the work, to agree on the documentation deliverables the process is expected to furnish. In every such case, the developer has appreciated the practical guidance that has been given which has aided him or her, to not only produce a better and more supportable product, but to enable the costing of the process to be more accurate, and thus to increase the developer's confidence of actually making an acceptable profit!

However, caution is still needed. In a recent purchase of a Microsoft Access®–developed application, enquiries with the development team unearthed the possibility that if used in a particular manner, the application could crash the network, a state of affairs hitherto believed to be impossible in such circumstances. This alarming scenario arose from the large number of locks set per connection associated with the application. It was found necessary to install certain patches into the network to avert this danger.[3]

If a quality review is used rather than an audit in procurement, it does not dispense with the need to record the decision and its grounds. This should be done briefly and concisely, to provide the necessary reassurance both to purchasing department and to the IT group committed to managing the product subsequently.

AUDIT TEAMS

There is no hard and fast rule regarding the composition of the purchasing firm's representation on the audit team. Some firms send an individual auditor, others a multidisciplinary audit team. There are two factors of central importance: the nature and scope of the audit enquiries, stemming from the standards expected, and the competence and expertise of the auditor to understand and interpret the responses given.

For audits carried out against the guidance provided in the GAMP guide (1996), the auditor(s) will require broad experience in the application of the principles of good manufacturing practice to the use of computer-related systems, as well as some practical experience in the creation of software and the special challenges it presents. Since there are very few individuals who possess such a spectrum of skills to a sufficient degree, a multidisciplinary team of two or three is usual. If, however, a single individual can be found within the purchasing company with experience both in quality-related areas and in software engineering, an audit by a single *accredited* auditor becomes practical, with substantial cost reductions. Accredited is important; should the competence of the auditor ever be questioned, the entire value of the exercise in terms of the reliability or impartiality of the conclusions drawn, and their ability to withstand regulatory or managerial scrutiny, becomes suspect.

ACCREDITATION OF AUDITORS

Very few purchasing firms (one of which happens to be in the pharmaceutical industry) have so far addressed the issue of the *internal* accreditation of software QA auditors, though there may be others. A structured training course terminating in a test of competence is a prerequisite for qualification to conduct software engineering audits, whose findings form an integral part of computer-related system validation records under good manufacturing practices regulations. The implied standards against which such audits are conducted are those that have been published and accepted by consensus, both within the industry and the regulatory community, and appear in the documents mentioned in the introduction. There is a convergence occurring now between these standards and those applicable to the software industry as a whole. An example of this is the inclusion in the purchasing guidance section of the TickIT Guide (1995, appendix 4, page 5) of a reference to the GAMP guide (1996) published by the UK Pharmaceutical Industry Computer Systems

Validation Forum. However on a much broader front, for audits of software in general against the TickIT standards, a mature scheme of auditor training and accreditation has been in place for some time. Appendix 2 of the TickIT Guide details the academic requirements, attributes, training and experience required for lead, senior and provisional TickIT auditors. The attribute standards described therein are extracted from a booklet[4] obtainable from the International Register of Certificated Auditors.[5] It is interesting to note that the academic qualifications cited mirror the balance advocated earlier between academic, IT or business experience on the one hand, and a recognized QA qualification on the other.

Since the TickIT scheme is relatively mature, should not all software houses seek accreditation from TickIT accreditation bodies, 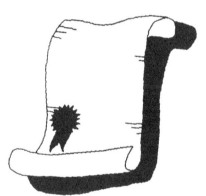 and should not purchasers confine their software acquisition to that from TickIT-accredited software vendors? In an ideal world, the answer to both of these questions would be yes. The fact is, however, that despite the excellence of the TickIT scheme and the success of most of its accredited companies, they represent only a small fraction of the total software industry. The vast majority of software vendors, many of them very small, are nowhere near the TickIT standards either in life cycle methodology or in documentation. Many of them have only an instinctive idea of good software engineering practice and need a great deal of help to improve their quality and productivity. The prospect of this is only likely to be entertained under the sanction of the possible loss of business. It is not likely to be practicable for the foreseeable future to confine purchase of software in general to certified, accredited vendors. In the meantime, enlightened purchasers are well advised in their own long-term best interests to help their suppliers in the ways described in this book. Vendors following this advice set their feet firmly on the high road toward ISO 9000-3 (TickIT) compliance and can move smoothly toward formal certification as and when the business environment becomes insistent on this as an indispensable and recognized badge of competence.

ESTABLISHING A RELATIONSHIP
WITH A SOFTWARE VENDOR

The importance of the initial contact that the auditor makes with the vendor is hard to overemphasize. Vendors vary enormously in their initial attitude to a software audit. This reflects to a large degree their approach to quality, but it would be misleading to imply that this is the only factor at work. Size is also of crucial importance; many small vendors with a programming team of two or three have few, if any, formal procedures; they tend, therefore, to fight shy, feeling instinctively that an audit is certain to cast their business in an unfavourable light. For very small software development teams, written procedures are less vital in preserving a quality culture than in a larger organization. Closely knit groups are quite able to work to very high standards with a minimum of documentation, although in such cases the auditor will need to exert greater effort in unearthing evidence for this. Since the auditor cannot and must not prejudge the issue, it is essential to reassure the vendor staff of these realities and to put them at their ease.

Since the inception of the UK Medicines Act in 1968, pharmaceutical companies have been obliged to ensure that their manufacturing operations comply with the principles of good manufacturing practice, described in official publications such as that known familiarly in the United Kingdom as the Orange Guide (from the colour of its cover) and in the Code of Federal Regulations in the United States. Experience with good manufacturing practice audits within the industry, both external (i.e., by regulatory authorities) and internal, have shown that it is vital to elicit the full-hearted co-operation of the audited department or group from the very outset if the audit is to prove to their long-term benefit. Failure to establish this atmosphere, when the audit is first arranged, makes it far more likely that an adversarial atmosphere will be created. As a result the audit tends to degenerate into something resembling a police action (see figure 2.1) where defensive attitudes are adopted by those being audited in an effort to conceal unpalatable truths. The auditor is regarded as interested only in defects and instinctively viewed with hostility and suspicion.

This principle applies equally forcefully in the case of software vendor audits. The vendor must be convinced that the audit represents a real opportunity to improve the development process and, in so doing, increase long-term profitability. At the same time, it

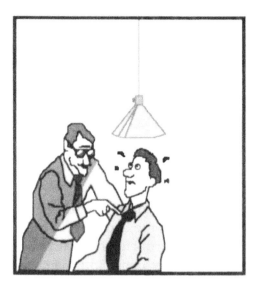

Figure 2.1. Police Action!

allows the purchaser to assess the risk inherent in acquiring the particular software product and version. The interests of both parties lie in establishing long-term relationships with one another.

In broaching the subject for the first time, the auditor must exert a high level of personal communication skill in assessing very quickly the likely attitude of the vendor's representative to whom he or she is speaking—usually the managing director, president or a senior sales manager of the company. The auditor must stress very early on in the conversation the benefits of the assessment to the vendor and allay any underlying misgivings. It has not been our practice to charge, or allow ourselves to be charged, for the visit. We shoulder the cost of travel and invest our time, while the vendor company invests its time, thus sharing the cost of the process between both parties—an equitable arrangement since both stand to gain equally from the exercise. Experience has shown that with tact and sensitivity, the vast majority of vendors with initial reservations can be reassured successfully. Once this happens and everyone relaxes over the objectives of the process, experience has shown in every case that the audit becomes a profitable and also, incidentally, an *enjoyable* experience for all those involved. Furthermore the friendship established during the audit can long outlast the visit, with informal discussions and advice being exchanged over the telephone between auditor and vendor for months afterwards. Many large corporate organizations who have already implemented quality management systems or have obtained TickIT certification are immediately and instinctively receptive to the concept of an audit (because of their familiarity with surveillance audits), and a positive relationship arises here quite naturally from the start.

CONFIDENTIALITY

CONFIDENTIAL A common misgiving among vendors is the concern for secrecy surrounding proprietary techniques within code on which the value of the software turns, and the perceived threat that this will be compromised through an audit inspection. Great care is needed to reassure vendors that the nature of the code and any clever techniques that may have been created within it are not the focus of the inspection; rather, the focus is on the engineering disciplines used in the development. Although source code will be inspected, this activity will confine itself to compliance with declared in-house standards, good programming practice and *nothing else*. The auditor must also make it abundantly clear that whatever emerges in the audit, whether favourable or otherwise, will not be divulged by the purchasing company to any third party under any circumstances, except with the express written permission of the audited firm. Frequently, the signing of a nondisclosure agreement is an essential prerequisite for the audit to proceed, and the auditor should show no hesitation whatsoever in entering into such an agreement, subject to routine legal scrutiny. It has been interesting to observe the much greater emphasis placed on the completion of nondisclosure agreements by vendors in the United States than is commonly the case in the United Kingdom or throughout Europe. This may simply be a cultural phenomenon, or it may reflect a greater competitive spirit among companies within North America. Whatever the reason, such emphasis should never be treated by the auditor as being in any way unnatural.

THE AVOIDANCE OF SURPRISE

One of the most important elements in fostering the team spirit on which all successful auditing depends is the avoidance of surprise. The department or function being audited relaxes and benefits most if they understand fully, in advance, exactly what the audit is about, the questions that will be asked, and the documents that will be required. Cynics might at once object that this is a deceiver's charter, allowing the clever manager to pull the wool over an auditor's eyes and get away with murder! Although there is no doubt that an unscrupulous minority exists in a few organizations in this fallen world, practical experience shows that this is very rare indeed. Most people have a positive and constructive attitude if treated kindly and competently, and wish to promote their company's best interests with integrity.

The auditor should, therefore, send to the vendor's nominated representative, with whom he or she has initiated contact, a comprehensive list of the areas to be examined, and provide the vendor with every opportunity to openly share and resolve any concerns and misunderstandings in advance of the audit. Trust is thereby established and strengthened as the process continues, and nothing in the audit comes as any surprise. Even so, it is extraordinary how effective a competent auditor can be in bringing to light features of the organization of which even the management were unaware. Indeed, this is one of the principal benefits that the auditor, an impartial outsider who can be seen to be ignorant of the company's practices without shame or embarrassment, can bring to the vendor—he or she can ask the so-called *idiot questions* that no one else had ever thought to raise. The auditor can also contribute further by sharing experiences of previous audits (on a completely anonymous basis of course), in the sense of suggesting practical improvements in the process that have been found worthwhile in the software industry as a whole.

THE RECALCITRANT HARD CORE

Sadly though, it has to be admitted that there remain a few vendors who cannot or will not recognize that their own vital interests are at stake in this process. Some refuse even to countenance an audit visit, caricatured by figure 2.2, on the grounds that their processes are above criticism and beyond any possibility of improvement,

Figure 2.2. No Entry

implying a degree of impertinence on the part of the auditor for having the audacity to suggest otherwise, however tentatively! Others allege the cost of the audit (five to six hours of time from one or two managers or other representatives) simply cannot be afforded in today's competitive environment, leaving the auditor wondering how delicately the company's finances and future must be balanced if this were really so! Others seek to equate the value of the audit with the profit to be reaped from the sale of this one licence, and refuse the audit on the grounds of the sale being of insufficient worth to justify it. It has proven difficult to convince several vendors who have adopted this position how meaningless such an equation is, since the potential benefits of the audit to the vendor are quite unrelated to the profit from any one sale. Regrettably, once an entrenched attitude has been expressed or a negative atmosphere has been generated, it has proven extremely difficult to dispel it, a situation often aggravated by a lack of willingness on the part of the senior company representative involved to lose face, and admit he or she might have been misguided, acted hastily or with prejudice, or just to have taken the wrong end of the stick.

LOCATION, TIMING AND DURATION

The audit must be conducted at the premises where the software has been developed and where it is maintained (invariably one and the same). This may seem too obvious to need stating, but the situation has occurred in the past where maintenance and development are organized out of different offices on opposite sides of the world, and the auditor has discovered on arrival at the premises that the staff cannot furnish the information required. It is vital not just to send in advance the list of the areas to be examined, but also to discuss exactly what the information means with the company representative who has been nominated to act as host. This will avoid the cost and embarrassment of an abortive visit.

Experience has shown that an audit conducted along the lines described in this book takes about 5–6 hours. If the audit begins on the agreed date at 0900 it is usual for the summary or wrap-up meeting to take place no later than at 1500. This has the three following advantages:

1. It limits the audit to a crisp, disciplined examination of the important areas of software development in an efficient manner, without an undue sacrifice of productive time for the vendor.

2. After the departure of the auditor, it gives the vendor sufficient time on the same day, while the memory is still fresh, to discuss the findings internally.

3. It gives the auditor time either to travel home, avoiding additional accommodation expense, or if far from home, time on the same day to consolidate the notes in preparation for composing the report.

THE STRESS OF TRAVEL

Developer locations are seldom nearby for the software QA auditor. Fortunately, many will be no more than a few hours' drive from home. Regardless of the effort directed toward combining multiple audits into a single trip, and the work shared among auditors domiciled in different countries, intercontinental travel is an unavoidable necessity from time to time.

Many who have never travelled abroad on business seem to envy what they regard as the *glamorous lifestyle* (whatever that means!) of the regular executive traveler. As those who fly long distances regularly will testify, such idyllic views, coloured as they often are by happy memories of holidays, are a far cry from the reality of business travel. However seasoned he or she may be, once away from home, the traveler becomes subject to a set of anxieties regarding deadlines, missed connections, loss of passport or money, and meeting and interacting with strangers in an alien environment. All of these combine to impose a level of stress over and above the normal requirements of the job. Moreover, travel and accommodation increase the cost of vendor assessments, and it is in the firm's interest to ensure the maximum return on the considerable investment involved. Thus, both company and employee have a stake in reducing the additional burden of stress and ensuring, as far as possible, the auditor's optimum effectiveness when working far from home.

Travel predisposes an individual to work stress, lack of exercise and obesity. It constitutes a hazard and an accident risk merely as a function of the distance flown or driven. Travel fatigue arises from repeated short journeys or time zone changes. Disturbance of the body's circadian rhythms (or *jet lag* as it is commonly called) during east-west travel varies widely between individuals and predisposes to fatigue, disorientation, lack of concentration, appetite loss and gastrointestinal symptoms to varying degrees. During the adjustment period, which again varies widely, performance is poorest and fatigue is most pronounced at times corresponding to night on "old" and "new" times. There are also insidious and possibly more serious health implications for the frequent flyer, which are explored, together with suggestions to mitigate them, in appendix 13.

Recognizing this, it is clear that sensible planning of schedules and the choice of transport to be used is the foundation of any successful business trip. For example, not all auditors will be permitted first-class travel with a chauffeur-driven car to and from airports. Driving oneself compounds the stress of travel with that of the driving component and its risks. Some companies wisely forbid driving after long-haul flights for this reason. The auditor needs to learn quickly from experience how long it takes him or her to recover from particular time changes, and to adjust schedules accordingly. The aim is to strike a balance between an overpressured timetable, when performance will be affected, and too slow a pace, which breeds boredom while away from familiar surroundings and increases costs needlessly. In my experience, one day (including the travel day itself) seems to be required, on average, for every four hours of time change to readjust adequately, although sleep patterns can take much longer to normalize. Discovering one's own limitations is essential to successful cost-effective forward planning.

Occasionally, last minute changes in business arrangements make an ordered period of readjustment impossible. Under these conditions, it is important to realize that the most appropriate time for work immediately after a flight is when it is daytime in both the old and new time zones (i.e., the evening after flying east, but NOT the evening after flying west). Schedules of trips for multiple audits should be structured to allow sufficient time for the composition in full (and ideally also typing up) of the audit report prior to travelling to the next vendor location. Such discipline is essential to avoid the fatal disease of mental confusion between successive audits that is likely to arise if such a precaution is ignored, for whatever reason.

THE SELECTION OF AUDITORS

The foregoing paragraphs have already implied certain personal characteristics desirable in candidates to be appointed as QA auditors. These need to be explored in more depth.

Quality assurance auditing is, as we have underlined, as much about providing consultancy as auditing per se. Since the vast majority of vendors today fall far below the standards exemplified by ISO 9000-3 (TickIT), most of them solicit practical guidance as to how to improve their processes to achieve the benefits reaped through compliance with standards. The auditor, therefore, needs not only to be thoroughly familiar with the technical principles of good software engineering; he or she must also have sufficient awareness of currently available guidance material, such as that in GAMP guide (1996), to be able to recommend practical and cost-effective measures.

No better summary of the academic requirements and the attributes and aptitudes needed to become a successful auditor can be found than that in the TickIT guide (1995) for provisional, senior and lead auditors. The TickIT auditor is required to be educated to first degree level, preferably in a numerate or technical discipline, or a holder of a recognized qualification, Higher National Diploma in the UK, or its equivalent. However, candidates who have substantial IT and software experience can be considered for registration without these qualifications. This type of experience is essential even for candidates with distinguished academic qualifications, since there is no substitute for the depth of insight gained by actually having written software oneself, facing the mental disciplines it demands, and learning through bitter experience the dreadful consequences of attempting to create software without adequate quality assurance. The guide goes on to express much the same requirement under its provisions for required experience: "at least five years practical experience of technical development life-cycle work for complex information systems". TickIT also requires a recognized quality assurance qualification, such as Member of the Institute of Quality Assurance (MIQA) or Fellow (FIQA), or other foreign qualifications recognized by the International Register of Certified Auditors. Such qualification could have been acquired in an environment far removed from practical software experience, such as pharmaceutical industry quality control. The significance of this requirement lies in the relevance of compliance with procedures within a controlled process, and in that respect is indispensable.

The guide goes on to require personal as opposed to academic qualities. It requires "demonstrable evidence of mature interpersonal skills and adaptability with the ability to handle tactfully and constructively contact as an equal with the most senior levels of client staff". The predominant element of consulting in the audit process amply justifies this qualification. Furthermore, the audit requires the ability to assimilate rapidly a vast amount of information about a vendor's processes in a very short period of time, and to form a sound and mature judgement on their strengths and weaknesses extremely quickly. The guide expresses this reality in its requirement of an "advanced technical solving ability . . . handling issues of complexity within the software and IT sector . . . with above average attention to detail". In some cases, vendor representatives will be unwilling or unable to understand, or worse still be unwilling to face up to, identified weaknesses in processes and the need for corrective action to effect improvements. The auditor needs "skills of observation and persistence", "the ability to influence through persuasive argument in the context of", "meetings at the highest level", a truth thoroughly endorsed in my experience. The audit wrap-up meeting is usually conducted in the presence of the vendor's chief executive, whose wholehearted endorsement of improvement actions must be secured.

We live in an era of so-called ageism, where youth is idolized and the experience and maturity of late middle age is undervalued.[6] The average retirement age in the Western world continues to fall, with the pace of change and business downsizing and delayering acting as stimulants to increasingly early retirement.[7] But the principles of good software engineering practice are not changing at anything like the rate of the evolution of technology. This stability, coupled with the personal requirements that have been described, suggests that the role of auditor is ideally suited to the senior executive of more mature years, able to work almost entirely unsupervised, and to whom the solitary nature of the work, with its extensive travelling, is not uncongenial.

THE AUDIT REPORT

We have examined the business case for a purchaser's software quality procurement strategy. The audit business process, the outworking of that strategy, furnishes as its final deliverable the *audit report,* which will be discussed in detail in chapter 14. This is intended to give future prospective purchasers of software from the vendor in question an insight into the level of structural integrity that can reasonably be expected in the product as a result of the vendor's engineering process. It also gives a good indication of the quality of other products produced by the same vendor, since it is extremely rare that products are engineered to different standards.

This report is provided not only to enable the immediate purchaser of the software to draw conclusions as to its suitability and fitness for purpose, but also for the guidance of other prospective purchasers within the organization months or years later. Since such individuals may only have a superficial acquaintance with the vendor, they will need, and benefit from, as much background information germane to the technical data as the auditor can usefully include. Accordingly, the auditor also needs to include *brief* information about the company in general, its history and its finances, as well as other products in its portfolio. He or she must not omit information on the market exposure of the product, since this gives an indirect indication of the level of in-built quality and residual defects, and complements the specific technical findings.

The remaining chapters of this book are devoted to describing exactly those characteristics of the software engineering process which are examined during the team's assessment—what is sought and what is its significance for software quality. The chapter arrangement reflects my experience of a wide variety of vendors of all types and sizes, and also corresponds to the structure of the final report. Doubtless there are many other approaches of equal value, but the methodology implied by this book has been shown to be comprehensive, thorough, and a searching evaluation of a vendor's capability against the consensus of the software engineering standards of today.

Notes

1. This term, not perhaps so familiar to non-British readers, is borrowed from the world of tailoring. It describes something designed and made to **exactly** fit the customer's **specific** requirements, and which is therefore unique, or *one of a kind*.

2. While outsourcing can often be highly advantageous for peripheral activities, such as, for example, travel offices, corporate restaurants or office cleaning activities, it poses great dangers when applied to critical areas of corporate infrastructure such as IT, which is now so intimately related to the core activities of the business.

3. PRB: "Record Lock Threshold Exceeded with Large Action Query". PSS ID Number Q102522 (Microsoft Corporation).

4. *Requirements of the National Registration Scheme for TickIT Auditors*

5. Telephone +44 (0)171 401 2988

6. Although age discrimination in employment recruitment was outlawed in the United States and Canada some years ago, it remains endemic elsewhere, particularly in the United Kingdom. In a recent study by the UK *Institute of Management*, 60 percent of vacancies were found to carry an age-related restriction. In another survey, job applicants over 45 were automatically sifted out by a third of employers.

7. According to the UK-based *Association of Retired and Persons over 50*, only 50 percent of men aged 60–64 are now working, a figure down from 80 percent just 25 years ago.

3

Company Organization and Project Management

*New ideas hurt some corporate minds rather
as new shoes hurt some feet.*

Anon

In order to fully realize its potential to benefit both the purchasing company and the vendor, the assessment process must address the needs of key individuals in both organizations. From the purchasing company's point of view, the intended beneficiaries are not only the immediate prospective purchasers of the software under review, but also others in the company who in months or years to come may be seeking software in the same application area. Since the principal deliverable item from the process in the purchaser's eyes is the audit report, this must address the needs of both sets of readers, today's and tomorrow's. Although today's reader will already be familiar with the vendor company (since they are likely to have requested the audit in the first place), this will not be the case with tomorrow's. Reading the report perhaps months or years after it was issued, they may have little or no knowledge of the vendor in question. The first section of the audit report, therefore, should contain a few brief informative paragraphs on the company's history, financial state of health, its prospects and its whole approach to the management of software development projects. The audit assessment should commence with the acquisition of this information.

HISTORY

Company history is vitally important because it affords a sensitive barometer to the *culture* of the company. Culture is that indefinable set of assumptions and values that underpins all policies and activities and heavily influences an organization's behaviour especially in unexpected situations. The auditor can save much time and effort by requesting from the vendor any publicity or press releases that describe the company's evolution to date. All but the smallest organizations can usually produce this at the drop of a hat. Further information, sometimes of a less complimentary nature and highly relevant to the purpose of the audit, often emerges in discussion at this point. For example, one company had been bought and sold like a second-hand automobile several times in a three-year period, and had only recently achieved what it reckoned was an ownership of reliable financial status. How hard it is for a quality culture to take root in such shifting sands! At the other end of the spectrum, there are long-established companies being overwhelmed by the flood tide of technological change for which they are technically and psychologically unprepared, resisting the advance of the inevitable in a manner reminiscent, once again, of King Canute. Many companies adapting well to the changing environment are failing to distinguish technical principles of good practice that are unchanging and, therefore, need to be permanently established, from the details of moving technologies that are fleeting and transient. The company's history, then, is quite a reliable indicator of what is likely to emerge later on in the audit.

SIZE

Size has a huge influence on the weight and interpretation to be accorded to much of the evidence uncovered during the audit. Many of the requirements of good software engineering practice have evolved from the recognition of the difficulties human beings have in communicating with each other to the standard of precision required in software development. Computers, being utterly unintelligent and remorselessly logical devices, are only capable of doing exactly as they are programmed with virtually absolute accuracy and repeatability. In this sense, they are immensely superior to the human mind. In another respect, however, they are incomparably *inferior* in that they entirely lack the huge potential of the imagination that confers on human beings their enormous creative ability as well as their adaptability, their capacity to respond to changing circumstances. It is extremely hard for the human mind to stoop to constrain itself to think like a computer. Indeed, a little thought will show that to boast of being as logical as a computer, far from being something to be proud of is, on the contrary, demeaning and dehumanizing. To be condemned to such a state would rob us of much of our God-given potential and reduce us to the level of automatons. But here is the irony—to think like a computer is exactly what is required in software development! In software-related activities, we must define what we mean so clearly that even a *stupid computer* can understand it unambiguously!

This truth has profound implications in relation to the size of a software development group. Within a small, tightly knit group of two or three like-minded and gifted individuals well versed in the technology, it is perfectly possible to establish technical assumptions verbally with a high degree of precision. This usually happens over a period of years, and can blossom in the development of one or perhaps two complex software products of considerable sophistication, and a high level of in-built quality. There are tens of thousands of such small companies thriving at the present time, on whose creativity and flair the explosion of today's technological revolution has been based. Such companies are extremely lean, able to respond to technical advances with great rapidity and agility and to bring a new idea for a niche market from conception to profitable product very quickly. Many of the packages purchased by my own organization, one of the largest and most prestigious multinational pharmaceutical companies, is from vendors such as these. But there are two problems from which vendors of this type cannot readily escape: the lack of clearly demonstrable evidence of in-built quality to enable purchasers to distinguish the pearl from the dross, and the inability to grow safely.

As any gardener or farmer will testify, when the wheat or plants grow, so do the tares or weeds. There are just as many small organizations producing poor quality software as good. A widely available and well-advertised package has been known to corrupt much of the data associated with it, due to some internal software defect (as yet unresolved in the current version). Software produced without an adequate level of in-built quality will possess a high level of unknown residual defects, many of which may never come to light, but which may cause disasters such as these without warning. The cost implications of such eventualities bear no relation to the original purchase price of the software. This is very hard for most purchasers of software to understand, since the assumption that the more you pay for an item the better the quality (a principle which holds good for many commodities) does not necessarily apply for software. In very small companies, there is rarely more than a fraction of the documentation disciplines in place which would be essential within a larger group to developing the software with the same level of quality. However, because communication is so much easier, this does not mean that the software is not of adequate quality. The purpose of the audit is to probe the manner in which the software has been developed by evaluating what evidence does exist. This necessarily involves a high degree of judgement, and hinges critically on the attitude of the developers, especially in the realm of attention to detail. Good disciplines, such as change control, audit trailing and the use of comments in source code, can demonstrate a good standard of software development in an informal atmosphere within a group of two or three, who know each other's strengths and weaknesses intimately.

The danger for these undocumented procedure-less organizations is the exponential increase in risk inherent when the group grows. A newly recruited programmer must be taught the culture of the group, a web of consensual assumptions of acceptable and predictable behaviour accumulated over a long period of time. The challenge facing the group is to explain all of these to the recruit, to ensure that he or she both understands them fully and the reasons behind them, and furthermore that he or she accepts them. It is well nigh impossible to ascertain with certainty whether these conditions have been achieved without a practical test in the form of a period of probation. During this period, the recruit joins the team in software development but under supervision. Imperfect and flawed as we all are, this can never be wholly effective. It is in this interval then, that the recruit becomes a *cuckoo in the nest* (figure 3.1), with misunderstood assumptions of one kind or another on his or her part leading to the incorporation of defects into the product which

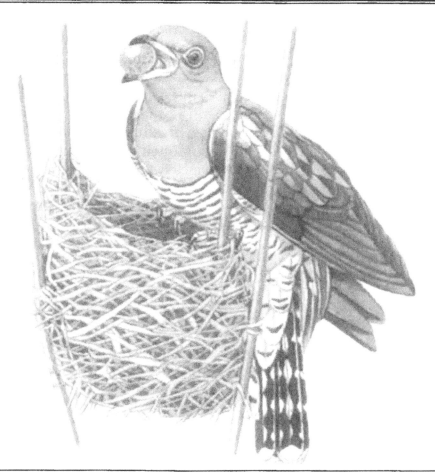

Figure 3.1. The New Recruit in an Organization Without Procedures! (© Helicon Publishing Ltd)

would never have occurred otherwise. Worse still is the fact that these misunderstandings are not amenable to any form of systematic search or discovery. But, bet your life on it, after a while these will emerge, but only after the damage has been done. The group thus reaps the bitter harvest of recruitment in an avalanche of field defects, dissatisfied customers and forfeited future business (costs unknown and unknowable).

The disciplines of documentation implicit in ISO 9000-3, the GAMP guide and similar standards or guidance are aimed at mitigating these risks. Complex information is transmitted much more effectively through the written word than orally. Many small organizations have never bothered to document their standards or procedures in the belief that there is no economic return for the cost involved. What they have failed to realize is that the unwritten consensus between them is seldom as watertight as they imagine. The discipline of documentation exposes this delusion which today is already imposing its own hidden cost. They have also failed to anticipate the need for growth whose advent is usually sudden, market driven and unexpected. The objection often raised against the introduction of documentation disciplines is that of *mindless bureaucracy* (paperwork existing for its own sake—an overhead and a drain on profitability). This is, sad to say, well founded but provides no excuse for neglecting the simple, straightforward documentation of what is done and why. *Common sense* is the moderating ingredient, as figure 3.2 illustrates.

DOCUMENTATION: THE PROBLEM WITH PAPER

The traditional means of storing procedures, standards and specifications is on paper within filing cabinets. Over the years, a plethora of systems of document control have emerged, reflecting the difficulties implicit in coping with the limitations of such a medium.

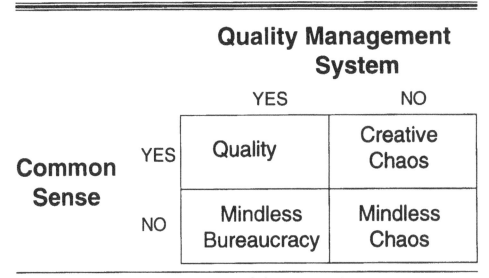

Figure 3.2. The Importance of Common Sense

Paper is bulky, which discourages fulsome recording; its management and handling is time consuming and expensive, and access is slow. The advent of the photocopier has made document control a nightmare. There is no completely reliable means of knowing from an isolated document whether it is the master or whether a later version exists elsewhere. The integrity of all paper-based systems is hostage to the compliance of others with document handling procedures.

Fortunately, such information need no longer be committed in the electronic age to paper (an information medium of the 1st century[1]), but stored, displayed and maintained within the medium of the 21st century, the ubiquitous desktop computer. Personnel in offices across the globe may access data from a single, updated source via replicated databases (a subject we will explore in greater depth in chapter 10). Groupware such as this offers the huge advantage of a single master source of a document. The medium need no longer constrain the availability or raise doubts as to the reliability of the message. If hard copies are taken for convenience, they are not to be regarded as the prime source of the information, but only as temporary walk away copies bereft of the status of a prime document. Another major advantage is the ability to relate different documents together so that disparate sources of information can be accessed simultaneously (another aspect explored in chapter 10 in the context of procedures). It is an issue that has relevance to all aspects of a business's operation, in fact, far beyond the immediate confines of software development.

FINANCIAL BACKGROUND

The reader would be forgiven for wondering why a section on company finances features in a book about developing good software. Why should a software QA auditor have any concern about the financial health of a prospective vendor? The ability to sustain a long-term business relationship as a quality-assured supplier implies the need for a sound business base, and it is to this matter that the auditor must at least direct some attention. Is it likely that the vendor will remain in business long enough to support the provided software over the duration of its expected lifetime?

The auditor must seek out whatever financial information is available. Some vendors will willingly disclose certain financial data to an auditor, though they are seldom likely to divulge anything not already in the public domain. In the United Kingdom, companies that have limited liability status are obliged to submit accounts to Companies House in London. Other traders, including individuals, partnerships and companies without limited liability status are *not* obliged to submit accounts in this manner although they must make returns to the Inland Revenue for tax purposes. Private *limited* companies above a threshold balance sheet total (£1.4 million at the time of writing) and with more than 50 employees must submit audited accounts in full to Companies House. Companies below this turnover and staff level are defined as "small companies" under the Companies Act. As such, they are still obliged to submit audited accounts, but these can be abbreviated in that they need not disclose turnover and are exempt from the requirement to include a Profit and Loss account. Should their turnover not exceed £350,000, they are not even obliged to have their accounts audited, though they must bear an accountant's report or certificate. Very small companies, meaning those below a turnover of £90,000, do not even have to obtain an accountant's certificate. All that is required of them is a balance sheet signed by a director. All accounts submitted to Companies House enter the public domain, and are thus available for inspection. Public Limited Companies, on the other hand, are obliged to register their audited accounts (which then become public, as their title implies) regardless of their size. They may also have to comply with stricter rules governing the disclosure of information imposed by the UK Stock Exchange. Foreign companies with a branch office in the United Kingdom are also obliged to make certain returns to Companies House.

If the accounts are in the public domain, the auditor will usually be given, or can obtain, the most recently published set in these circumstances. The situation in the United States is more complicated, in that the corresponding rules vary from one state to another. At one extreme, companies in one state, regardless of size, are free from the obligation to register any accounts whatsoever, a fact that has attracted some companies of UK origin to register there.

There is, however, a difficulty. Most QA auditors do not possess the financial acumen to interpret financial data reliably. Another more practical approach is to be recommended, therefore, which kills two birds with one stone—overcoming both the unavailability of data for small companies and the problems of interpretation in one. This technique involves the use of the service provided by one of the commercial credit reference agencies. *Dun and Bradstreet* is perhaps the best known; their name is now almost generic for this kind of enquiry; *Graydon plc* in the United Kingdom is another. These organizations are able to obtain a wide spectrum of useful information for a modest fee, either on public or private companies, from databases published on ViewData services, from public records of County Court judgements and from reference to a sample of suppliers for bill payment performance. On the basis of these figures, the agencies are able to build a profile of a company and compare it with its peers in its own business sector and allocate it to a risk category. These agencies are also able to search databases for information on overseas firms, though this usually takes a few days. Their report contains not only factual information, but also a measure of interpretation, some of which is, so to speak, hidden between the lines. Whilst the information primarily addresses credit risk a company that is judged to be a high credit risk will probably also be one in a more risky overall position anyway.

An auditor can make good use of this by including an indication of the company's financial health in general terms in the report to accompany and illuminate the technical findings. It is important to emphasize that, while such information is strictly speaking in the public domain, it is normally provided on the understanding that the data are treated with discretion. One way of respecting this is to shred the report once it has served its purpose.

FUTURE

Apart from strictly financial information, the vendor needs a viable business plan. In this connection, therefore, the vendor should be asked to state where the company's strategic future is perceived to lie. With the frenetic pace of technological change that shows no sign of slackening, there is a huge turnover of software companies, many disappearing without trace each year. Those that fail to survive can often trace their demise to a lack of flow of ideas to supplement their original business vision, failure to adapt to technological change quickly enough, failure to improve their processes cost-effectively (in which worthy objective the audit is aimed at assisting) beyond that of the competition, or failure to diversify in the face of a shrinking market.

ORGANIZATIONAL STRUCTURE

Control within the software development process relies critically on the various players knowing exactly what they are responsible for, what their authority is, and what they are expected to do. Project management is essential if costs are to be controlled and the company is to continue to trade profitably and to prosper. Thus, every company should have some kind of organizational structure diagram (known as an *organigram*), showing the chain of authority and responsibility. Very small companies sometimes excuse their lack of such a document on the grounds that everybody knows what the structure is. This is sophistry since close questioning among staff will usually highlight at least a few misconceptions. The value of the document far exceeds the cost of producing it and is a basic sign of a well-run organization.

The next documents which should be sought are the job descriptions of all employees engaged in some way with software development. In a larger firm, the auditor would not attempt to inspect all such documents, but might review a sample of one or two for content. The objective is to ensure that as far as possible each member of the staff has a written record of his or her areas of responsibility in the company. For small firms where staff tend to be multiskilled and are required to perform various roles at different times, the job descriptions should reflect this. A job description should neither be too detailed as to be unwieldy, nor so brief as to be meaningless. It should as far as possible refer to the tasks involved in the software life cycle methodology in use, and, therefore, bear some relation to the life cycle description document discussed in chapter 8. A suggested layout for an old-fashioned style of job description is provided in appendix 11.

QUALITY ASSURANCE

We have already established that high quality software, defined as software doing what it purports to do and not doing what it purports not to do, cannot be built without a set of formal, organized arrangements directed to this end. These arrangements, whatever form they take, will be ineffective unless

- They are endorsed wholeheartedly by senior management as a central part of the company ethos.

- They are implemented and managed by a least one individual of adequate competence and authority.

- There is a degree of independence on the part of quality assurance from both developers and management to ensure that procedures are followed.

All software firms, however small, should have at least one competent individual formally appointed to carry out the responsibility for quality assurance. In larger organizations, this will usually be a full-time role and may involve subordinate staff. Even in the smallest company, someone should be appointed. It might be the head of development; in these circumstances, the element of independence must be preserved, at least in the testing function. Ideally, it should be an individual from another group, frequently the support group, who can monitor the project process as a part-time role and ensure that procedures are being followed, milestones reached, documents approved and signed off, and so on. In a number of successful small companies, the managing director has assumed the responsibility for quality assurance as a part-time role. Another major benefit, a by-product so to speak of a QA presence, can result from the enhancement of the effectiveness of staff, in that the formality of simple controls and procedures can be understood and handled by a staff member of lesser knowledge and experience. This is an ideal role for a junior member of staff to learn good practice whilst releasing experienced, high flier programmers for the tasks requiring their skills, an approach that has been successfully implemented in several firms. This individual must not be responsible to the head of software development in this role; he or she must report at a higher level in the company for QA matters to ensure that he or she cannot be overruled when the heat is on, and temptation to take shortcuts or implement what is pejoratively known as a *quick fix* becomes irresistible.

Transforming a software development group to adopt standards and incorporate methods to assure quality cannot be achieved without initial cost, and it is disingenuous to imply or suggest otherwise. Exactly what these costs will be will vary enormously from one organization to the next. The economic case for going this way is that as time passes, the support costs will decrease as the development process improves, more than compensating for the QA overhead cost. These matters are discussed in more depth in chapter 5. The overriding principle is to keep the quality procedures as simple as possible to facilitate understanding, demonstrate tangible benefits, and maximize prospects of improving processes.

THE IMPORTANCE OF INDEPENDENCE

Developers are notoriously incapable of testing their own code with any degree of impartiality. This is understandable, since the demanding disciplines of creativity make it impossible to stand back and challenge one's work from a critical standpoint. (The author's own efforts to proofread this manuscript have been hampered for precisely the same reason!) Module testing among peers is the very minimum level of testing that should be conducted, supplemented by overall system testing by someone unconnected with development but intimately aware of the intended functionality of the product from the user's perspective.

THE NEED TO INVOLVE EVERYONE

Quality assurance can only be successful when everyone in the organization is committed to it as a business-critical issue. In immature companies where quality consciousness has not been part of the historical culture, quality assurance tends to be seen initially as imposition of external control, carrying with it overtones of constraint on creativity, impediments to making money, and police action! These juvenile instincts, products of the *cowboy culture* which will be mentioned again in chapter 11, must be dispelled through enlightened leadership, education and training, the foundation of which must be that quality assurance and future employment are inextricably linked. No self-respecting purchasing company committed to its own future prosperity should touch software produced in this atmosphere if at all possible.

PROJECT MANAGEMENT

The last aspect of the company's operation to be explored in the first section of the audit is the management and control of projects. The need for effectiveness in project management applies with equal force in any collective team activity, conducted within strict constraints of time and budget, and which is aimed at producing a discrete product. The most effective framework for such control is that of a life cycle. Since the critical need for a life cycle for successful, cost-effective software development has already been described, why should there be a need for a second life cycle?

This question is frequently raised and betrays a misunderstanding of the distinction between the project process and the software development process. Although intricately intertwined they are, nevertheless, separate. Project control disciplines are necessary for making anything, and focus on the coordination of the contributions of various members of the team. They always involve the creation of a *project plan*, since without a plan a project is unmanageable. They are concerned with ensuring the completion of set tasks at certain milestones, the reporting and handling of slippage, and the control of finance. Software development disciplines, on the other hand, focus on the definition and documentation of requirements, traceability, compliance with work standards, correlation of test activity and its results against the specification at the corresponding stage, and so on. They involve an analysis of risk and uncertainties. Confusion of the two life cycles often results in awkward and cumbersome procedures being developed, albeit under a quality culture with the best of intentions. Being poorly focussed, the quality management system becomes a target for criticism, usually under the dreaded epithet *bureaucracy*! Nevertheless, in a software house the two sets of disciplines run side by side in parallel and link together at all points. However, their separate spheres of application and direction must not be confused.[2]

It is vital that a vendor has a clear methodology for addressing project control issues. Most successful vendors use one or other of the most popular project management software tools as an aid, such as Microsoft *Project*™; another which is in widespread use and whose development, interestingly, has been inspired by experience derived from the enormously complex U.S. space missions, is *Schedule Publisher*™ (Advanced Management Solutions, Inc.). Projects can, of course, also be managed and tracked with pen and paper charts, but most firms have already progressed beyond this. What is essential is that no project should be undertaken unless it is subject to a clear project control methodology from conception to completion supported and endorsed at the highest level within the company.

The reason for this is clear. Projects constitute risk. They expose the organization to a hemorrhaging expenditure over months or years, where the probability of payback is never 100 percent (i.e., entirely certain). Some risks cannot be contained, even with the best industrial intelligence (e.g., a competitor simultaneously introducing a superior product, though industrial espionage should not be countenanced under any circumstances!). The most serious risk, though, is that of uncoordinated and haphazard effort, ill-defined personnel responsibilities, untracked and cumulative slippage in performance against estimates, both on the timeline and the budget, leading to runaway and potentially ruinous cost, with an ever-diminishing prospect of an *economic* return. A full treatment of risk in software development and how to reduce it has been published by Ould (1990), who has given the following summary of typical areas in which risk and uncertainty can be found:

- User interfaces

- Performance

- The use of new software

- The use of new hardware

- Interfaces to other systems

- Poorly defined requirements (the most common source of major faults in delivered systems)

- Novel problem domains

Experience shows that projects do not suddenly overrun by a year or so. They creep out of control one day at a time. Scores of software houses have disappeared without trace, for no other reason than from being overwhelmed in the calamity of ineffective or nonexistent project control. The auditor's concern must be that the vendor should at least remain in business long enough to support the product acceptably, and ideally grow and prosper. Project management methodology is the best assurance that can be given that business continuity will be maintained.

An example of a project life cycle approach is shown in figure 3.3, based on the diagram provided in the STARTS guide (1987). It shows the relationships between technical development and quality assurance, as well as the critical role of project management in the initiation and control of the whole process. It also distinguishes the activities relating to development from those relating to released product, known as configuration management.

There are now signs of increasing awareness among both purchasers of IT and within the UK government of the critical importance of effective project control on the part of software developers. The *BuyIt Guidelines,* first mentioned in the introduction and

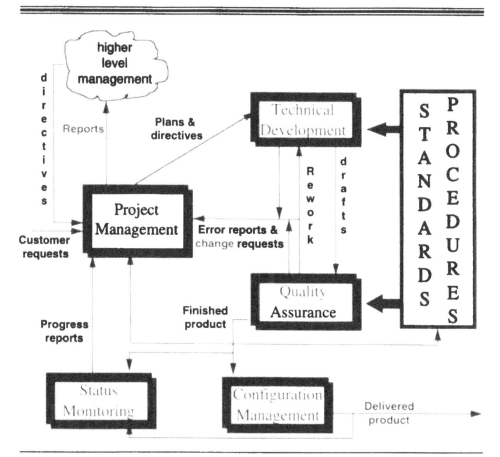

Figure 3.3. A Project Control System

unveiled in June 1996 by the then Science and Technology Minister, Ian Taylor, are intended to provide a checklist of management issues that senior executives can address to keep projects on the right lines, and also a set of warning signs that give telltale signals of things drifting out of control. Launching the guidelines, Mr. Taylor is reported to have said,

> *It is urgent that senior management are able to exploit the potential of IT if we are to exploit the opportunities emerging from the information society.*

To be fair, the guidelines do not claim to be the panacea for all project ills. Just ticking boxes is no substitute for capable and competent leadership from the project manager. However, they reinforce the importance of what the auditor is seeking in order to be assured of the vendor's long-term viability. Because they reflect a rising sophistication in the understanding of project management by purchasers of IT and, therefore, what they will increasingly expect to find in vendors, a summary of the guidelines has been provided in appendix 12. The guidelines have been backed by a prestigious list of organizations, including Barclays Bank, Shell, the Confederation of British Industry, the Computer Software Services Association, the UK National Computing Centre, and Uniforum, as well as the UK government itself.

In a study, Coopers and Lybrand found that two thirds of UK firms have suffered at least one project that failed to deliver business benefits, with 20 percent suffering actual financial loss. Across the Atlantic in the United States a third of an estimated 250,000 projects were canceled in 1995 at a combined cost of $80 billion (£52 billion).[3] The case, therefore, that help is needed in this sphere is unanswerable.

KEEPING PROJECTS UNDER CONTROL

We have examined the ease with which projects drift out of control. Since this phenomenon is widespread, what can be done to prevent it?

Documentation is crucial. Firstly and fundamentally, there must be a written statement of the company's approach to project development. It should comprise a description of the project life cycle—the successive steps of a software project and how the project is to be managed. We have already acknowledged the common mistake of confusing the project life cycle with the software development life cycle. The former is concerned with managing the process (making sure the deliverables appear on time and within budget), while the latter is concerned with the technical and quality aspects of the product itself. Certainly, they are closely related, but they are conceptually distinct.

For instance, one would need a project life cycle if one were developing, say, a potato peeling machine from scratch (the example most far removed from software development that sprang to mind!). How can it be ensured that everyone on the team knows what they are expected to deliver and when? What management aids (e.g., GANTT charts) are in use? What reporting mechanisms are in place for reviewing progress? Three separate tools are indispensable for project control:

Practical Guidance

Create a document describing the company's project life cycle approach (how we manage and control projects around here so that they deliver the product on time as expected and within budget, enabling us to have a sporting chance of making a profit and staying in business).

1. **Project plan**, which primarily defines both the objective and scope of the project. It then defines the roles, responsibilities and tasks throughout the project, and the expected timetables and costs.

2. **Quality controls** (to be discussed in detail in chapter 5), since they are by far the best means to maintain control of a project. They speak more convincingly and reliably of the true status of a project than the apprehension of any individual. These provide the essential brakes in the process, complementary to the drive to get the product out, which can restrain a project running out of control at an early stage before unacceptable abortive expense has occurred. Their effective presence has saved the bacon of many a company, while their absence has lain at the root of the demise of many others.

3. **Quality plan**, defining which controls are to be effective at which stage. It describes the quality deliverables that *prove* quality is being built into the product.

All three should feature prominently in the documentation of the project life cycle process in general. By documenting the approach taken to project management, the firm can ensure that everyone's understanding of how the project is to be managed, and how it will be costed, will be the same. Now it must be stressed here that no two projects are the same, and that any generic approach to project management is limited in usefulness. Thus, when a project is initiated, the general life cycle will be adopted, but any departures from it in the special interests of this particular project will be noted on the project plan. The plan can, therefore, assume the general (and be more concise as a result) and concentrate on the particular. By balancing the general and the particular in this way, the firm derives the benefits and security of established best practice without sacrificing the flexibility needed to accommodate special circumstances.

PROJECT CHANGE CONTROL AND
SECURITY MEASURES

"The best laid plans of mice and men" so the saying goes. If only life were like that in a small town in Nevada where so little ever changes that the local radio station is said to be still running last year's weather forecasts! On a more serious note, though, change is a fact of life, and as we have seen constitutes in connection with projects a major source of risk to software companies, both large and small (especially the latter). How can that risk be managed and mitigated?

Keep It

Simple

Practical Guidance
Create a procedure that describes exactly how changes within projects will be managed so that whatever happens, we will stay in control of our destiny and deliver our product on time (even if later than originally forecast) and within (perhaps a revised and higher) budget.

There must be a documented procedure describing what will be done when changes are imposed on projects for whatever reason. This procedure will detail the mechanisms by which the team recovers the control that the change either threatens to undermine, or even blow away altogether. It will describe how the effect of the change will be reviewed and what mechanisms will be effected to revise the schedules and costings for the project, how each person involved will be kept informed, and so on. It will enable management to foresee and plan for the consequential changes in other operations of the company. Once again, these are usually simple, practical measures in the main.

The benefit of documenting the actions is that in the heat of the moment when the pressure is on, management will know exactly how they will respond. They are much less likely to react hastily, unadvisedly and capriciously.[4]

PROJECT REVIEW OR POST MORTEM

We have already noted the Japanese experience with *kaizen,* or continuous improvement, in the context of statistical process control.

Exactly the same principle can be applied to software development and lies at the heart of the concept of Total Quality Management.

As the process is improved, the few major causes of failure will become quickly apparent. It is perfectly possible in these circumstances for a firm to respond like the foolish man who looks into the mirror, sees what is wrong with himself and what needs improving, but goes away and does nothing about it. This is fatally easy to do at the end of a project, when the immediate interest of what happened is waning, because it is now history and there are more important fish to fry.

But as we have noted elsewhere, those who ignore the mistakes of history are condemned to repeat them, so it is vital that time is found for a dispassionate and reflective review of the project to take place with one overriding objective: to address the systemic weaknesses of the process. By holding on to the gains we are able to make from correcting the process, we can ratchet up the profitability, productivity, quality and speed of the project process in the future. Quality is all about satisfying customer requirements, while Total Quality is all about achieving a quality product for the lowest possible cost and involving everyone (totally) who participates in any way in the project process.

In doing this, it is common for the small number of major problems to become occluded or swamped by the mass of trivial mistakes that pose little threat to the profitability of the business and whose amelioration will deliver little financial reward. Concentrate on the one or two major issues that have emerged.

Some of the best vendors carry out this exercise with a *project improvement team,* which might consist of one of the project team members, the QA manager, and perhaps a project sponsor, such as a senior manager in a larger company, to add weight to any putative process changes. They begin by selecting the key subprocesses

Keep *It* Simple	**Practical Guidance**
	Create a procedure describing the project review process aimed at improving the process and avoiding the repetition of past mistakes. Include the method of evaluating the improvements and their incorporation (hopefully) into company standards.

in the overall process that need attention, then defining the improvement objective for each one and a timetable for implementing it. Once implemented, the effectiveness of the improvement is measured, perhaps on the next project. At that point, the improvement is incorporated into the company's standards and procedures. These activities, shown in figure 3.4, exactly match the Shewart cycle discussed in chapter 1. This is the *virtuous circle* of process improvement, the Holy Grail of quality assurance, measured in real, tangible, bottom line profitability, in customer satisfaction, and in the long-term resilience of the company. It is what this book is intended to promote. Once the quality circle is being completed on a regular basis, project after project, the company is really on the move toward maturing in its software engineering capability.

Finally, in the interests of improving the company's profitability and its ability to respond rapidly to fleeting market opportunities, the team might begin to consider addressing the thorny issue

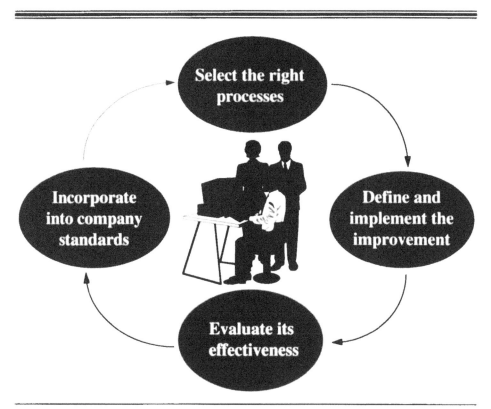

Figure 3.4. The Process Improvement Team

of how programmers spend their time. Time is one of the largest components of project cost, but also perhaps the most difficult to contain. How can the time taken to deliver the software, using the controls that we have identified and implemented, be further reduced? The key to any process improvement strategy is the ability to collect meaningful and accurate process data. Perry (1996) and his coworkers have described their experiences, drawn from the insights afforded by the behavioral sciences, in designing and conducting experiments intended to show exactly where the time of software engineers, involved in a major project, actually goes. It will probably not come as a complete surprise that this does not always agree with the information recorded on time sheets, if these are used. Their findings will be of value for project improvement teams wishing to go beyond the purely systemic improvements alone into the realm of the cultural.

This concludes the team's assessment of the company's general state of health and approach to projects. The next chapter addresses the entire range of software produced by the vendor and how it is supported, with special attention being given to the particular product of interest to the prospective purchaser.

Notes

1. According to tradition, paper was first made in 105 A.D. by Cai Lun, a eunuch attached to the Eastern Han court of the Chinese Emperor Hedi.

2. The process of writing this book offers an instructive illustration. A target date was given by the publisher for the final draft—the last deliverable. Since the two reviewers would each need a month, reviewing concurrently, this fact dictated when the first draft manuscript would have to be completed. Copyright permissions also needed to be organized and to be available along with the final draft. A notional budget had also been set for copyright fees which could not be exceeded. None of this had anything directly to do with the *content* of the book or of the creative activity needed to produce each chapter. The *project management* process and the *production* process, then, although related, were thus quite separate.

3. News item in *Computer Weekly*, 13 June, 1996.

4. In a much loved classic British TV comedy series on the role of the Home Guard in World War II the platoon's corporal, an elderly butcher, can be entirely relied on to react to a crisis with a total, pathetic, and, of course, quite predictable loss of self-control, prancing around while frantically exclaiming *Don't Panic!! Don't Panic!!*

4

Products and Their Support

Tell me, my friend, not what you wish me to hear,
but rather that which I need to know.

Anon

Although the focus of the QA audit is the engineering process used to develop the software rather than its functionality, the team must understand at least to a superficial degree what the software is designed to do. Since the auditor may be the only member of the assessment team not intimately familiar with the software, and subsequent readers of the audit report may be similarly ignorant, a little time will be needed to appreciate other products that the vendor has created and the overall relationships one to the other. Thus, there must be at least a cursory examination of the vendor's *software portfolio*.

THE PRODUCT PORTFOLIO

Information should be made available on each of the various products in the portfolio. There are usually at least three or four, although in a few cases these may be little more than clones or minor variants of the principal product. This is the stage of the assessment in which the vendor representatives on the team tend to feel the most comfortable, and therefore why it is beneficial to place it early on in the audit. They are normally very proud of their software products, understandably so and thus intensely keen to discuss their merits at length. Now although information is precisely the commodity the auditor is seeking, a difficulty can arise at this point. Unless this enthusiasm is gently but firmly restrained, the entire audit process can be innocently hijacked into becoming a sales presentation! Despite careful preparation over the telephone, a misunderstanding of the true nature of the audit has arisen occasionally. It has then been discovered, to the profound dismay of the auditor, that an elaborate and fulsome presentation, expounding the incomparable virtues of the products, has been prepared in advance. In these circumstances, it is essential in the most tactful and gracious manner possible to steer the proceedings firmly back onto the path of righteousness, however unappreciative the auditor might be perceived to be. The lesson these circumstances teach is the importance of the auditor ensuring that the vendor *really understands* the objectives and scope of the audit team exercise in the terms outlined by the list of the areas of interest sent previously. In most cases, extensive conversations will ensure that such a tacit assumption is not misplaced, but this has not always been so. The auditor is well advised to double-check the vendor's measure of understanding before the visit should any residual doubt remain.

Vendors always seem more than willing to provide brochures of their portfolio on request. These can be useful in summarizing portfolio functionality in the final audit report, rather than attempting to rely solely on notes taken contemporaneously.

PRODUCT BACKGROUND

Longevity in the marketplace and the number of licences sold provide important pointers to a product's quality. Unlike old cars (or, for that matter, elderly auditors!) software does not wear out or deteriorate with age. Providing it is being maintained in accordance with good software practices, it actually *improves* as it gets older (perhaps like a fine wine), with critical defects being brought to light and corrected. If this is not the case, or if the software is being extensively changed over a very short period of time (the so-called *exploding requirements* scenario), there is every likelihood that each defect removed will be replaced by another (or several).

Great care is needed in weighing this information, since a widespread temptation to place far too much weight on very limited market success can be detected. This has been particularly common in relation to the many specialist and niche software packages whose engineering has been examined, and especially so when the technical findings have been unfavorable. "But there are 100 people using this software, so it must be all right!" has been the typical cry of protest from a disappointed prospective purchaser. Sadly, 100 people using the software is no safeguard against the pernicious effects of critical shortcomings in the development process, such as the absence of structured test plans. These 100 users may all be executing the same 0.1 percent of the possible pathways through the code and, therefore, their combined activity reveals very little of the software's potential behaviour. Unlike mechanical or electromechanical systems which tend to give warning of impending failure, software failures occur completely without warning and are related only to the occurrence of the circumstances necessary for their appearance. These bring to light the programming or design errors that have always been there, but have remained dormant until now. A software product may contain hundreds of such hidden defects, waiting invisibly in the wings for the moment to pounce on the unsuspecting user.

CUSTOMER REFERENCE LIST

Apart from the number of licences sold, another important exposure parameter is the type of customer which constitutes most of the users. If a considerable proportion of the users of a product are in organizations capable of exercising the software to close to its fullest extent, defects are far more likely to emerge. Most vendors are willing to make a customer reference list available on request, although the auditor should exercise great sensitivity here. Some vendors regard this information as of the highest commercial significance and are extremely reluctant to reveal it, while others are much more relaxed. As has been hinted already, the auditor's interest is mundane and straightforward, without any overtones of industrial espionage, glamourous and exciting though that might be! The auditor's interest is confined to simply ascertaining the degree of external exposure of the software. He or she should make no reference in the report to specific customers without the vendor's express permission, confining comments in this area to generalities. On no account should a list of software customers be removed from the vendor's premises, unless there are compelling reasons for so doing and the vendor's specific approval has been secured.

FREQUENCY OF REVISION

The rate at which new versions of the software have been appearing since its launch is an excellent indicator of the quality of the initial requirements and the vendor's understanding of the market and its evolution. The ideal state at which to purchase software is when no more that one or two releases are appearing each year. After launch software has a market life cycle whose stages can be described in similar terms to our own: birth, adolescence, maturity, senility and death.

Launch is synonymous with birth. **Adolescence** is the phase of exploding requirements mentioned earlier, which ought to be brief, but is frequently embarrassingly extended, with perhaps four or more releases per year. This usually indicates that the functional requirements were incompletely understood, either because the users were insufficiently deeply involved, or that the market trends had been inadequately perceived. It has been said that the most successful companies are those that discern market movements earliest.[1] The auditor should probe the reason for a rapid series of early releases. These are usually to be found in two areas. The first is that of poor requirements definition early in the life cycle, leading to an avalanche of enhancement requests from initial users to amend or extend the functionality. Such requests are often for features that ought to have been foreseen and included, but were not either because of carelessness, or because of pressure to complete the project. The other frequent cause is weak design and coding disciplines that fail to remove defects which have appeared in the code, either from a flawed design, or from poor or nonexistent programming standards. Acquiring such software may result in pressure from the vendor for frequent upgrades, which may bring their own crop of new defects and interruption of business continuity if the life cycle is out of control.

The stage of **maturity** is reached when the product is largely meeting the entire need of the business application for which it is intended, and that the level of emerging defects has dropped to a low level. In these circumstances, the trickle of enhancement requests reflects not misunderstood or ill-defined requirements, but the slow evolution of the business application itself. This is the ideal stage at which software should have arrived at the time of purchase.

Senility occurs when the application is totally stable and the software extremely closely matched to it, so that no further changes are required and the emergence of defects has finally petered out. It is in this restricted sense that software improves with age. However, better approaches using newer technologies are suggesting that in the foreseeable future, this software will be superseded by a new and maybe radically different product that will render this product obsolete—the terminal stage of **death.** There are occasions when a sound business case can be made for the purchase of senile software, which can be implemented cost effectively and is likely to be highly reliable. Its stage in its life cycle and what that implies must, however, be thoroughly understood.

The number of staff working on the product should correspond to the software's stage in its life cycle. Any evidence of reluctance on the part of the vendor company to fulfill its obligations to support a released product adequately should be viewed as a serious cultural flaw. A laboratory automation system from a major international vendor will serve as an example. This software, installed some years ago in a number of laboratories which became dependent on it to a high degree, was riddled with defects. Regrettably, the vendor firm had decided to direct almost all its resources to new product development, leaving users of the existing product stranded high and dry with dozens of unresolved defect repair requests. Much long-term damage to the vendor's reputation was the inevitable result—no one will ever know what this cost the supplier in terms of lost potential business.

USER COMMUNITIES

An active user community for a software product or suite is a sign of good health, both for the product itself and for the vendor's future. The benefits from the group's activities work in two directions. Firstly, by sharing practical experience of using a product, users are able to explore the strengths and weaknesses of an application in far greater depth than can usually be documented by the vendor firm, however assiduous it may be in the production of manuals. In the case of large applications, user groups have often been able to discover esoteric product functionality of which even the vendor was scarcely aware! It is also quite common for workarounds for frequently encountered defects to be developed and disseminated among users far more quickly than if users were reliant solely on the vendor's own resources.

Another major asset in participating in a user group applies especially to highly configurable products, such as laboratory information systems, whose functionality and usefulness can be extensively enhanced by macros or native language code programs written by users themselves. These bolt-on routines can be invoked from hooks[2] provided in the standard application. The creation of such a *contributed software library* under the auspices of the user group enables members to avoid reinventing the wheel for software for common tasks associated with the application. Caution should be exercised, however, as the innate quality and reliability of such additional supplemental code can become an issue for all but the simplest routines.

The second principal benefit from these groups accrues to the vendor, who is able to receive a much more reliable measure of the product's quality level, as perceived in the field, and a clearer view of the required direction for future enhancements. User groups will frequently meet once or twice annually for two to three days, during which members give presentations on the joys and sorrows of using the product, and from which a prioritized wish list often emerges. Therefore, it is in the vendor's interests to give every encouragement, both organizational and financial, in ensuring the viability of such groups. However, user groups should operate as independently as possible from the vendor to ensure an atmosphere where both praise and constructive criticism of the product and the vendor's support performance may be fully and freely aired. With a realistic member subscription and a vendor subsidy, the annual meeting (in a congenial but not overly expensive location) of the most successful groups can, in my experience, become the highlight of the year for both users and vendor staff alike.

VERSION SUPPORT

There seems to be much confused thinking and a lack of clear policies on the issue of version support. Most suppliers tend naturally to fall over backward in offering to support all released versions of their products, but often fail to foresee adequately the implications and costs of their support policy, especially if this has never been expressed clearly.

For mature, standard products, it is a mark of weakness if a vendor is attempting to support more than the current version, and perhaps also the preceding release. Supporting previous versions from a misplaced sense of customer service involves considerable cost and is, to say the least, unwise. It smacks of confused thinking and misplaced altruism, a lack of clear perception of how the customer's long-term interests may best be served. As long as backward compatibility has been maintained in product development, these are better safeguarded if the advantages of migration to the current version are clearly explained and advocated, and a financial incentive attached to induce the customer to upgrade. Vendors should not flinch from the withdrawal of support for earlier versions in these circumstances, since the elimination of avoidable cost is in everyone's long-term interest, customer and vendor alike.

A difficulty arises when an erstwhile standard product has been extensively modified for individual customers, thus creating a set of essentially bespoke products. This desire to satisfy the needs of specific users is, regrettably, frequently accompanied by a failure to foresee the ongoing support costs of such a policy and to realistically include these in the cost of the initial customization. This situation has been found to be common in very small vendors without user groups, where there has been a marked failure to filter out the desirable from the essential, and who do not possess the commercial maturity to resist the temptation to satisfy every short-term market possibility. This millstone around a growing company's neck is hard to shed without some very tough and courageous decisions. These matters will be raised again, but from another perspective, that of version control, in chapter 11.

The auditor should record the mechanisms by which support is proffered to customers. Practically all vendors operate a telephone

Keep *It* Simple	**Practical Guidance**
	Include in the quality management system simple, concise procedures describing the processes involved in supporting released product in the field.

hot line. Whether the customer's experience of using the hot line turns out to be pleasant, or on the contrary *infuriatingly frustrating,* is quite another matter. For many vendors, the poor quality of the development process, and the defect-ridden products that inevitably result, mean that the limited human resources that can be devoted economically to operating a telephone hot line, quickly become overwhelmed. The use of automatic call handling facilities in the form of polite recorded messages, inviting the caller to hold on until an agent is free, is widespread. While the technical features of such systems are impressive and undoubtedly advantageous, they have serious disadvantages. Customers frequently find themselves left waiting in a queue for an indefinite period of time while soothing music is played, this presumably being intended to dampen the customer's justifiably rising level of anger at the appalling quality of service provision! Since most of such calls will have originated from product defects, the lack of adequate telephone support facilities rubs salt into the wound, with the inevitable consequence of lost potential future business. Many poorly performing companies who have installed a *toll-free* telephone support line (where the vendor company itself foots the bill for customer call waiting time) have had to withdraw it smartly on cost grounds, but this avoids addressing the fundamental process issues to which these costs are a pointer. The customer's realisation that his or her firm, rather than the supplier, is now incurring this charge, which for overseas calls in business hours is not trivial, adds insult to injury and exacerbates their sense of disillusionment.

It is therefore vital to know the average and maximum residence times for support calls held in the automatic queue. Are the technical arrangements in place to obtain this data? Such data should be reviewed by quality assurance and management on a regular basis as a key company performance indicator.

Quite a number supplement these arrangements with the good offices afforded by dealers and value-added resellers through whom their products are distributed. Dealers contribute to support by providing a first line response to users, thus relieving the supplier of many enquiries of a more trivial nature. They may also assist in the initial prioritization of enhancement requests and defect repairs, although their capacity to do this is often severely constrained, and the feedback given can be wholly unrepresentative. Some of the smaller vendors whose products have not attracted the formation of a user group have begun to use the Internet as an inexpensive substitute, dubbed by one comedian as the *poor man's user group*. This takes the form of a bulletin board to which all users may gain access, and on which defect reports and enhancement requests may be posted. However, there is no substitute for in-depth face-to-face contact between users over the course of a two-day meeting, where the *culture* of a software application can be thoroughly explored (discussions which are invariably lubricated with generous quantities of ice-breaking, inhibition-releasing beverages, usually available in the hotel bar!).

There should be a specific procedure, if relevant, describing how emergency releases are distributed to customers in the event of a serious fault emerging from released product that requires the immediate notification of every user site.

Keep *It*

Simple

Practical Guidance

Create a document describing the company's procedure in the event of a critical fault developing in released product that requires the immediate notification of every user.

ESCROW AGREEMENTS

For many years, the arrangement of escrow has been a condition of many major contracts in the computer industry. This is the formal lodgment of source code and development tools with a third party, and which are to be made available to customers in the event of the insolvency of the vendor firm and its cessation to trade, and only in these circumstances. Even today, many smaller vendors have made such arrangements, usually with a local solicitor, bank, or even the UK National Computing Centre.

There is no objection whatsoever to such arrangements, though it is quite clear that the notional benefits of escrow are now being widely discounted. In all the cases save one of vendor bankruptcy and business wind-up which have been made public, customers have not attempted to take advantage of the escrow to obtain the application's source code and tools. The reasoning behind this appears to be the belief that to attempt to support and maintain code of other authorship is unrealistic from both technical and financial viewpoints. Source code and life cycle documentation in the best of environments is rarely of a depth and comprehensiveness to enable total strangers to begin to support, let alone enhance for the longer term, an application of any complexity without enormous risk. On the other hand, seldom is the application sufficiently business critical and so unique as to preclude other less risky and cheaper alternatives. This usually leads to the freezing of the code while plans are conceived to replace the application with a competitive product, hopefully offering other business advantages and effectively bringing forward a migration of the application that would have occurred anyway.

SUPPORT CULTURE

Finally, the auditor should form an impression of the vendor's underlying attitude to customers and their interests. Is the vendor in business just to make a *fast buck* from the sale of licences, or does the vendor aspire to forge a long-term business partnership with each customer? There is no prescriptive formula that can be advanced for arriving at this assessment, although the information already gleaned from the enquiries outlined in this chapter should, by now, have removed most of the doubt in this matter.

Having gleaned at least a reasonable knowledge of the vendor's product range and an understanding of the place occupied within it by the product of interest, together with an appreciation of the depth to which it can be supported and its current stage in its own life cycle, the team is now ready for the next phase of their examination. This is the critical and searching exploration of the extent, if any, to which quality is actually being built into the software as it is developed. It is to this that the next chapter will be devoted.

Notes

1. The example of the attitude of IBM and Hewlett Packard in the 1980s to the appearance of the personal computer is instructive. Their perception of the emergence of the client-server and open systems environments at that time triggered HP's fundamental change of strategic direction, on which the company's enormous subsequent growth was based. IBM, on the other hand, languished through a traumatic period from which it has only recently emerged, being left behind almost completely by the personal computer revolution, of which with foresight and imagination it might have had the lion's share.

2. A *hook* in a standard, configurable software application is used here in the sense of a entry of some kind, designed to allow the standard software to temporarily suspend its execution, and invoke another program entirely designed by

or for the user. Such a *bolt-on* program would perform some related processing task, either on information passed by the calling program or derived from another source, and return information back to the standard application. This design feature has been used frequently, and highly effectively, in scientific software packages to promote both user customisation, and the interfacing of standard applications software to legacy systems, without compromising the integrity of the standard application.

5

Quality Assurance and Configuration Management

Everyone wants to go to heaven, but no one wants to die.

Anon

THE VALUE OF QUALITY IN THE BUSINESS

The purpose of this chapter is to explore the role in the software development process of quality assurance, which is defined by IEEE (ANSI 730) as follows:

> *A planned and systematic pattern of all actions necessary to provide adequate confidence that the item or product conforms to established technical requirements.*

The place of quality within the business as a whole is vital, as we have already seen in previous chapters. If quality does not lie at the heart of the organization's culture at all levels, then any attempts to impose quality assurance are bound to fail. They will simply be regarded as impediments to the *real work* and ways will be found to circumvent them—people are hugely resourceful given the determination. The fact that the *real work* may be something that no one will buy and which may, therefore, sink the business is beside the point under this kind of thinking.

Companies are composed of people pursuing processes to make a profit. In most companies, a total quality initiative starts with a single individual committed to quality, sometimes referred to as a *champion*. He or she may be a new recruit or an existing member of staff who has become aware of the hazards to which an uncontrolled organization is exposed. But having a champion is not enough since money must be *invested* to introduce quality assurance, an investment expected to repay itself handsomely in the medium to long term. For this reason, total quality must start at the top of the company, for without top level endorsement, money will not be forthcoming. In most of the best companies, the board of directors or, in a small company, the managing director, has issued a mission statement defining both the place of quality and the centrality of the customer in all of the company's activities. Once this is established, then it becomes possible to define the *processes* needed to fulfil the mission. Each *process* must be documented in a *procedure* describing how the process is executed. The collection of procedures together with the associated company standards, guidelines and forms (all of which can be in electronic form), is known as the *quality management system*, and is the essential tool for moving an organization from the Capability Maturity Model's repeatable level to the defined level. The relationship between these is illustrated in figure 5.1.

A mission statement might run something like this:

> **Purpose**: *We provide . . . services that contribute to the success of individuals, businesses, communities, and countries around the world. By creating software solutions for our customers . . . we help them achieve their goals.*

> **Mission**: *Our mission is to be the premier . . . company in the markets we serve.*

> **Values**: *Our behaviour is guided by fundamental values which flow from a total commitment to integrity: customer focus, respect for one another, teamwork, initiative, professionalism and quality.*

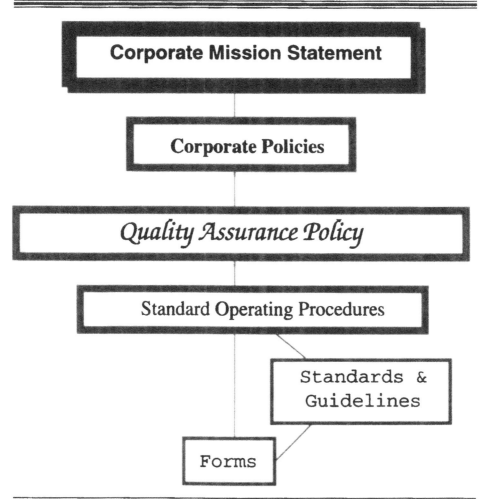

Figure 5.1. Quality Assurance in the Corporate Framework

QUALITY MANAGEMENT SYSTEM

The quality management system essentially describes *the way we do things around here*. It is absolutely fundamental to building quality into software for several reasons. Because it is the encyclopedia of how we do things around here, it ensures that a particular process is repeatedly conducted in the same way, and that this way of working is known by everyone, is amenable to inspection by both management and visitors, and therefore is amenable to systematic improvement in the future.

If the quality management system is to deliver its intended business benefits, it must be followed. A quality management system gathering dust on a shelf is of no use to anyone. It must be kept up-to-date and rigorously enforced. Resistance to the whole concept of a quality management system has frequently been encountered on the grounds that it will constrain the creativity of the gifted people on whom the company depends. Now let no one deny that there is truth in this! Any system worth having is deliberately designed to constrain individuals, but only (and that is the operative word) from pursuing practices that threaten the success of the development process. To be specific, software development depends critically on the controlled flow of information between the players. While this flow remains verbal and informal in nature, it is vulnerable to lapses in memory, misunderstanding of the message and loss. Documentation of the critical information ensures a safe and secure flow. Once this is recognized to be the best way of working, it is essential for everyone to abide by it if the benefits are to be reaped and the potential losses avoided.

In organizations still at the Capability Maturity Model's initial level (creative chaos), management must be aware of the probable prejudice against the constraint of a quality management system. It is frequently initially perceived as stifling of initiative, bureaucratic and repressive of personal responsibility, and project managers and programmers usually seem to be the ones most entrenched in their opposition. To counter this, management will need to explain the hidden costs and risks inherent in the present way of working and the need to improve business practices and, in turn, the company's profitability. Constructing the quality management system in such a way so that each standard it contains describes the defects that it is aimed at avoiding assists this education process, which can be powerfully assisted if the highly skilled programming staff (from whom, as we have noted, the most vociferous objections usually arise) are genuinely empowered to participate in the ownership of the system. Thus, all the experience and judgement available in the programming team has been publicly recognized in support of the company's standards. In this connection, systems and procedures that are quite new to the current way of working ought to be avoided where possible, because where written procedures are based on current practice, acceptance is secured much more quickly. Where the quality management system has been introduced sensitively in recognition of these principles, acceptance both of the concept and of its QA disciplines has usually been rapid and complete.

Every quality management system will contain standards that are common to every project, such as particular language standards. However, no two projects are identical, so a project manager must have the freedom to adjust the details of the system to suit the needs of a particular project, in consultation with the team, by choosing those that are relevant. Some may need strengthening; others can be omitted as irrelevant in this case. Failure to accommodate this flexibility is one of the principal reasons for the failure of Total Quality Management initiatives in software houses, and one of the best ways to express it is to draw up, for each project, a *QA plan,* described in more detail below. This relationship is shown in figure 5.2.

Some small companies seem hardly aware that they have a quality management system at all. Some procedures have been recognised and documented to varying degrees, but the term *quality management system* has never entered common parlance. The recognition that an embryonic quality management system has been in operation tends to come as rather a pleasant surprise, and has been a powerful stimulus in its further development. In the more mature companies, a number of common benefits have been apparent. Mobility of staff becomes easier when less reliance is placed on head knowledge and skill in one specialist area. With documented procedures and standard ways of doing things, the capacity of a company improves, since software development becomes more efficient. Customer requirements, being more central, cut the level of complaints regarding incorrect or inadequate functionality. Together with a lower level of residual defects, this feeds through to a reduction in the effort required in the support area, which more than repays the cost of the system in the medium term. Finally, management has become more aware of the strengths and weaknesses of the operation. Because these are now much more visible, management is able to distinguish the small number of vital issues from the many trivial ones. This enables them to initiate the really important process improvements more quickly and more informedly.

To summarize, a quality management system can be introduced quickly by documenting current practice, but it must be flexible and preserve the centrality of the customer's needs, as shown in figure 5.3. It ought to constrain the creativity of the staff only in the sense of outlawing sloppy and undocumented practices that fail to preserve vital information and which, therefore, jeopardize the process.

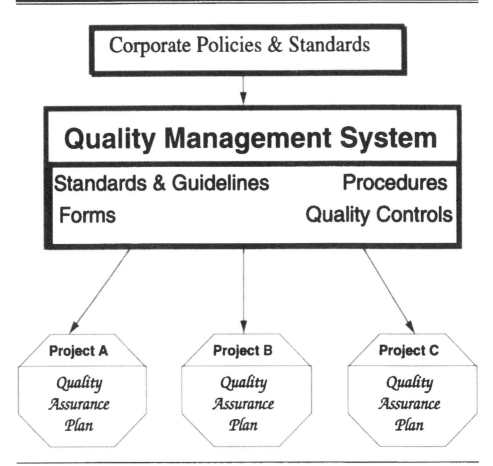

Figure 5.2. A Quality Assurance Plan for Each Project

QUALITY ASSURANCE PLAN

The sequence of steps for all sound technical planning is as follows:

- Say what you are going to do in advance.

- Do it!

- Record that you have done it.

- Assess how well it went and take corrective action.

This is, of course, just a rehash of the *plan-do-check-act* Shewart cycle. The place of the *QA plan* is in the first quartile (i.e., to define in advance what we will do, how we will check that it has been done

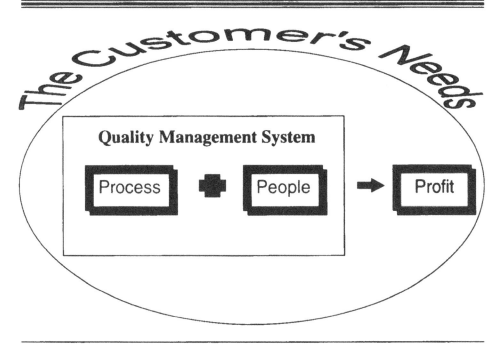

Figure 5.3. Relationship Between the Quality Management System and the Customer

and how we will act if it goes awry). Our plan will state this for every deliverable expected from the process. It will state those activities and controls that are to be effected to ensure that the developed software product is fit for the purpose for which it was intended and meets its design requirements. In other words, for every deliverable, we need to state what the quality features will be and how we will assess their presence. The project team should work out together how the project is to be tackled on the technical level, the methods that will be used, the intermediate deliverables, the resources that will be required, any specific training, and how configuration management will be handled (see below). These, together with any agreed variations from the "official" quality management system forms the foundation of the quality plan. Next, it should identify the documentation governing the development, testing and maintenance of the software. This documentation must include at a minimum the following:

- User requirements specification: what the system is expected to do from a user's perspective

- Software design description: how the system will be designed to achieve the requirements

- Structured software test plan: the tests that will be conducted to prove that the requirements have been met and the results that ought to be obtained

- Software test report: the results of the tests, with special attention to nonconformities

- Installation document: how to install the software at the user's location

- User manual: instructions to the user on how to use the software

- Software configuration management plan (discussed below)

To many small companies yet to adopt formal quality assurance, the above list may seem intimidating and unnecessary. However, a number of small software houses are implementing a software quality plan along these lines in a simple way, producing the documentation above as a natural result of a controlled, methodical life cycle approach. The benefits they have found are a major reduction in risk in the project, a closer approximation between projected and actual time to delivery, a reduction in cost by the avoidance of overruns common in earlier times, and the elimination of a high proportion of residual errors in delivered code. These savings have greatly outweighed the cost of the quality plan itself and its associated measures, the effects eventually feeding through as increased profitability. They are, therefore, determined never to look back.

The quality plan should specify the company's standards and practices to be followed in the project. These would normally include standards relating to documentation, logic structure, program coding and comments (described in more detail in chapter 8). It should define the *reviews* to be conducted to safeguard the company during the project process. Why have reviews? What purpose do they serve? No one individual, however gifted, should be expected to produce technical documentation free of error. We make mistakes, we overlook important details and we make unconscious assumptions that trip others up. It happens constantly, everywhere and under the pressure to innovate and deliver it creeps in with increasing severity. A company interested in survival (an acutely important issue for the small company) and intent on reducing the ensuing risk to its future will seek to remove these defects at the earliest possible opportunity. This is the purpose of the reviews built into the quality plan.

The review would be formal in a large organization, but in the small company, it could be simply the study of a document by another competent and qualified individual for the purpose of identifying errors, followed by a signature and date on the final document (which could, of course, be just as easily in a Lotus Notes® database or in other electronic form rather than on paper) recording that the review actually took place. What is most important is that the defects that might have caused havoc at later stages are no longer present, and the ensuing losses will not be incurred. Such a review is not expensive, but the potential for making savings is substantial. Who would defend omitting it knowing these exigencies, other than someone with a corporate death wish?

At a minimum, a review should take place of the following:

- User requirements document—where the majority of foundational errors occur and whose careful review is likely to be, by far, the most cost-effective of all

- Design specification

- Structured test plan

- Source code

It is most important that the plan describes the techniques to be used to ensure traceability. Without this essential safeguard, there is no certainty that either the design will lead to a system that meets the user requirements specification in a particular detail or in its entirety, or that the structured test plan will include all of the functionality (both positive and negative) incorporated into the design. There are many different techniques by which traceability can be ensured, but one of the most effective is the simple proviso of *paragraph numbering*. Each paragraph of the user requirements specification refers to a paragraph in the design specification that addresses those requirements. Each individual test featured in the structured test plan refers back to a paragraph number in the design specification. A check can be made in the test plan review whether every paragraph in the design document receives a mention, and so on. The quality plan should, therefore, specify the traceability approach to be used, and the quality assurance check that will ensure its effective incorporation before coding commences.

The plan should describe the processes to be followed for reporting, tracking and resolving software problems; any tools and methodologies to be used; and the way that the source code will be controlled. In this latter respect, there are a number of excellent products now on the market for this purpose, one or two of which will be mentioned in chapter 8. The plan will define what records associated with the development process will be kept and maintained and for how long. More detailed guidance on the components of the quality plan are available from the IEEE (ANSI 983). Finally, the plan must include the critical *quality characteristics* that must be met in the final product, and the *quality controls* that will ensure their presence.

QUALITY CONTROLS

The QA plan must include the quality controls that will ensure the incorporation of particular characteristics that have been defined as essential to the project. A control is associated with the *documentary evidence* proving that the characteristic has been achieved. It will be remembered that documentary evidence is the overwhelming theme of computer-related systems validation, and it is in this respect that the parallel between the two disciplines is most apparent. Here are few examples of quality controls:

- A test in the structured test plan that demonstrates that a particular function works correctly; **evidence: the test record**

- A review which was aimed at ensuring compatibility with the UNIX environment; **evidence: the minutes of the review meeting**

- The running of a CASE tool that looks at source code to see that it kept to the specified programming standards; **evidence: the tool's hard copy report showing the absence of any violations**

The first of these examples addresses the functionality quality characteristic, the second the UNIX compatibility quality characteristic and the third the maintainability quality characteristic.

Defining these tangible pieces of evidence in the quality plan at the outset of the process enables everyone to understand what is expected. It provides a safeguard against a key element being missed and no one highlighting the fact until much later, if at all. In this respect, quality controls are an important risk-reduction device. Their monitoring forms a critical part of QA activity.

CONFIGURATION MANAGEMENT

Configuration management is such a fundamental aspect of software development that it is frequently adopted unconsciously as part of the life cycle without being recognized as a specific discipline. It forms the subject of its own ISO standard (ISO 10007). It focusses on the many *items* that are produced and which need to be controlled within the project, an item being defined as an entity whose development must be controlled and tracked. The history of the development of each entity must be tracked so that it can be reconstructed at any future time in any of its former states. Items can be simple objects, such as an ordinary text file, or a more complicated one such as a library, either of routines stored on a computer or of files stored by other means, each of which may be an item in itself. As an item is developed, it evolves from one *variant* into another as functionality is added, until a particular variant is then declared to have become a *version*. Successive versions represent the progress of the item in time.

At some particular time in the life cycle, a collection of items may all conform to some defined state or exhibit some characteristic. This is called a *baseline* which could, for example, represent a particular build of a software product. A *configuration* is a collection of versions assembled with some common purpose, for example, for a software release.

"Why bother with all this?" critics might mutter. The purpose of configuration management (figure 5.4) is to make sure of the availability, consistency and accuracy of all the items being developed so that they can be changed as required in a controlled way. Management is thus kept abreast of progress in a secure manner, with less risk to the business. For example, in the event of some catastrophic failure, the current state of all items in the project can be accurately regenerated. Objects can be safely shared between programmers. Design corrections and enhancements can be implemented, tested and documented safely and securely according to well-understood

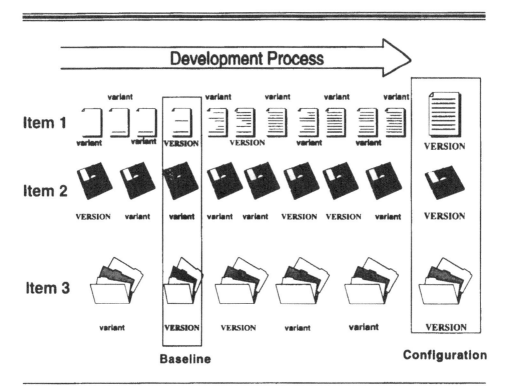

Figure 5.4. The Essence of Configuration Management

procedures so that prior to delivery the exact state of development and testing is known. Because of this, documentation can be readily assembled to accompany the delivery, and there can be absolute certainty that what was actually delivered to the customer was identical to what was thought to have been shipped (which is not always the case!). Subsequently, should problems arise (and they often do), these can be associated accurately with versions of each of the component items.

SOFTWARE CONFIGURATION MANAGEMENT PLAN

The configuration management plan should be drawn up at the commencement of a project. It need not be a long document and may be subsumed within the overall quality plan discussed above. It should identify the items (deliverable and nondeliverable) associated with the various stages of the project, defining any terms specific to this project and refer to any general company procedures. If one project follows the same lines as a previous one, the configuration management plan may be a simple revision of "one we made earlier".[1] It should name all members of the project team, who is responsible for what, and the resources to be used (e.g., existing software libraries). It should state who may authorize changes to items during the project. It should define the particular project milestones to be passed and the existing or new company procedures to be followed. The plan should define the naming conventions to be used for items, the change control procedure (described in more detail in chapter 11) to be used, and the review mechanism (which in a small company could be a weekly review meeting with someone recording the minutes, for example). The point here is that what is to happen is stated in advance, everyone knows it, and the group can collectively make sure it is followed. If any tools or methodologies are to be followed these should be mentioned, as well as the means by which items should be stored (e.g. a Lotus Notes® database could be used to record minutes of meetings, and a source code control system used to safeguard developed code). For a small company, such a plan can be quickly drawn up, circulated and approved, with significant reduction in later project risk, but at very little cost.

BUILDING QUALITY INTO SOFTWARE

Almost all of the preceding discussion has been directed toward one aim, to **build quality into software** through controlled processes designed **to avoid the incorporation of** errors and to ensure that the finished product **functions as originally intended**. All organizations that have yet to appreciate fully these principles labour under a common delusion: that testing is the means by which quality can be added to software (rather like the icing on a cake). The evidence for this becomes painfully plain early in an audit. The less mature an organization, the greater the reliance on testing and the greater the proportion of time and money devoted to it. As figure 5.5 shows in caricature, the old-fashioned uncontrolled empirical model ("put it together and see if it works") places an inordinate emphasis on testing, while the quality-assured process places all of the emphasis on the foundation stones of getting it right at the requirements and design stages before a line of code is ever written.

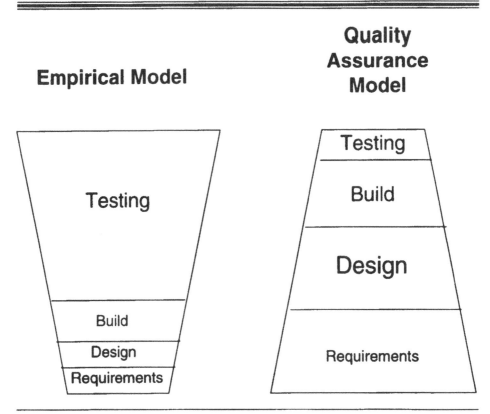

Figure 5.5. Models of Software Development

Testing then reduces to confirming the quality level *already present in the software.*

Why is testing incapable of building quality into software? Software in all but the very simplest programs is very complex. It may consist of thousands of lines of code with numerous paths and branches from instruction to instruction, or if event driven, be amenable to thousands of different combinations of execution sequences. We might suppose it possible for quality assurance or another independent agency to inspect the code when it has been completed. This issue became a hot topic in the late 1980s in the evolution of computer-related system validation standards by the U.S. pharmaceutical industry and the FDA, as documented by Chapman (1991b). He reports how the committees had found that for all but the smallest programs this was totally impractical. It could be imagined that a low level line-by-line inspection of code would best be conducted by a team of specialists, working for no more than 2 hours at a time because of fatigue. This implies a maximum quota of only 150 lines per day and leads to the extraordinary but inescapable conclusion that a 1.5 million line product (not uncommon) would require almost 40 worker-years of inspection effort!

Exhaustive *dynamic path analysis* was another testing technique discussed whose impracticality was exposed by Myers (1979). He showed that for a simple If-Do loop using only 10–20 statements with 20 iterations of the loop, there were about 100 trillion possible pathways. If someone were to try to write, execute, and verify a test case every 5 minutes, the task of testing every path would take 1 billion years (not taking account of coffee breaks!). Therefore, testing of software only exercises a small proportion of the possible pathways through the code, and is only capable of bringing to light a very small proportion of the total number of errors buried in the software.

This is commonly known as *black box testing* or *functional testing*, since it concentrates on measuring functional behaviour only (output versus input), with no knowledge of how the program is designed or works internally—the program is regarded like a mysterious black box that cannot be opened and whose contents therefore remain enigmatic. Clearly, therefore, the only practical approach to ensuring the reliability of software is to implement measures to avoid putting errors into the software in the first place, and to take steps to remove those that slip through the net systematically, and at the earliest opportunity. This can only be done, as we have seen, by using an organized development process consisting of a series of distinct phases collectively referred to as a *software life cycle*, three models of which were examined in chapter 1. The existence of these phases enables reviews and tests to be conducted at discrete points, making control and traceability possible.

It should now be apparent why companies still operating on the old, semichaotic empirical model derive so little benefit from their huge emphasis on finished software testing. When fully brought home, this truth hurts, because companies sincerely believe they are doing the right thing and are behaving from the best of motives. Despite spending vast sums of money and other resources on testing the product to death, the support desk telephones still glow red hot from one fault call after another. Everyone is running round frantically trying to get the released software established in the marketplace and contain the resulting hemorrhage of business inherent in a damaged reputation. But integrity is no substitute for knowledge, and well-meaning delusion is no basis for business success. Far be it from me to deny that integrity is indispensable *par excellence,* but so also is technical competence and the wise use of resources.

Failure to understand that a quality product can only result from a quality-assured process was exemplified in a painful letter sent by a chief executive after that company's rejection as a software supplier through a software QA audit. He wrote,

> *It may seem contradictory that we have a quality product yet fail a quality audit, but this arises from the fact that the audit reviews the processes involved in the software pro-duction, rather than on assessing the end product . . . we can provide a quality product but at present we are unable to fully prove it.*

If a quality product emerged from a uncontrolled process, it would be as miraculous as water running spontaneously uphill. Nature is not like that, as experience of life abundantly demonstrates. The un-derlying plea seems to be "never mind the quality, look at our lovely glossy brochure"!

SOFTWARE INSPECTION

An attempt has been made to show that dynamic path analysis is hopelessly impractical when used as a testing method at the com-pletion of the life cycle. However, at the proper time, the technique comes into its element. When used at the early stage of coding by programmers, checking each other's work on a module-by-module basis, it has been shown to be an extremely powerful and *cost-effective* means of removing errors. Defects removed at this stage are found much more easily and in far greater numbers than if left until later stages. Furthermore, the cost of removing them here is only 1–10 percent of the cost of removal later on, as Boehm's data (1981) in figure 5.6 based on the analysis of 63 projects shows.

Therefore, it is used most successfully if modules are kept small and within strict size boundaries. Because it involves a close in-spection of the structural logic of the software, it is known as *struc-tural testing* or *white box testing* (a white box being one capable of being opened and its contents examined in detail). The term *inspec-tion* is now commonly used and has been officially incorporated

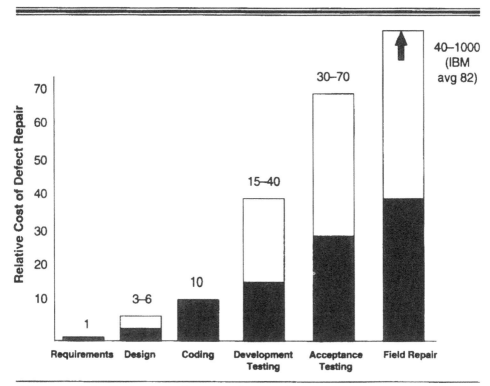

Figure 5.6. Relative Costs of a Defect Repair

into the ANSI/IEEE standards (ANSI 610) for software engineering, being defined as follows:

> *A formal evaluation technique in which software requirements, design or code are examined in detail by a person or group other than the author to detect faults, violations of development standards and other problems.*

This definition shows that the technique is not confined to source code, but can just as usefully be deployed on the documents from which the source code is derived and from which most of its defects arise. It can, in fact, be applied to any life cycle document, a subject to which we shall return in chapter 10.

The formal technique of software inspection supported by numerical metrics was pioneered by Michael Fagan, a quality control engineer at IBM's Kingston, New York, laboratories in the 1970s. Known as Fagan's Inspection and first published in his now famous paper (Fagan), it owes its origin to the principles of statistical process control adumbrated by Deming and Juran, which was explored in chapter 1. Until that time, the concept of zero defects in software had been regarded as the unachievable Holy Grail of computing. Now there was a practical and *measurable* method to begin to approach it. A detailed description of the technique is beyond the scope of this book, but has been thoroughly explored in the excellent work by Gilb and Graham (1993) with a foreword by Watts Humphrey, father of the Capability Maturity Model. A brief summary of the technique now follows, although readers intent on implementing this powerful technique are urged to obtain this book for detailed study, rather than relying on the brief appetizer given here.

The technique is illustrated in figure 5.7 and begins with a request for inspection by the *author* of the document or code. The author gives the material to be inspected (the product document or code) to the *inspection leader* who has been appointed to supervise the inspection. The leader makes sure that the *product document* meets the general entry criteria already defined for that kind of product document to avoid wasting everyone's time if basic rules

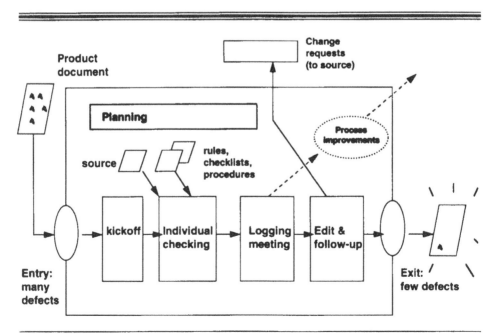

Figure 5.7. Software and Document Inspection Technique

have been violated (e.g., has the author of code abided by the company's established programming standards?). The leader then convenes a kickoff meeting to distribute the following:

- The *product document* (which is to be inspected)

- The *source document* (on whose basis the product document was drafted; e.g., in the case of source code it might be the design specification that the code is supposed to implement)

- Any *reference documents*, such as rules, procedures and checklists that relate to the product document

This package is given to each of the *checkers*. These people will each work alone, seeking discrepancies between source and product documents, and by using the reference documents try to find the maximum number of potential defects. The checkers record these as *issues* as objectively as possible, ready to report them at the *logging meeting*. It is important to note that these issues may not be actual defects in the product document itself, and even if they are the word *defect* has critical and pejorative overtones, which are not in keeping with the spirit of the exercise, so the word *defect* is, therefore, avoided at this stage.

This meeting is convened by the *moderator* for three purposes:

1. To log the issues found

2. To discover more major issues during the meeting, stimulated by peer pressure

3. To identify and log ways of improving the inspection process itself

At the end of the meeting, the *editor* (usually the author) is sent away with the list of the issues to resolve them. Issues may be a defect, a lack of explanation or understanding on the checker's part, or a defect in the source document which may require rectification by someone else. The inspection leader subsequently follows up with the editor that effective action has been taken on **all** logged issues.

Because considerable statistical data exists relating the number of errors found on each inspection cycle to those that yet remain to be found, an estimate of the latter can be made. If this exceeds predefined *exit criteria*, another inspection cycle is ordered; otherwise, the code meets the quality standard and can qualify as the source document on which the work of the next life cycle stage can be safely based, albeit perhaps with a warning label of the estimated number of remaining defects.

The most powerful aspect of the technique is its potential for improving the software development process itself, since this implies that defects are prevented from recurring, so ratcheting up the capability of the organization. This can be facilitated by a *process brainstorming meeting,* an optional adjunct to the basic technique, where up to 10 of the major issues identified are selected for analysis. Those with the greatest severity and potential loss are chosen first. Once the root causes are brainstormed, the log of the meeting is passed to the *process change management team* charged with effecting the improvements in the software development process itself.

Where inspection is in use, it has been very successful. It does not seem to be in use to any significant extent in enterprises where the programming staff numbers less than six; in these companies, the approach of peer review or code walk-through (known as *the poor man's inspection!*) is very common. This is a pity, because the principle of inspection is at heart straightforward and can, in fact, be operated quite successfully by a small group. Ignorance of its potential benefits and an exaggerated impression of its cost lies at the heart of this reluctance.

CODE WALK–THROUGH

Walk-through is defined in the ANSI/IEEE (ANSI 610) as follows:

> *A review process in which a designer or programmer*
> *leads one or more other members of the development*
> *team through a segment of design or code that he or she*
> *has written, while the other members ask questions or*
> *make comments about technique, style, possible errors,*
> *violation of development standards and other problems.*

Clearly, walk-throughs are far less rigorous than inspections. They are only capable of highlighting a fraction of the errors that inspection is capable of identifying, and give no indication as to the level of remaining defects. Thus, serious flaws can, and commonly do, escape detection causing havoc later on in the life cycle. Furthermore, there is no formal means of addressing the inherent weaknesses of the process that are giving rise to the errors that are discovered;

hence there is no systematic assurance that the organization is improving its performance.

Having said that, walk-thoughs are a great improvement over conducting no reviews at all, a situation still to be frequently found today. They are best conducted by a small group meeting for no longer than two hours at the most to review a strictly limited amount of code or documentation. The composition of the group is usually the author, a peer programmer who can understand the code while forswearing ownership of it, and a representative of quality assurance (to follow up any issues). If the author's *manager* can be **dissuaded** from attending, so much the better! The meeting must be firmly chaired to keep attention focussed on the job, with all attendees having the materials to be examined beforehand. The objective, as with formal inspections, is to highlight potential problems rather than argue about solutions. The results of the walk-through should be minuted (either by a secretary or by the QA representative) so that defects can be eventually discussed at the project post mortem (discussed in chapter 3) in the interests of identifying fundamental *process* defects. Some of the most successful software houses (which are, as it happens quite small) run repeated program code reviews and walk-throughs spanning the whole duration of the programming phase, although they are always completed well before formal integration testing commences (though not necessarily before module testing).[2] Testing phases are discussed in chapter 9.

Keep *It* Simple	**Practical Guidance**
	Create a document describing the procedure to be followed for structural testing of all source code modules by means of a formal inspection or code walk-through. Include how the minutes of the meeting will be recorded and how identified defects will be followed up.

What should be examined in a code walk-through? The group is best advised to concentrate its attention on the most critical parts of the software in relation both to the design on which it is based (which should by this time have already been formally reviewed and approved) and the functional requirements specification. The group should ensure that programming standards (addressed in detail in chapter 8) have been followed. Care should be taken to scrutinize the logical flow to ensure not only that it is in accordance with the design but also that no code has been left unreachable. Any code that has been rendered redundant by changes that have been made to the design while the coding has been progressing should be removed. Critical algorithms as defined in the user requirements specification should be exhaustively checked.

A BLACK AND WHITE ISSUE

As an organization improves its capability the emphasis on testing should shift from finished product (black box) testing to structural testing (white box testing, either code walk-throughs or, even better, formal inspection as depicted in figure 5.8). However, the two classes of testing must not be thought to be mutually exclusive. It is not being suggested that an organization could ever become so skilled and thorough at inspection as to be able to dispense legitimately

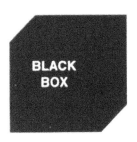

Functional Testing

No knowledge of what goes on inside

Confined to outputs versus inputs

Performed on finished system

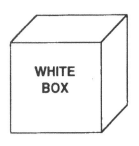

Structural Testing

Detailed knowledge of how it works inside

Line by line inspection or review of source code, including programming standards, style, database design, control methods, etc.

Figure 5.8. Two Complementary Test Approaches

with finished product testing altogether. Neither testing approach is able to detect all of the defects in a system, and both methods remain important. Black box testing can be usefully applied to the system as a whole, while white box testing should always be applied in-depth to software modules. Taken together, the total assurance delivered is greater that that of the sum of each approach considered separately.

It is on this principle that the validation of computer-related systems in regulated industries rests. The value of functional testing during system validation by the user critically depends for its significance on the level of structural testing carried out during system development by the vendor. Only when both are taken together and indicate a high level of system compliance with requirements and a very low level of residual defects can reliance be placed on the system to be fit for its intended purpose.

INTERNAL AUDITS

Once a quality management system is in place delivering the benefits it was designed to deliver, it may be thought that no further activity in relation to it is needed. If only this were true! Human nature being what it is, there is always the temptation to adopt a short-term perspective under the pressure of deadlines and to believe that the undocumented quick fix is the best action for the moment. As any probation officer will testify, apparently reformed criminals are always prone to recidivism. Recognition of the weaknesses of human nature lies at the heart of the surveillance audits that are an integral part of the obligations shouldered by software houses certified under ISO 9000-3 (TickIT). Indeed, the concept of the internal audit has long been common in all regulated industries. It is the process of periodically ensuring the standards and procedures are being complied with, in the long-term interests of the company's well-being. The success of the internal audit depends critically on the culture within the company and the degree of recognition of the value of the quality management system. In a healthy organization, the quality management system must not be regarded as an unchanging edict inscribed on tablets of stone and which can *never* be changed. It must be subject to intelligent evolution and development as technology improves and the needs of the organization change. This flexibility has already been emphasized in connection with staff empowerment and morale. Notwithstanding this, there will be certain principles that do merit the permanence of being set in stone. For example, one such edict might be as follows:

> *Thou shalt never change a segment of code without complying with Change Control Procedure C12345*

although procedure C12345 **may** from time to time be modified.

To deliver its full benefit to the company, the internal audit must be seen as a *team activity* between quality assurance and the development group, aimed at identifying the level of compliance with standards and procedures, the reasons for noncompliance, and the scope for improving the quality management system. If attitudes do not mature, or deteriorate so that the audit becomes a police action, then the value is almost entirely lost from the outset, and the organization has serious problems. The reader will recognise these considerations as exactly the same as those that apply to the external software QA audit, as we have seen.

The frequency of the internal audit must be set sensitively. If conducted too infrequently, this can lead to an ossification of the system, with obsolescent standards being flouted and discredited. Over frequent audits become burdensome, not cost-effective, and can lead to friction between development and quality assurance. With these realities in mind, the audit frequency can be adjusted as time passes to reflect the rate of change of technologies and commercial activity.

DEFECT REPORTS AND ENHANCEMENT REQUESTS

Almost all vendors operate a formal system for the receipt of reports of defects in released code and requests for its enhancement, and store these in a database of one kind or another. Although there are a number of commercial products on the market to meet this need, some vendors will incur the cost of designing their own, usually as it happens using Microsoft *Access*™. A good reason why this was done is still awaited, fueling the suspicion that at heart there has been a lack of awareness of the various commercial software packages available for this purpose.

Prioritization of defect reports and enhancement requests is a vital discipline to ensure that development effort is wisely directed for the long-term good of the company. Many individuals find it extremely hard to disentangle the urgent from the important, expressed cogently by the old adage that when one is up to one's neck in alligators, it is difficult to remember that the original objective was to drain the swamp! The belief that meeting the immediate short-term need is *always* commensurate with the much larger, long-term strategic aspirations of the company is as common as it is misplaced. Another tendency is to concede automatically the immediate demand of the client with the loudest voice.[3] An awareness of management's weakness to communicate strategic thinking clearly enough to those *at the coal face*, to enable development managers to allocate programming resources in the most effective manner, is unavoidable. There is often a conflict between further development of an existing product arising from client pressure, and development of a totally new concept of which the market is as yet unaware and on which the company's future may critically depend. It is very hard to resist demands for changes which will have immediate impact on customer satisfaction, when effort ought to be concentrated on an innovative product of which no customer is yet aware. Missing a launch date by as little as a month in a highly competitive market area may mean the difference between making a fortune and failing even to recover development costs. The users of a series of well-known laboratory analytical systems in the late 1970s became contemptuous of the vendor's parrot like response "we do not support this" to requests for crucial enhancements. In that situation, many of these users were not only dependent to a large degree on those systems for the running of their laboratories, but also constituted the core market on whom the success of that vendor's replacement analytical systems depended. This is a good example of the dilemma sometimes faced by successful software companies, and it is foolish to pretend that there are any slick and easy answers. No wonder development managers often feel caught between rock and a hard place in circumstances where the only beneficiary appears to be their competitors.

In certain circumstances, it may be prudent to leave some defects unresolved where there is a satisfactory workaround. Great care needs to be exercised here, however. Users thereby receive a subliminal message about attitudes that are the very antithesis of a customer-centred approach. This may be very unfair to the vendor if the decision to devote resources to innovation ultimately stems from a desire to meet the future needs of those *same* customers.

The team should seek evidence that whatever tool is used to record, there is in operation a unique indexing system through which changes in source code can be tracked back to the request or report that originally gave birth to it. This ensures that the company is capable of reconciling all the defect reports and enhancements with changes actually effected in software or, in other words, of knowing which defects or enhancements have not, in fact, been dealt with.

CERTIFICATION

The next QA issue that the auditor should address is whether or not the organization has achieved TickIT certification and, if not, whether the firm aspires to do so. It is vitally important in this connection, however, to make a clear distinction between operating in accordance with the ISO 9000-3 standards (which this book is advocating) on the one hand, and being *publicly certified* as doing so on the other. Why should a company go to all the trouble of transforming the business through effective quality assurance and not automatically proceed to advertise this fact to the world through certification?

It has already been shown in chapter 3 that while transforming the software development process involves an initial overhead cost to the company, this is more than repaid, once the quality management system is firmly established, by much greater savings accruing in perpetuity from lower defect rates and a closer match between functionality and requirements. When it comes to certification, however, the cost-benefit issues are completely different.

Certification is only of benefit to a company if business is likely to be lost without it. In many business sectors where large software projects are involved, ISO 9000-3 accreditation is already a mandatory requirement for the selection of firms to be invited to tender. Uncertified software houses in these markets are, therefore, at a crippling disadvantage. At the present time, however, there is a huge spectrum of business where TickIT accreditation itself is not seen as a critical asset. This is certainly the case with most of the business software that has been audited so far. This is to be regretted, but it is a fact of life. Software firms in this category need to consider carefully whether they would be likely to see any economic return from the considerable cost of obtaining and keeping accreditation as a separate exercise, following on from installing a quality management system. In short, the badge may be dispensable even if the realities that it signifies are not.

Certification involves assessment of the software house by an accredited certification body in two stages:

1. The quality management system is judged against the TickIT standard.

2. The organization is audited to check day-to-day compliance with the quality management system and that the standard is effective.

Corrective actions may be required and these must be verified before the certificate is issued.

The fees charged for these activities are considerable. At current rates, the initial assessment fees are in the order of £4000–£7000 for a software house of 50–100 employees operating on one UK site. In addition, some certification bodies charge a one-off application and certificate fees of about £500 for each certificate. On top of this, there will be further charges for the regular subsequent 6-month surveillance visits likely to cost about 30 percent of the initial assessment cost per year. It is also important not to overlook the internal costs directly related to the assessment process, which might typically be as follows:

*   Preparation for the assessment, 15–30 person-days

*   Assessment, 10–12 person-days

*   Surveillance, 5–10 person-days for each visit

Although these figures may be less for a smaller company, the cost is likely to be higher as a proportion of turnover.

There is already a large body of evidence to show that companies that have obtained certification have shown a consistent pattern of commercial success. This success arises both from the innate benefits of operating in a quality-assured manner (which a noncertified company can obtain just as well), and also from the *marketing benefits* accruing in its particular sector from certification. Thus, if these latter are unlikely to be significant, it is essential that a company carefully weigh the prospect for any economic return before embarking on this kind of investment. Furthermore, as the maturity of purchasers improves, it is essential to keep an open mind on this issue, since what is expensive and of no practical use today may become business critical and indispensable tomorrow.

THE COST OF QUALITY ASSURANCE

So far, no detailed attention has been paid to the cost of quality assurance. To suggest or imply that quality assurance itself comes free would be both foolish and disingenuous. To develop and operate an effective quality management system represents an additional overhead cost for a software house of any size. The actual percentage of development cost that the additional overhead of quality constitutes ought not to vary much with the size of the company. The best estimates of the detailed contributions from different quality-related activities that have been published are those included in the Price Waterhouse report (1988) mentioned in the introduction. A table of the individual QC activities, in terms of percentage of total development time, required to meet the ISO 9000-3 standard for a typical project appears in table 5.1.

Now, of course, all software developers already spend a considerable amount of time on activity, principally in retrospective testing. In the majority of organizations, and especially the smaller ones, where the capability maturity is that of creative chaos, or perhaps occasionally between this and the next, repeatable level, the proportion of system testing already well exceeds the 7–10 percent

Table 5.1. Estimated Quality Control Effort (reproduced from Appendix VI of the Price Waterhouse report by permission— see Acknowledgements)

Activity	% Total Development Effort
Planning	2–4
Progress meetings	4–6
User sign-off	—
Configuration management	1
Change control	1
Documentation control	—
Design reviews	2–4
Code walk-throughs	2–3
Error logging	1
System testing excluding rework/retesting	7–10
Acceptance testing excluding rework/retesting	3–4
TOTAL	23–24

of development effort included in the above. Hence, for many such firms, the additional overhead of migrating to a quality-assured process would be well under 10 percent. The Price Waterhouse authors estimated 5 percent as a general guide.

The most important principle that must be kept constantly in the forefront of all thinking when constructing a quality management system is the KISS principle (figure 5.9), which addresses both style and content. The simpler a procedure is to adopt and follow, the more likely it is to be effective. It should be expressed succinctly, with as few words as possible, avoiding irritating tautology, repetition, redundancy and verbiage. Furthermore, every quality management control, constraining as it does the activity of programmers or others in some way, must be demonstrably directed at avoiding a particular bad practice or a recognizable cause of defects. As mentioned earlier, the things that programmers *most detest* about the job is often an excellent starting point for constructing the first few procedures. It must, therefore, be quite clear that each and every procedure offers a financial saving to the company, so that ignoring or circumventing it is tantamount to feeding pound notes, dollars, or whatever your currency is, through the grille of the drain in the street outside, as illustrated in figure I.4 on page 15. If procedures become needlessly complex, the quality management system will degenerate into a bureaucracy (self-perpetuating procedures with no cost benefit) and will impose a very different KISS principle—the kiss of death to quality and improvement!

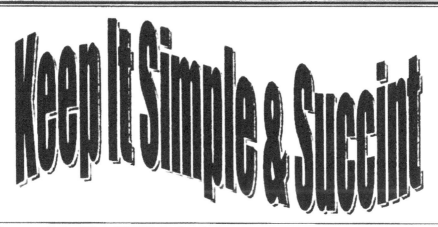

Figure 5.9. The KISS Principle

It is necessary to make one final point of political significance in regard to implementing a quality system. The cost of the quality system is immediate, tangible and measurable. Therefore, it offers an easy target to its detractors, who can gleefully point to the costs as another example of bureaucratic lunacy impeding the profitability of the organization to satisfy some external standard. The difficulty is compounded by the fact that the overheads inherent in today's chaotic modus operandi are hidden, unknown and unknowable, as we saw in our discussion of statistical process control in chapter 1. Since these cannot be quantified with any certainty, the debate is very hard for the apologists of quality assurance, for which the personal attributes of courage, conviction and steadfastness will be required, until the practical benefits of fewer defects and lower support and maintenance costs feed through. It is the overwhelming consensus among those that have approached or achieved an ISO 9000-3 (TickIT) compliant methodology that the savings accrued from an effective quality management system vastly outweigh the costs of the quality system; companies following this route have shown a consistent pattern of commercial success irrespective of their size or market area. The relationship between costs and benefits, and the time delay between them are portrayed in figure 5.10 reproduced by permission from the TickIT guide (1995).

CONFOUNDING THE SKEPTICS

In most companies, where the adoption of a quality assured development process is advocated with evangelical zeal by a champion of quality principles, there is usually, as has just been hinted, a caucus of irredeemable unbelievers. Resistance arises in the face of change despite the patently obvious fact that the exhaustive testing effort is proving incapable of detecting more than a fraction of the latent errors in the products. How are the skeptics to be converted to realizing that a quality management system will be a worthwhile investment if they have yet to be convinced of its business-critical importance?

The best tool to achieve this is a *quality policy*, a document that sets out their covenant with each other in the corporate team, with rather the same flavour as a mission statement. If the policy is to have any credibility whatsoever, it must be endorsed at the very

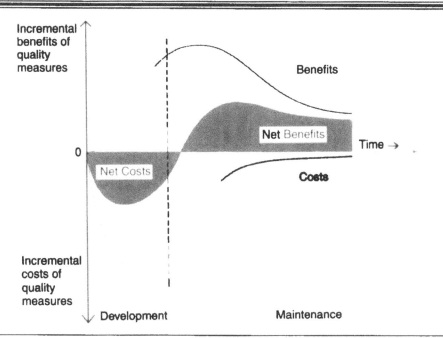

Figure 5.10. The Costs and Benefits of Software Quality Assurance

highest level in the organization, thereby constituting a tangible expression of senior management's commitment to a quality culture. Occasionally a firm has been visited which has already had a quality management system in place for some time, but has never secured this high level endorsement, without which the quality management system is severely handicapped. A prestigious symphony orchestra of talented players, each capable of making a virtuoso contribution is crippled unless someone, whom all respect and to whose authority all willingly submit, decides what page of the music is to be followed and what tune is to be played. By thus setting the atmosphere, the conductor is able to draw forth the full talents of each musician, blending them all into a harmonious whole. Thus, the quality policy can be compared to the conductor's baton.

What then ought the policy to contain? One way to start is to focus on the five features of software quality (Price Waterhouse 1988) that we considered in chapter 1, and show how a quality management system promotes the attainment of those features in the product. As we look at each feature in turn, there is bound to be considerable overlap between them, but a section of it might read something like examples 5.1 to 5.5 inclusive. Each example is presented in the slightly light-hearted context of an imaginary software house, Stupendous Software Inc. This, however, is intended to underline the deeply serious principle that the Quality Policy must reflect the company culture and must be "owned" by all of the staff. The importance of this vital theme cannot be overemphasized.

THE FIRST TENTATIVE STEPS

If an organization has no quality management system whatsoever, there is no better place to start than by defining the quality policy, since all the procedures and disciplines inherent in a controlled methodology are derived from the firm's approach to quality as described in the policy. Often companies dither for a long time before getting started, mainly through ignorance of where to begin. Another cause of failure is the fear of making mistakes, a weakness to which many of us are subject. In this respect, we need to learn the lesson of the proverbial *tea bag*: it is that we will only discover our innate strength when we get into hot water! On a more serious note though, failure is something we can only avoid by saying and doing nothing. This is surely utter defeatism. Every parent can remember their children's early attempts at walking, and the scraped knees and tears that were the prelude not just to the achievement of walking, but of running also!

Let us see initial failure or setback, then, as just a delay and never as a defeat; just a detour rather than a *cul-de-sac*, because failure is often the first step on the road to success. Henry Ford, mentioned in the introduction, encountered much frustration and discouragement in his early days, but subsequently changed the world for ever through the motor car. We could cite many other examples of early pioneers who overcame discouragement—Thomas Edison with the incandescent bulb, Alexander Graham Bell with the telephone, the Wright Brothers with powered flight, and a host of others. All of these changed the world they knew beyond their wildest dreams. Changing the culture of a company may appear to be as impossible and intractable as trying to eat an elephant. Elephants, though, *can* be eaten (though the author cannot personally vouch for the taste!), provided this is done by means of a *large* number of very *small* bites. Thus it is with the creation of an effective

Example 5.1. A Sample Quality Policy for Cost

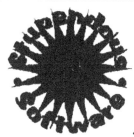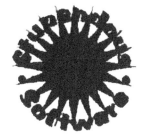

Stupendous Software Inc.

Our Quality Policy: Cost

Objective: That software will be delivered within the budget and will be financially viable

We will adopt standards by writing procedures that define exactly how we work. We will improve them in the light of experience to institutionalize what we have found to be the cheapest and most productive way (from the point of view of the operation **as a whole**, development **and** support) of doing everything. We will adopt simple, yet formal, configuration management and change control to avoid the unnecessary costs of uncoordinated changes to source files, libraries and any other item in the development process. We will adopt simple yet formal document control to ensure that no document is changed capriciously (on someone's whim, however exalted), and that every document is checked for quality before it is issued. We will subject code to peer review and release (because we are a small company) / formal inspection with metrics (because we are a big company and the large risks of our projects demand the thoroughness and rigor of formal inspection to remove defects)[i] so that we can scale down our expensive and inefficient testing effort and save money by reducing the level of residual defects. We will thus build quality into software rather than try to test it in. By reducing the level of errors in the product, and in more closely meeting what the market wants, we will be enabled to make more profit and have a better chance of long-term prosperity.

[i] Delete as appropriate

Example 5.2. A Sample Quality Policy for Timeliness

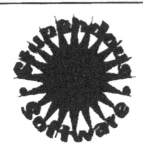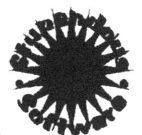

Stupendous Software Inc.

Our Quality Policy: Timeliness

Objective: That software will be delivered on time

We will document as simply, but completely as possible, our approach to projects
and we will stick to it. We will describe and use the most appropriate project
management tool available (Microsoft *Project*™, AMS *Schedule Publisher*™, etc.)
to record our expectations of how long steps are going to take. We will write a
procedure requiring the composition of a simple project plan. We will always
make sure that every team player has an agreed (with himself/herself), written
(paper or electronic) document stating what he/she is to deliver and when. We
will acknowledge the relentless operation of Murphy's Law (what can go wrong
will go wrong) and include how we are going to maintain control when that
happens. We will have formal procedures describing how we monitor and review
progress. We will write down what we will do when the users (who have
solemnly promised that the documented requirements really are now, at last,
correct) belatedly discover for the umpteenth time that there was, after all,
something else they had forgotten to mention!

Example 5.3. A Sample Quality Policy for Reliability

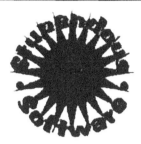 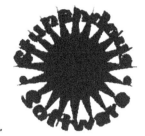

Stupendous Software Inc.

Our Quality Policy: Reliability

Objective: That software will be accurate and correct

We will always draw up a simple, yet formal, quality plan at the outset of a project defining the quality controls we are putting in place. These are intended to ensure that we develop what we plan to develop, rather than the brilliant and innovative masterpiece that nobody will actually buy. It will define the pieces of documentary evidence that will prove that our product is emerging as the design document intended. Our configuration management and change control procedures will ensure that no unintended or uncontrolled changes slip through the net. Our procedure for code walk-through / formal inspection ensures that defects in code construction are spotted at once. Our design review procedure ensures that at least two knowledgeable individuals have ensured that our design is fully traceable to the user requirements specification in all respects, both in what the user wants the software to do and what the user does NOT want the software to do. Our structured test plan procedure will ensure that our testing plan is already in place before testing commences, that it is comprehensive, covering all aspects both positive and negative, and that it is fully traceable back to the design document. Thus, if we change the design, we can safely and exactly make just the required changes to the planned testing to provide proof that the intended design change actually occurred. We will use automated test tools where possible to avoid the carelessness that boredom breeds in humans charged with the unenviable task of the repetitive testing of software.

Example 5.4. A Sample Quality Policy for Functionality

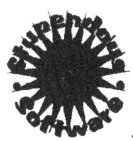 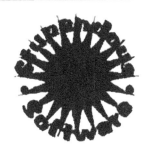

Stupendous Software Inc.

Our Quality Policy: Functionality

Objective: That our software will meet the users' requirements in terms of function, ease of use, efficiency, portability and security

We will adopt a formal, stagewise approach to software development with a clear delineation between each stage, and describe it in a life cycle description document. This formal methodology will ensure that we develop a product that closely matches the users' expectations, to be proved by a satisfactory user acceptance testing report. We will predefine design criteria based on user requirements; review our design for testability, traceability and suitability; review any changes we subsequently make to it. We will follow our procedure to develop structured test plans to ensure the achievement of intended system behaviour versus design. We will make sure our beta testers follow our procedure written for their use to record compliance of product with requirements.

Example 5.5. A Sample Quality Policy for Maintainability

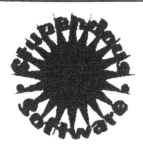 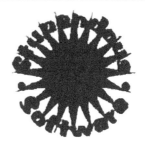

Stupendous Software Inc.

Our Quality Policy: Maintainability

Objective: That defects that survive undetected at earlier stages of development should be readily identifiable and easily correctable, and that the software should be safely extendible to a predictable degree

We will institute written design and programming standards and techniques to ensure that unintended behaviour in the software results in a clear unambiguous message to the user and comprehensive, detailed technical information to support personnel. These standards will direct the construction of software in a modular fashion with copious documentation enabling the safe reuse of modules, libraries and objects in future products, thus contributing to an improving level of quality in products as the company matures. Our configuration management and change control will ensure the safe, secure modification of software without the incorporation of a dozen further adventitious errors, each change in software source code being easily and unambiguously traceable to the support call or request that spawned it. Our methodology should enable us to enhance the software at minimum cost as and when the market demands it, in the direction and to the extent that could have been reasonably predicted at the time of its inception.

quality management system. This monumental and intimidating task suddenly begins to look easier when a draft quality policy, and the first tentative procedure, have been drafted, even if both may subsequently require heavy revision to get them to a useful stage.

This completes the examination of the QA approach element in the software development process. The next chapter switches the spotlight to the programmers themselves and the standards which guide their work.

Notes

1. A well-known catch phrase in Britain coined from the handicraft demonstrations in the *Blue Peter* children's TV program.

2. A detailed document and software review procedure can be found in the GAMP guide (1996).

3. Redolent of the public speaker whose habit was to mark in the margin of his notes at appropriate points *"case weak—shout loudly"!*

6

Human Resources

Are not five sparrows sold for two farthings and not one of them is forgotten before God? But even the very hairs of your head are all numbered. Fear not therefore; you are of more value than many sparrows.

Luke 12: 6–7

THE IMPORTANCE OF THE STAFF

So far, we have concentrated on the process of software development, the customer and the sometimes conflicting demands of maintenance and development. The reader might be forgiven for assuming that these were all that successful software development was about. The truth is, of course, that people make up companies. Their skills and attitudes are critical to business success, and any improvement initiative that does not regard the needs of the staff as of the highest importance will fail. Therefore, it is to this aspect of the company that the auditor now directs his or her attention.

The way that people are treated in the workplace and the cultural atmosphere set by the chief executive and, in the larger concern the board, can make or break a firm. This is especially important in the IT industry, since software development is, as we have seen, a highly creative affair. Creativity is a delicate flower which blooms only in a climate which encourages the cultivation of skills and competencies. It needs the sunshine of encouragement from the company's decision makers and the rain of technical training to make the most of the fertile soil of methodologies, tools and languages.

THE PSYCHOLOGY OF CHANGE

How can a software house transfigure itself to adopt a software process possessing the five attributes described in the suggested quality policy in the last chapter if it is not doing so already (and very few firms in today's software industry are)? The organization's IT capability needs to *mature* and that implies *cultural change*. But this is nothing like as simple as it sounds.

It is a fact of life that while some people seem to thrive on change, others find it difficult, threatening or even traumatic. Change exacts an economic and psychological cost on an organization, and will not happen until the pressure to maintain the status quo is outweighed by three other factors. These factors, originally identified by Professor Trybus of MIT and shown graphically in figure 6.1 are as follows:

1.   A level of dissatisfaction with the way things are now

2.   A clear and positive conception of the ideal solution to current problems

3.   Knowing what steps (particularly the first steps) are needed to achieve it

These factors must combine to overcome the inertia acquired by all organizations, especially those with staff of long-standing. Opposition to change expresses itself in all sorts of epithets, many of which reflect a deep fear and insecurity over the loss of the familiar. For example, it is extraordinary how in so many organizations there is never time to do things as well as everyone would like, but always abundant time available to correct them. Here are the most common objections to quality improvement that we encounter:

•   "We haven't done it like that before!"

•   "That will never work in this company!"

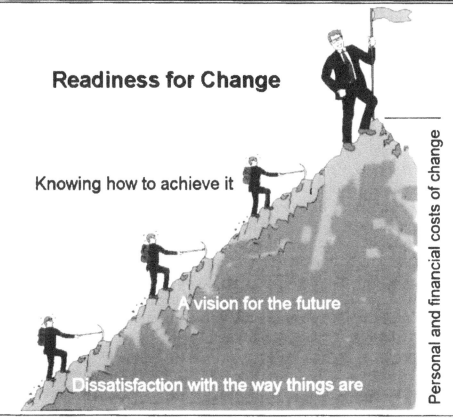

Readiness for Change

Knowing how to achieve it

A vision for the future

Dissatisfaction with the way things are

Personal and financial costs of change

Figure 6.1. Readiness for Change

- "Well, it sounds impressive, but . . . "

- "If it was such a marvelous idea, we would have done it earlier . . . "

- "It's all right in theory, but it won't work in the real world!"

- "We haven't budgeted for it."

- "There's no time for all that . . . "

- "We just don't have the people to make it work."

- "That sort of thing only works in small companies."

- "Management would never be convinced . . . "

For change to be successful, it needs both a sponsor and a champion. The sponsor is one who has the power and authority to ensure the public endorsement of top management. The champion has the clarity of vision to manage and implement the changes themselves. Both of these individuals, working together in a pull and push fashion ensure that movement eventually happens.

Fowler and Rifkin (1990) believe the most difficult aspect of communicating the nature and implications of change to those most affected is that of bridging different frames of reference. These frames are the ideas, theories, beliefs, feelings, values and assumptions which together allow people to interpret their experiences meaningfully. A clash between the manager's frame and the engineer's frame is a frequent cause of friction and an impediment to change. They outline a brief tutorial on implementing technological change, including how to overcome resistance and how to pace change within people's capacity to cope with it. They continue with an analysis of the context that surrounds and pervades the organization in which modern technology is implemented, critical for identifying tactics for specific process improvement activities. They describe a method of mapping to determine in advance how likely a particular technology is to succeed in a given organization. For example, why is the mature technology of UNIX easier to implement than newer technologies, such as Ada? Finally, they describe the role of people comfortable in more than one frame of reference (redolent of linguists fluent in more than one language), whom they term *boundary spanners*—people able to facilitate the transfer of new technology and skills from developers to users.

Care, patience and counseling are sorely needed when working with those most resistant to change. They need reassurance of their continuing value to the organization and the contribution they can make under the new arrangements. Since the qualities of patience and enthusiastic drive are seldom found in a single individual, the commissioning of a change management team is often more successful where different members of the team can focus on the separate challenges to be faced. Tact and diplomacy are of inestimable value. People must not be rushed, but on a happier note, very few ultimately refuse to respond to care and consideration.

THE DEARTH OF LEADERSHIP

We examined in chapter 1 the principles of statistical process control on which the revolution in the productivity and quality performance of Japanese industry after the war was based. We saw that it was in-built defects in the process or the system that were responsible for most of the faults in the product, and that the product could never exceed the capability of the system or process that produced it. We have reflected this thinking in the realm in software engineering by our emphasis on a life cycle approach. It was also apparent that the operators of a process were incapable of improving the quality of the product just by working harder. The process itself had to be improved and it was the responsibility of management to do this. Their leadership was crucial.

But real leadership in Western industry is a scarce commodity. In many industrial companies, the staff are assessed by an annual performance review which focuses on the outcome of the process—the worker's perceived productivity. But the worker is not responsible to a large degree for the productivity on which he or she is assessed. Differences that are caused entirely by the system he or she works under are ascribed to the worker himself as if he or she were in control. The assessment then assumes the nature of a lottery. Doing one's best is praiseworthy, but it is not enough. Luck is needed. Poor assessments under these conditions leave staff bitter, crushed and depressed, mystified as to why they are inferior. In intellectual areas of work, such as programming and research, a system of annual assessment encourages a *management by fear* culture, nurturing short-termism (the quick fix for this year's bonus), rivalry, political in-fighting and the triumph of individualism (figure 6.2), destroying long-term planning and teamwork. The manager becomes a manager of defects, and the staff propel themselves forward at the expense of the good of the company. Everyone considers only their own interests, with scant regard for those of others.

The culture of the promotional lottery is hard to shift, since most of today's senior managers are just yesterday's lottery winners. They are anxious to take the credit for winning, but are only willing to concede with some reluctance that the dozen other competitors who lost were in fact equally talented. Thus, they have a vested interest in proliferating the arrangement. What is desperately needed is leadership to address the weaknesses of the system. This will mean changing the way we do things, *rocking the boat*, subordinating personal goals in favor of the good of the organization. It means addressing the problems of people head-on, to foster pride in the job, and switch the focus from the self-centredness of the individual (what can I **get** for myself) to altruism for the team (what can I **give** for the good of all). How can we be trained to behave differently?

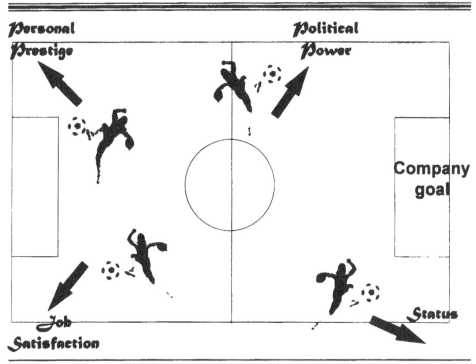

Figure 6.2. The Triumph of Individualism

THE PREVALENCE OF AMATEURISM

But this is only part of a broader picture. The competitive advantage of companies, and at a higher level nations, depends on the skills, resourcefulness and creativity of its people. This is especially important in the intellectually intensive world of software engineering. There has been a shortage of IT skills in the United Kingdom for many years. As early as 1986, the Advisory Council for Applied Research and Development (ACARD 1986) had drawn attention to the warnings of the Institute of Electrical Engineers the previous year that since some 10–20 percent of business expenditure was devoted to computers and related equipment (7 percent of the UK Gross National Product at that time), their optimum use was highly determinative of the prosperity or downfall of the enterprise. In the light of this, the lack of understanding of good software engineering practice in the industry at the highest levels was a cause of serious concern. Such concern was well founded since a widespread lack of competence in IT continues on the part of both developers and users of software. Still today, starting salaries for new graduates in computer science and related subjects in the United Kingdom are elevated over those of their colleagues in other disciplines because of the continued imbalance between supply and demand.

But the problem extends far beyond graduate recruitment and over industry as a whole. The ACARD report was emphasizing as early as 10 years ago that all those involved in IT (and that included almost all managers) needed a coherent and contemporary appreciation of the subject. The IT management of my own company deserves particular credit for the remarkable foresight it has shown in transforming IT in recent years from an organization on a local basis to one on a global footing, thereby reaping a much better return from its IT investment than many large organizations. But the challenges that must be faced in IT restructuring are formidable, and underlie the widespread awareness within industry and commerce in general that the benefits of IT are not yet commensurate with the enormous investments that have been made. Matters are aggravated by the widespread tendency to underestimate the complexity of the technical challenges posed to IT by business process re-engineering. The need today for technical competencies is even greater than at the time of the ACARD report and applies at all levels in industry,[1] both producers of IT products and services and their customers. Why then are so many of today's industrial and commercial managers across the entire industrial spectrum, who are now responsible for IT, so conspicuously ill-equipped to deal with the technical demands that its management presents?

We believe that the recognition of IT as a *technology* (i.e., applied *science*) sheds light on one of the major causes. In any of the pure sciences, or in medicine, it would be unthinkable for anyone without formal college education to at least the baccalaureate level, supplemented by appropriate post-graduate professional qualifications based on technical competence and awarded by a recognized qualifying body, to assume supervisory responsibility for the pursuit of the discipline to professional standards. In many critical fields such as healthcare, qualifications such as these are even enshrined in statutory requirements. Now, over the last two decades, the explosive growth in computer technology has led to the creation of huge, networked empires whose level of complexity calls for at least a similar level of professional skill as that of the scientific spheres for its effective management. The growth in technology has overtaken everyone and elevated many to levels of responsibility far beyond the intellectual capacity of all but the most exceptionally gifted to cope. Yet many managers who find themselves in this position today have not enjoyed a college education, let alone the benefit of subsequent in-service specialist training of the necessary breadth and depth. On no account should this be construed as an unflattering reflection on those caught in the midst of this dilemma. It is as much an accident of history as by design, since education and training has little chance of keeping abreast with technological development at today's meteoric pace. But intelligence must be trained to be useful. In the face of relentless pressure for systems of technical excellence, exerted by those driving forward the re-engineering of business processes, often on a sizeable scale, many flounder, unable to translate the business demands coherently into practical service solutions. Their dilemma is heightened by the widespread perception of the technical possibilities with today's hardware and software, but without a realistic appreciation of its limitations. In the smaller concerns, many IT managers have come from commercial backgrounds, and are thus bereft of any formal training in mathematics or logical thinking.

It is this lack of competence which is widely perceived at lying at the heart of the crisis in today's management of IT. This seems to be most commonly manifested in two ways:

1. In purchasing companies, there is no awareness of the critical importance of in-built quality to the secure implementation of acquired software, often purchased without even a semblance of structural integrity, at considerable risk to the business.

2. In vendor companies, there is no appreciation of the tremendous losses inherent in a chaotic development process, where information flows are uncontrolled, and a refusal to countenance the cultural and structural changes needed to build quality into the product to ensure long-term survival in the marketplace.

The establishment of standards and certification schemes itself testifies to this widespread lack of professionalism within IT as a whole, accompanied by a lack of understanding of the mathematical principles on which IT ultimately rests, as the authors of the ACARD report implied. The emergence of computer science as a discipline in its own right is belated recognition of the need to introduce academic rigour (figure 6.3) into the theory and practice of a subject now so critical to the world's economy.

TRAINING

Thus, the rapid pace of technical change imposes a critical need for regular in-service education and training, to update obsolete skills on the supply side (software developers) and general awareness of IT and its potential on the demand side (purchaser management).

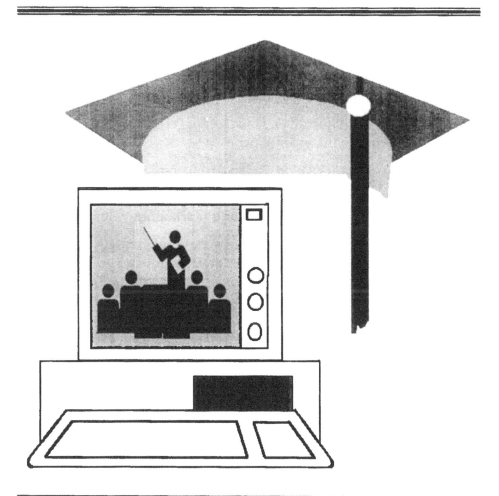

Figure 6.3. IT Needs Academic Rigor

Although the increasing trend toward short-term contractual employment in IT in the United Kingdom at the expense of the recruitment of permanent employees (converging to conform more closely with the United States picture) is undermining job security; the improved level of job mobility is encouraging the development of skills in this, the most innovative of industries. A change of job breeds a more open, less insular attitude. However, managers need to address the related personnel issues, such as portability of pensions, if this trend is to continue. The cost of education is one of the principal elements of capital investment in the development of software. It must not be confined solely to technical issues for programmers; there is also a need to inculcate an appreciation of the fundamentals of the business, the marketing of software, and its place in the business of the customers.

The ACARD report recommended that all sections of industry using software increase their provision for in-service training to meet the following *annual* targets:

- Directors, executives and senior managers receive one week of technical training.

- Managers receive two weeks of technical training

- Technical IT staff receive three weeks of technical training and one week of business and marketing training.

These recommendations have not been implemented across the broad spectrum of demand-side purchasing industry to any appreciable degree. Managers on the whole making software purchasing decisions still entertain a childlike faith in the assumed structural integrity of the software they buy, believing it to somehow match the opulence and quality of the glossy advertising brochure.

THE HUMAN FACTOR

For companies on the supply side, there appears to be a yawning gap between recognizing the critical importance of training to competitiveness, and actually getting around to doing something about it. Companies which show by their practical behaviour—in terms of how they recruit, motivate, and retain their best people—that they value them highly are the ones that will survive today's frenzied climate. For small companies, it is especially important that the investment made in the training of staff is not lost through needless hemorrhage of personnel before a reasonable period for an economic return has elapsed. Staff morale is vital.

STANDARDS

The ISO 9000-3 (TickIT) standard's requirement for training is as follows:

> *The supplier should establish and maintain procedures for identifying the training needs and provide for the training of all personnel performing activities affecting quality. Personnel performing specific assigned tasks should be qualified on the basis of appropriate education, training and/or experience, as required.*

> *The subjects to be addressed should be determined considering the specific tools, techniques, methodologies and computer resources to be used in the development and management of the software product. It might also be required to include the training of skills and knowledge of the specific field with which the software is to deal.*

> *Appropriate records of training/experience should be maintained (ISO 9000-3, paragraph 6.9).*

These requirements are further elucidated in the TickIT Guide (1995), which describes typical training activities and commends the "retention of records showing the relevant education, training attended, experience, skill levels and qualifications achieved by each employee".

What seems to be needed, then, is a process improvement standard that does for *people* what the ISO 9000 standards do for *systems and processes*. Such a standard would provide practical guidelines to bring the common business objectives to the center of the thinking of each individual and foster his or her continuous improvement in the performance of one's job. Such an approach for **people** would complement what the life cycle does for the **process**. Such a standard for industry as a whole has already been developed in the United Kingdom since 1993 and is known as *Investors in People*.

INVESTORS IN PEOPLE

The Investors in People Standard provides a framework for improving business performance and competitiveness, through a planned approach to setting and communicating business objectives and developing people to meet these objectives. The whole thrust of the exercise is to ensure that what individuals can do and are motivated to do is directed or channeled into what the organization needs them to do. In this sense, the aspirations of the individual are subordinated to those of the business, as illustrated in figure 6.4. The outcome of this approach is to drive the organization to higher levels of performance and to a greater degree of competitiveness.

The standard rests on the foundation of a company commitment to maximize the skills of all employees to achieve business goals and targets. It seeks to relate training and development activity directly to business objectives. It then provides a means of

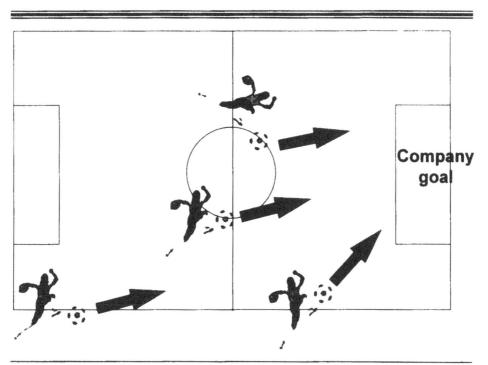

Figure 6.4. Aiming Toward a Common Goal

ensuring that adequate resources are devoted to training and development, and that these are used in the most effective way. Finally, it provides a good practice benchmark against which the organization can measure its progress toward improved business performance.

Investors in People[2] is a cyclical process consisting of three stages:

1. The **review** of existing skill levels and, therefore, training and development needs now in the context of the business.

2. **Action** within the individual's employment to provide suitable and relevant training.

3. **Evaluation** of the effectiveness of the training both for an individual's development and for the organization's benefit.

A company can implement these principles without proceeding to an assessment under the scheme with a view to certification, just as in the case with ISO 9000 compliance. Since assessment costs money, smaller companies may choose to do this, although the actual cost depends on the size and structure of the company and the number of employees. Everyone in the company must be committed to achieving the standard, especially senior management and the chief executive who must approve the organization's commitment to the employees and review how the business is actually benefiting from the training program.

Happily, the standard is not prescriptive in the sense of insisting that employers approach training and development in a particular way. Like the ISO 9000 family of standards, it respects and encourages individual approaches that comply with the standard. Ideally, these ought to be as close to a company's existing practices as possible, thus making use of the best that currently exists. The standard provides a refreshingly long-term view of the organization's aims, in contrast with the short-term myopia which handicaps so much management thinking. As its name implies, it gives the investment in people, a company's most expensive and valuable resource, a greater focus.

The standard's benefits can be summarized as follows:

• Ownership by employees of their training and development program. Of special importance in IT, the program brings greater acceptance of new technology, changing now at an ever-increasing rate, and greater job satisfaction.

- The likelihood of reduced staff turnover and absenteeism.

- Focus on the training needs of senior managers to improve business planning, for the benefit of all employees, and increasing the awareness of the company's strategic objectives at all levels. For purchasing firms the centrality of IT will figure prominently.

- Legitimizes the use of work time for training.

- Emphasizes the centrality of quality assurance, complementing the ISO 9000 thrust.

- Improved competitive advantage through greater employee productivity.

If a company decides to pursue assessment, the additional benefit of public recognition can be realized. This process takes between 6 and 18 months, dependent, naturally, on how much is to be done and what attitudes (!) and systems need changing. Clearly, a careful evaluation of the actual benefit in relation to the market should be made before the assessment process is initiated.

The audit team should therefore ascertain the vendor's approach to training and how far this accords with the Investors in People principles, and whether training records are kept. These are vital not only to ensure the staff have the skills and competencies to be productive, but also that in the event of new recruitment becoming necessary, the organization has an exact picture of what skills are required. This ought to be happening irrespective of whether the firm has any intention of involving itself in an Investors in People initiative or not, and is the very minimum requirement.

Another record of great value in this connection is the maintenance of a *skill needs profile* for every post in the company. An example of such a profile is provided in appendix 9. Living in the fast-flowing white water of technical change, a company must know at any time exactly what skills, in terms of formal qualifications and experience, would be required to fill any of its key positions. By maintaining these contemporaneously with job descriptions (to which they are complementary but by no means identical), a company can confidently send the skill needs profile to an employment agency or headhunter in the sure knowledge that it accurately represents the contemporary needs of the firm for that position.

BEING A CARING EMPLOYER

So much for the positive side of Investors in People. Are there any potential drawbacks? Yes, there are and it is important to recognize them. By placing the emphasis on the organization rather than on the individual, the program is underlining the harsh economic facts of life. These remind us that in today's shrinking global village, the world owes no one a living. Although diligent employees fully deserve their wages, those who refuse either to pull their weight or identify wholeheartedly with the aims of the company are more readily identified within this framework. This usually arises when an individual perceives a conflict between the manner in which the company wishes to develop them and their own personal interest. In these circumstances, the program makes it easier to frame a case for dismissal, since the evidence of an irreconcilable divergence becomes naturally available in the process. In days when security of employment is a cause of concern to almost everyone in the Western world, the introduction of Investors in People may exacerbate this anxiety unless it is handled with sensitivity. It is in a company's long-term interests to be seen as a caring employer, particularly for those who, as we have noted in chapter 1, find change hard to accommodate. Wise firms will wish to err on the side of compassion, and assiduously avoid the temptation to use the scheme aggressively to retire or dismiss such individuals prematurely.

This is especially important to employees over about the age of 45; not only are their prospects of re-employment at this time of life now vanishingly small, but also their readiness to learn new skills and their adaptability to change are decreased as a rule. Companies exist primarily to make a profit rather than to be altruistic, although the most enlightened companies pride themselves on their loyalty to their staff, particularly long-standing members. The manner in which such employees are treated has an impact on morale far beyond the confines of the individual, and is a critical indicator of overall company values. The introduction of an Investors in People or similar program will be a mixed blessing unless the long-term interests of all employees are visibly safeguarded.

PERSONAL EMPOWERMENT

Deming's experience in Japan, and in Western industry since, has underlined the critical importance of the care of personal relationships within any team-based human endeavour. Each individual must feel valued as a person and belong within the group. The transformation of the organization is everyone's responsibility. The atmosphere and culture must be conducive to junior staff feeling empowered to express themselves constructively, even when their views may differ markedly from more senior staff. This might be particularly valuable if the working of the quality management system is reviewed from time to time. Everyone has their own contribution to make, although for some, their full potential within the company may not yet be apparent. The great benefit of Investors in People is its ability, when carefully implemented, of discovering and exploiting this potential to the enrichment not only of the organization but also of the individual's own life.

One particular software company is accustomed to setting each member of the programming team separate objectives related not only to software development but also to the company's mission as a whole. These are usually on quite different timetables but broaden the individual's horizons and widen his or her vision. For example, he or her might be assigned the objective of writing a précis of the progress of a project for the in-house magazine within three months, together with that of completing the coding of a module by the end of the week. Two objectives, one narrowly focussed, one more broadly so, both complementary to the other. This same company also insists on each employee having their own personal career development plan within the training program. The employee is thereby empowered to maximize his or her own potential in the direction of the overall company objectives.

OLD DOGS AND NEW TRICKS

The concept and practice of personal empowerment, to maximize the potential contribution of every employee for the prosperity of the business, is frequently a central objective of company restructuring and the re-engineering of business processes. What is often not widely appreciated is an enormous contrast between the management style required of managers within this type of culture and that of the traditional hierarchical approach to management, as caricatured in figure 6.5. Based on the military model and the exercise of power, management expected each employee to function only within the confines of the job description and no further. The manager's sense of identity was inextricably bound up with power, authority, and the implied omniscience associated with it—management's exclusive possession of the knowledge of the best way forward in all circumstances. Any subordinate criticism of management was regarded as insubordination, while the exercise of initiative from below, which might advertise the weakness or even incompetence of senior managers, was systematically stifled. It is almost impossible for managers of the old school, steeped in the power pyramid approach to subordinates, to switch over to a management style that positively empowers juniors to limited decision-making. It inculcates within many an overwhelming sense of insecurity and an inability to adapt which, though understandable, is to be regretted. It leads to early retirements and redundancies in large numbers that account for much of the cost of corporate

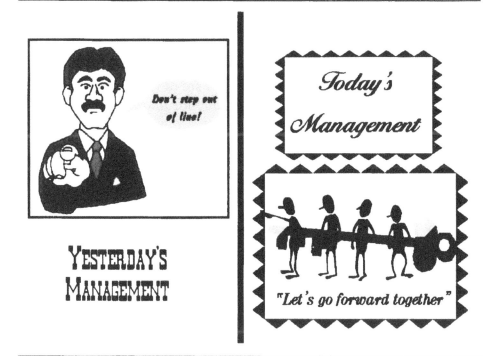

Figure 6.5. Changing Styles of Management

restructuring. This is a pity. Many traditional managers never come to understand that the risk in delegating responsibility down to juniors is largely mitigated by the added value released into the business and the focus on the customer. If the customer's needs are driving the business, then it is these that will dictate the decisions and circumscribe the actions of juniors.

Management, therefore, has little cause for anxiety that the wrong decisions will be taken. The customers are now the sanction that exerts the control which was once the sole province of managers. As a result, less managers are needed—*less chiefs and more Indians*—with a hands-off lighter touch, leading to "flatter", more cost-effective and competitive organizations. Moreover, the manager's role has changed to that of a facilitator, serving the needs of subordinates, who have become service providers to customers, by providing them with the environment and support to function effectively. Obviously, authority still exists in the background for disciplinary situations and the like, but the day-to-day atmosphere is based on mutual trust. In this sense, it is far more demanding of managers who need to exercise a delicate trapeze act, a balance between securing the full-hearted commitment of subordinates on the one hand, while unobtrusively leading from the front on the other. This is never easy since, when a disagreement arises, a knee-jerk relapse into the *might is right* attitude can terminally destroy **at a stroke** the mutual loyalty on which the success of the business now critically depends. Furthermore, the new set of values implicit in the new style are very far reaching, especially for managers as we shall see at the close of this book.

HOMEMADE TASTES BETTER

It has been emphasized already in chapter 3 that quality assurance can only be successful when everyone in the organization is committed to it. Skepticism over the introduction of standards and procedures often arises from the experience of standards developed externally and imposed. If staff are empowered to develop the quality management system themselves, based on their existing practices and procedures as far as possible, the chances of a successful transformation are greatly improved. As has already been suggested, a good place to start is to ask programmers what they like about their job and what they loathe. This frequently highlights bad practice and the areas where change is most sorely needed. For example, one might hear complaints about poorly commented code, or the lack of traceability of test plans back to the design document. An interesting common characteristic is that lack of discipline in development methodology usually falls most heavily on those who have to maintain the software. The loathings expressed have already gone a long way to gaining acceptance of the standards aimed at avoiding the particular evil in view.

Another policy occasionally seen is the practice of rotating staff between the development and support functions. While central to the idea of the Investors in People approach (equipping staff to perform more than one role), it also powerfully reinforces the legitimacy of the quality management system.

SMALL SOFTWARE COMPANIES

What are the elements of good practice in relation to programming staff in small companies for whom a formal Investors in People program would be inappropriate? In even the smallest concern, a simple record should be kept of the skills and experience obtained and any specific training undertaken for each programmer. This is not expensive or time-consuming; it should be reviewed at least once a year. This might be on the occasion of the annual review and development interview if that occurs formally, but ought to be reviewed in any case if the culture among the group is informal. Recruitment of new staff can then be based on this information.

LONGEVITY OF STAY

The auditor should record the average longevity of stay of members of the programming team. Although the implementation of a QA methodology is aimed at ensuring code written by one individual can be safely maintained by another, it is vital to ensure an adequate level of continuity. It is far better if, in practice, the maintenance of code remains in the hands of the original authors, who remain in the employment of the company long enough to see the product right through its shelf life of successive versions to maturity and senility. Coupled with this, most of the software portfolios examined are of closely related products addressed to a particular market or business area. Authorship of one provides fundamental expertise that is critical to the development of another. Continuity of the membership of the development team is, therefore, vital to the whole company's operation, and is not confined to the successful maintenance of one product.

On the other hand, all companies need a timely injection of new blood. Ideally, this ought to be contained within the capacity of the training program to bring novices up to skill levels before they can be trusted to work safely and competently on "live" work. The Investors in People standard is of enormous assistance in this regard, since through it the company will have the necessary knowledge and resources in place to bring recruits "up to speed" as quickly and as thoroughly as possible. Problems occur when companies experience meteoric growth due to the unexpected success of a new idea and engage a flood of new staff as an almost panic reaction to overwhelming development and support demands. In the absence of a tightly controlled methodology, this constitutes a period of high risk for software quality.

PERSONAL PERFORMANCE GUIDES

The classical job description is still used by many companies (though regrettably even today, still not all) as a means of ensuring that their employees know what they are supposed to deliver. This should be the very minimum the company ought to provide. However, in a true quality culture, enlightened by the insights derived from statistical process control, there are better ways of ensuring the confluence of the employee's own interests with that of the company. As we have seen, this is the principle at the heart of the Investors in People Standard. One of the best approaches[3] is something called the personal performance guide which, like all good educational traditions, is based on the three R's:

- Requirements statement: What does the company require of me?

- Review statement: How will my contribution be reviewed objectively?

- Reward statement: How will I be equitably rewarded?

Not only are these consistent with the Investors in People Standard, they are also aimed at engaging the employee's commitment and are focussed on satisfying the customer's needs, since in the final analysis it is the customer who pays the wages. The scheme, which must be implemented at all levels in the company if it is to be successful, is illustrated in table 6.1.

The categories of the guide are as follows:

Prime Purpose

The prime purpose must be a precise statement of what the individual is paid to deliver. For a programmer, it might be as follows:

> *To produce code modules in accordance with the in-house programming standards, to the appropriate design specifications, on time tables outlined in project control charts.*

For a finance manager, it might be as follows:

> *To provide accurate and timely information to the board on a weekly basis for strategic financial planning.*

The style of an achievement-oriented statement contrasts with the usual task-oriented job description. It is achievements that we should be focussing on since these earn the revenues that finance the wages!

Critical Success Factors

There are usually several critical attributes in any job that must be present for the outcome to be achievable. These critical success factors must be favourable. While they are not in themselves tasks, they are outcomes that must be achieved. The factors are expressed

Table 6.1. The Structure of a Personal Performance Guide

Feature	Description
Prime Purpose	What am I here for?
Critical Success Factors	What outcomes are essential for me to achieve my prime purpose?
Key Tasks	What must I do to bring about the outcome?
Performance Standard	How will I know when I have done it well?
Improvement Objective	What are the milestones on the road to doing it well?

in two parts: the desired outcome with a descriptive sentence. For example, a project manager might have the following factor:

Motivated and skilled programmers—a team that is trained, committed and enthusiastic to give of their best to get the job done.

A programmer's guide might have the following factor:

Competence in C++; the ability to develop code of adequate quality in C++ cost-effectively.

Most guides would have about four or five factors.

Key Tasks

Key tasks are the activities that must be carried out for the critical success factors to be achieved, and it is only at this stage, the third in our guide, that we actually start to describe activities. This again contrasts with a conventional job description. The key tasks use verbs rather than nouns and are intended to portray responsibility. For example, the project manager's guide might have the following key tasks:

Ensure that each of the programmers has had adequate training in C++.

Ensure the programmer understands his project deliverables timetable.

A QA officer's key task might be as follows:

Ensure quality controls in the life cycle are produced and delivered on time.

Most guides seem to end up with about 6–10 key tasks.

Performance Standards

But how would we know whether the task had been done well enough to ensure the achievement of the critical success factors? We need an **impartial measure** of success and failure (as Lord Kelvin's dictum reminded us), and this measure appears as the performance standard. Another way of expressing this would be to describe what excellence would look like when the task was completed. For example, the programmer's guide might state the following as the performance standard:

When the module I have created successfully passes the entire suite of tests specified for it at the design stage.

A project manager's might state the following standard:

When I have agreed to and documented a development plan with each team member.

We would expect one performance standard for each key task. Confusion over defining the tasks tends to result in difficulty in defining the performance standard, but if defined clearly, the latter just falls out naturally.

Improvement Objectives

As a personal performance guide is likely to be drawn up no more frequently than annually, the holder may need to define some shorter-term targets so that progress toward achievement of the longer-term objectives can be monitored. These milestones will represent partial rather than complete compliance with the objectives, and their achievement will provide some early indication that the individual is on the right track and serve as an encouragement. For example, a help desk manager might have as an objective a performance standard for customer support as follows:

100 percent of support calls will be actioned within 4 hours.

But at the moment, the level of calls being dealt with in this period is only 20 percent. An intermediate target might be as follows:

50 percent of support calls being actioned in 4 hours.

A guide developed along these lines can be a valuable asset for an individual's future development, a tool for management to groom someone for future promotion. The beauty of the system is that it applies right up to the top, the managing director starting out with his or her guide, then immediate subordinates drafting theirs to be consistent with the managing director's guide, and so on. This is not done behind closed doors. It should be worked out in an open meeting or workshop, peers and subordinates contributing to the objectives of their boss(es). Little imagination is needed to appreciate what strong meat this is going to be to many companies! A model guide thus emerges in an atmosphere of consensus. Subsequently, everyone's else's guide, completed by working with their boss and then discussed with peers will fall naturally within the objectives of the organization, just as the Investors in People standard intends.

A major advantage with this scheme is that it enables defects in the process, rather than in the contribution of individuals, to be highlighted. This works towards the avoidance of the evil of the performance lottery mentioned in chapter 1, when individuals are rewarded not on the basis of their own unique contribution but on the strengths and weaknesses of the process for which only the management is responsible. At the same time, each team player feels valued in that personal interests and aspirations are being recognized, self-improvement is encouraged and latent potential is developed, all the time within the overall company objectives. The emphasis is not on formal annual reviews but on regular informal reviews, building and consolidating personal relationships so that once the annual review does arrive, there are few surprises in store. This is a practical way not only of being a caring employer but also of maximizing the company's most expensive investment—its people.

So much then for the people, both those who produce and those who purchase software. This brings the first part of our examination to a close. The second part addresses the practical issues of the software development life cycle itself, focussing on simple practical recommendations for good practice compliant with ISO 9000-3 (TickIT) that are to be seen in one company after another. I shall include particular comments relevant to the challenges faced by the small software house, a category of vendors from which the bulk of software is now bought.

Notes

1. According to a recent survey published in *PC Week* (10 Sept. 1996), 43 percent of IT professionals feel their manager does not understand what they do, while 32 percent feel senior management has little or no understanding of the role of IT. Although 95 percent of employers recognize IT as business critical, only 54 percent have IT represented on the board. These findings should be cause for great concern.

2. More information on the Investors in People standard may be obtained from: Investors in People UK, 4th Floor, 7-10 Chandes Street, LONDON WIM 9DE. Tel: (+44) (0)171 467 1900; Fax: (+44) (0)171 636 2386

3. Described as the system in place at AT&T Istel (as it was then known) and published at the conference *TQM in IT* sponsored by AIC Conferences, London, February 1994.

Part 2

The Process

7

Software: Requirements and Design

Some of the language in requirements specifications is used to express thought, some is used to conceal thought, and some is used as a substitute for thought.

Anon

An understanding of the requirements of the potential user is the foundation of all successful software development. Few it seems would want to question such an obvious statement. Yet industrial history testifies to the fact that defining what a system is supposed to do has been, down the years, not just the most important step but extraordinarily the most neglected. From visiting vendors and following the IT press it is abundantly clear that, whereas there is intellectual assent to the importance of having requirements clear, the implications of this simple truth for the software development process (and the apportionment of effort it implies) have scarcely begun to be understood throughout large parts of the software industry. It is widely recognized that misunderstood requirements are the explanation for the spate of early enhancement releases that follow the first major release of a new software product as regularly as

181

night follows day. No one would dispute what an expensive exercise this is, but few seem to understand how it can be avoided. This chapter is intended to shed some light on the issues raised with the aim of helping firms to start off their development process on the right foot.

Requirements may originate either from a specific customer or a set of customers known by name and with whom the software house has established a commercial relationship, or they may be the software house's own perception of a market need that it intends to fill. The latter case requires market research and an acquaintance of the needs of potential customers at a very intimate level. Given that a group of users is available, whose written expression of the need for the application is to be the basis for the project, why is the accurate and comprehensive elucidation of requirements so vital to eventual success?

The answer to this question could be given in 6 ways:

1. **Cost:** Requirements form the foundation on which all project costings and scheduling rest, without which it is nearly impossible to estimate and plan the necessary resources, both human and material. In one vendor after another projects are running late or over budget, arising from evidence of failure to estimate the costs of the project as implied by the requirements adequately or competently.

2. **Functionality:** Requirements establish the basis for what the software is supposed to do. It enables users to agree with the developers so that necessary modifications can subsequently be made in a controlled fashion. This is easier said than done, as we shall see in a moment.

3. **Quality Assurance:** It provides the basis for judging the three fundamental yardsticks of quality assurance: *validation* (whether what we **intend** to develop is what is actually required), *verification* (whether what we **are in the process of** developing is what we intended at the outset to develop), and *testing* (showing whether what we **have** developed is what we actually intended to develop). Since validation, verification and testing are the three core activities of quality assurance, it is clear that the requirements are fundamental to all quality assurance activities throughout the life cycle.

4. **Productivity**: By enabling the requirements to be rigourously explored, the dreadful haemorrhage of cost due to later changes in design or, worse still, in developed code can be avoided. This enables the enterprise to produce the maximum amount of deliverable software for a given investment of time and money.

5. **Portability**: By knowing exactly what the software does, it may more readily be transported to other users or environments.

6. **Adaptability**: If the limitations of the software are clearly defined, enhancements and modifications can be made more safely and quickly, or planned enhancements which are too fundamental to be cost-effective and feasible can be identified before abortive effort is expended.

HUMAN LIMITATIONS

From an intellectual standpoint, computer programmers are, as a group, very different from the average computer user. Programmers are accustomed to subjecting their natural thought patterns to work within the restrictions imposed by the remorseless logic of the digital computer, a machine totally without imagination and completely constrained by the instructions given to it. As a result, they are at home with concepts expressed in a level of precision commensurate with this environment. In contrast the ordinary layman thinks on another plane altogether. The human mind has a fertile imagination that is capable of an almost infinite degree of adaptation and flexibility. This is so much part of everyday thinking that it is difficult for many to recognize how fundamental this facility is. Lacking this ability, computers attract contempt when failing to deliver the day-to-day benefits expected of them, because some change has occurred in the circumstances which were not anticipated in the software. The man in the street finds this hard to understand and often even harder to accept.

Programmers and users often also differ on a personal level. Programmers, being highly motivated problem solvers, tend to become rather self-absorbed. As a group, they are often strongly individualistic and tend to be rather poor team players and communicators. Obviously these are huge generalizations and many exceptions may immediately spring to mind; nonetheless there is much truth here. Thus, we have two disparate groups, both with their own attributes, limitations and, of greatest importance in this context, *language*. For any successful computer project to come to fruition, these two groups must somehow communicate with each other.

It is at this point that the liaison service provided by the programmer/analyst is so vital. As the term implies, there are two separate roles here. The role of the analyst is to understand completely the business process for which a software solution has been suggested, and to express its underlying algorithm with the precision and logical integrity necessary to make a computer solution feasible. The exposure of illogical or conflicting requirements is, naturally, central to the usefulness of the role. The programmer role is to convert those requirements into practical, executable code. While conceptually separate, the two roles are so intimately inter-related that they are often performed most effectively by single individuals. The challenge for such bridge-builders is to facilitate communication with the precision and depth necessary to ensure the comprehensive and accurate translation of requirements into product, without mutual misunderstanding and frustration between programmers and users. We have already seen that failure here is extremely common. What simple practical measures, therefore, can be adopted to aid this process?

USER REQUIREMENTS AND FUNCTIONAL REQUIREMENTS

It is absolutely essential that the user's requirements are written down and recorded so that both users and developers can ensure an adequate degree of understanding. But many companies are still not subjecting themselves to this discipline. Some are just ignorant both of the benefits of documented requirements and of the enormous hidden costs of attempting to work without them. Yet others believe that the capability of modern, fourth generation, rapid prototyping tools has rendered the need for this discipline obsolete. In both cases evidence can invariably be found at the other end of the life cycle (in terms of a late release or a cascade of subsequent corrective minor releases to repair misunderstood or incomplete requirements) to expose this delusion. As figure 7.1 shows, the user and

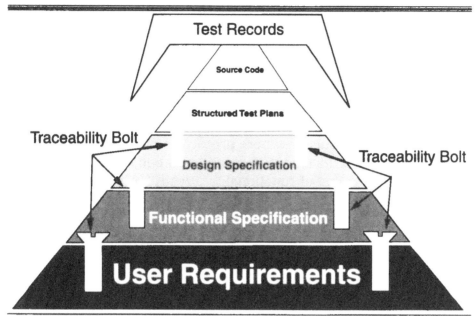

Figure 7.1. Traceability Promotes Stability in the Life Cycle

functional requirements occupy the indispensable foundation stone for all subsequent life cycle activities. It shows them both as discrete documents, a user requirements specification and a functional requirements specification.

Why have two documents when one might do, and what is the difference between them? A user requirements specification describes the needed functionality of a system, both what it is intended to do and what it is not intended to do, the data on which it will operate, and the operating environment in the common language of the user and appropriate to his or her application. It should also mention constraints, such as time and cost, and what deliverables are to be supplied. It should clearly distinguish between musts and wants, allocating some sort of priority to the latter, since every desirable but perhaps inessential feature carries a cost. A compromise will ultimately have to be drawn, perhaps eliminating some or all of the wants. It is important also that the user requirements specification concentrates on required functionality and not on how this might be developed. Once drafted and approved, the document would not normally be subject to further revision or formal document control.

The functional requirements specification, on the other hand, represents the developer's interpretation of the user's requirements in the developer's own language, suitable for use by a system designer on which the design specification can be based. In many cases, these two documents are combined, frequently because of the contribution afforded by rapid prototyping tools to the elucidation and clarification of the requirements. However, as has been noted already in the introduction where prototyping was discussed, there is still a need for a *document*. A prototype's behaviour must be described both in terms of functionality already present, what is absent but yet required, and the relationship to other modules and systems.

The word *discipline* continues to reappear with its unwelcome overtones of the restriction of freedom it suggests to our fallen natures. However, discipline brings it own rich rewards, which in this connection are now well established. Effort in ensuring the comprehensive and unambiguous documentation of requirements is abundantly rewarded by the avoidance of the repair costs mentioned earlier. Spending extra resources of time and money on getting this foundational aspect of the life cycle right is one of the best investments that can be made in software development, yielding a handsome return.

What are the essential features of good requirements specifications? The STARTS guide (1987) gives seven criteria, taken originally from the IEEE guide and which cannot be better expressed. They are quoted verbatim in Table 7.1. Both the user requirements specification and the functional requirements specification should conform to these criteria as far as possible.

AMBIGUITY AND NOTATIONS

Notations address the problems of ambiguity presented by language. A *formal notation* is a means of recording information about a system that reduces the risk of ambiguity and makes it possible to prove that developed code carries out the function that was actually required of it. The need for notations arises from the fact that colloquial English is quite unsuited to these purposes, being vague, imprecise, and full of implied nuances that in terms of the precision required leave vast areas of uncertainty. Worse than that, colloquial English may seem plausible enough and give the superficial impression that structure and connectivity have been described, while shielding fundamental inconsistencies and ambiguities.

Table 7.1. Characteristics of a Good Requirements Specification

Characteristic	Explanation
Unambiguous	There should be only one interpretation of every stated requirement. The many ambiguities in natural language must be guarded against and may be avoided by the use of a formal requirements specification language (or a glossary of terms).
Complete	Every significant requirement concerning system function, performance, attributes, interfaces and design constraints should be included. Completeness also requires conformity with any specified standards. The terms and units used should be defined, and all sections of the specification should be fully labelled.
Verifiable	Requirements can be verified if they are stated in concrete or absolute terms and involve measurable quantities.
Consistent	Stated requirements should not use conflicting terminology when referring to the same system element or call for different forms of logical data structures.
Modifiable	The specification should be structured and annotated so that changes to requirements may be made easily, completely and consistently.
Traceable	The origin of each requirement should be clear, and the format of the specification should facilitate referencing both forward and backward.
Usable After Development	It should be possible to use the specification after the system goes into operation for identifying maintenance requirements and constraints.

Stories abound of the confusion and needless costs that have subsequently had to be shouldered when these worms have burrowed their way to the surface at a much later stage in the life cycle. Notations enable the relationships between the disparate requirements to be correctly and clearly expressed, and assist in expressing requirements in a hierarchical structure, which promotes comprehensibility. There are various types of notations that are suited to the expression of the requirements of particular types of software, but the most common are diagrams (Martin 1987) of data flow and of data entity relationships. Although the user requirements specification may be expressed in the vernacular, structured English ought always to be used for the functional requirements specification; a glossary of terms and a data dictionary are always beneficial and are often indispensable. If the two documents are to be combined, then the use of structured English is essential. However, care should be exercised in choosing a notation, since the more formal the notation (and therefore the more rigourous), the less comprehensible it is likely to be to the untrained layman who may well represent the majority of users. Since their informed input is critical to the success of the process, any decision to combine the two documents into one should be weighed carefully. The notation must enable all of the functions of the system to be defined by it, but there is no reason why more than one notation should not be used, providing the reasoning and the distinction are clear. For example a very formal notation may be used for definitive parts of the document, like a mathematical notation with a defined syntax for algorithms, and an informal notation for the nondefinitive textual parts.

Several examples of the pitfalls of the vernacular have been provided in the IEEE Guide to Software Requirements Specifications (ANSI 830, page 11), of which just one will be quoted:

The data set will contain an end of file character.

This expression might seem innocuous enough, until it is realized that it could mean any of the following:

- There will be one and only one end of file character.

- Some specific character will be defined as the end of file character.

- There will be at least one end of file character.

The use of a suitable notation would avoid this ambiguity.

OTHER CRITERIA FOR REQUIREMENTS DOCUMENTS

There are 6 further standards against which a requirements document should be judged.

Completeness

The documents should include all of the requirements of the proposed system, including performance, positive aspects (what the system should do), negative aspects (what it should not do), and external interfacing. It should describe all of the transformations of input data in all circumstances, including that of erroneous input data. If at the time of drafting the document, certain information is missing, this should be mentioned so that the document is less likely to be used until complete. This underlines the importance of a *document control system* which will be further described in chapter 10.

Verifiability

There is no purpose to be served by including requirements that cannot be verified. For example, the requirements statement *the system should be user-friendly* is meaningless since the term *user-friendly* can mean so many different things. Then again the statement *the system should usually respond to an interrupt within 5 seconds* is also meaningless since *usually* is hopelessly vague.

Keep It

Simple

Practical Guidance
Create a standard describing how the user and/or the functional requirements specifications will be drawn up, what criteria they should meet, what they should contain, and what notations should be used.

Consistency

How could requirements be inconsistent? Sloppy terminology is the most common cause, but by no means the only cause, of inconsistencies. For example, a *directory* in the context of Windows™ 3.x might later be referred to as a *folder* for use under Windows 95®. The term *directory/folder* would emphasize their interchangeability and avoid confusion.

Modifiability

Requirements should be drafted in conformity to good document control standards, which include the author's name, a revision date, a revision number, a note of the changes made from one revision to the next (an audit trail), and a table of contents. There ought to be no repetition.

Traceability

The concept of traceability through the major documents of the life cycle (requirements, design, and structured test plans) is a little more subtle and still foreign to many in the software development community. Therefore it merits a more detailed discussion. Figure 7.1 illustrates the foundational consistency reaped by ensuring traceability, symbolised by the bolts securing each document to its progenitor. Without traceability, it is impossible to ensure that each requirement has been progressed through the life cycle correctly, if at all. Additionally, traceability ensures that each aspect of developed functionality, both positive (what the system does) and negative (what it does not do), can be substantiated for functionality and budget purposes. The pernicious effects of a lack of traceability are illustrated in figure 7.2.

How may traceability be achieved? The simplest method seems to be used successfully in the absence of formal tools is that of

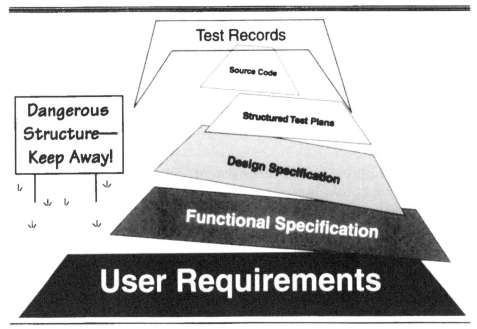

Figure 7.2. Life Without Traceability

paragraph numbering. Each statement within the requirements specification is numbered in some way. In successive documents, these paragraphs are referenced as the requirement is implemented in a design feature or in a test specification. A reconciliation may be conducted by quality assurance to ensure that all requirements paragraphs have subsequently been referenced. By this means, potential defects in functionality can be nipped in the bud cheaply before they become hideously expensive to correct.

Usability

The requirements document, and especially the functional requirements specification if the two are separated, should be laid out so that it can be used at all stages in the life cycle, especially the design stage (where it is the foundation of all work) and also in the post-release maintenance stage. Providing the criteria for modifiability have been met, the document should enable anyone with appropriate training to become fully appraised of exactly to what stage of development the product has been taken, in other words what changes have been made to the original requirements and why, and thus what the product in its present incarnation (i.e., as it is now) is supposed to do.

THE PROCESS OF DEFINING REQUIREMENTS

Regardless of the approach taken to elucidating requirements, the fundamental process involves four stages:

1. Getting the information from the users by asking the right people the right questions.

2. Expressing the answers using an appropriate framework or hierarchy.

3. Analyzing the information gleaned for completeness, consistency and precision.

4. Drawing up the requirements document meeting the characteristics defined in Table 7.1 and ensuring a formal sign-off of the requirements document.

This activity will rarely, if ever, follow a neat progression. Experience shows an iterative process is more usual, one set of requirements spawning another until the process becomes self-exhausting and the sign-off can take place.

There are, in general, three ways in which requirements are established. The traditional top-down analytical approach strictly follows the scheme of the classical life cycle models (Waterfall and V model) described in chapter 1, decomposing requirements layer by layer until the functions at the lowest level have been reached. This approach is gradually being eclipsed by two other methods, prototyping and incremental development both of which have already been discussed. However, it is vital that the requirements established by any of these three approaches culminates in a functional requirements specification that can be assessed by quality assurance as compliant with the standards, signed off, and which can then form the basis for defining the design objectives. It is failure to observe this discipline that can be seen time and time again in one vendor firm after another, as contributing heavily to the unknown and unknowable extra and avoidable costs of the creative-chaotic method of software development. One study by Boehm et. al. (1975) in the context of large projects showed that nearly two-thirds of program defects, and three-quarters of debugging effort, arose from a faulty design. The striking contrast thrown up from their project data was the large preponderance of design errors over coding errors, not only in terms of number, but also in the relative time and effort to correct them. We have already seen in the context of software inspection (chapter 5) that the earlier in the life cycle that errors are identified, the cheaper they are to correct. If the requirements as expressed are sound, then the design stands a sporting chance of also being sound. It is depressing to realize how little has changed in this respect in the 22 years since Boehm's paper was published.

The message is, therefore, to establish a procedure for elucidating and documenting requirements. Keep it as simple as possible, confined to the main stages that must be followed on every project, and do *not* try to specify aspects that will vary from one project to the next. Not only is this practice unnecessary (since these can be catered for in the project plan), it will bring the standard into disrepute.

CASE TOOLS: CAPABILITIES

The team should note any use of CASE tools to aid the development of software. The fundamental point about these is that they are only processing aids, and do not of themselves change the nature of the process in use. Using CASE tools in the context of a weak process

Keep It

Simple

Practical Guidance
Create a standard describing how user requirements information will be acquired, how they are to be analyzed and documented, and who will sign the document(s) off prior to use as a source for the next life cycle stage.

only results in the automation of the production of defective code. Whereas tools are common in more traditional, third generation language developments, they are rarely to be found used in the object-oriented arena. This is a pity because tools can still assist immensely in the requirements and design stages of the life cycle, even if few are yet applicable to object-oriented programming, since they are based on proven design technologies. They are capable both of greatly accelerating the architectural analysis stage of the design process and improving its innate quality by avoiding the in-built defects which inevitably creep in with manual approaches. An example would be the ease with which entity (a component or element of a design that is structurally and functionally distinct from the other elements and that is separately named and referenced) diagrams (ANSI 1016) showing data entity relationships can be produced. There is no tool yet available that encompasses all of the planning, development and maintenance needs of the life cycle. However, the march now stolen by hardware on software strongly indicates that tools are likely to provide the most cost-effective way of enhancing the quality of software development in the future. Their appropriate use can result in the generation of better quality software more quickly and at lower cost. However, great care ought to be exercised in committing the development group to any tool in this still inchoate technology before a thorough evaluation of its applicability to the particular techniques of software development in use in the firm has been made. The tool must be appropriate to the methodology.

CASE TOOLS: SHORT–TERMISM

The fact must be faced that in the short term, the use of tools may not effect a marked reduction in cost, and, in fact, may increase it slightly, reflecting the effort required to understand how to use to use the tool effectively within the company culture as it is. It is critical, therefore, that the staff, both within development and within the support group (if separate in the larger organization) are trained effectively both in the methodology that has been adopted and the tool that supports it. The major benefit from the use of tools is in software quality rather than in immediate productivity; therefore, the benefit of the tool will appear further down the line in savings in support costs. However, these can be enormous when taken over the lifetime of the system, so a blinkered, short-term view of tools ought to be avoided. Once a tool has been instituted and is working well, no decision to change it should be taken lightly, as the risk of magnifying overall costs will be high. The integration of CASE tools from different manufacturers offers one of the most promising advances for the foreseeable future.

THE CONTENTS OF A USER
REQUIREMENTS SPECIFICATION

Although it is impossible to be specific about the details of a user requirements specification since software projects vary so widely, there are certain broad headings that will be featured in most of them. They are given here as guidance on which the in-house standard for user requirements specifications can be based. The summary in the GAMP guide (1996) represents a broad consensus of thinking among today's IT customers in the pharmaceutical industry, but is applicable quite generally. For this reason, the GAMP material has heavily influenced the following suggested list:

- **Introduction**: author name, rationale for the project, nature of any associated contracts, relationship to other documents, key objectives to be met, benefits, and main functions and interfaces.

- **Functionality**: calculations, modes of operation (start-up, shut down, failure), security.

- **Data**: definition of types, valid ranges and limits, capacity requirements, performance and archive requirements.

- **Interfaces**: main user types, other systems (including computers or equipment).

- **Environment**: where it will be sited and any constraints this imposes.

- **Other parameters**: when required, compatibility with associated systems, required uptime, any legal or procedural limitations to be considered, other constraints (such as user skill levels).

- **Maintenance**: likely enhancements in the foreseeable future, ease of maintenance, expected lifetime.

- **Life cycle issues**: any purchasing company standards to be followed, QA standards or mandatory design methodology, special testing, delivery (training courses, data to be converted or transported, documents to be delivered, deliverable media format), and post-delivery support.

- **Glossary of terms**

THE CONTENTS OF A FUNCTIONAL REQUIREMENTS SPECIFICATION

The functional requirements specification is based entirely on the user requirements specification (if a separate document was assembled), and provides the definitive list of design objectives for the system. It describes what the system will do and what facilities and functions are to be provided in rigourous terms, meeting the characteristics defined in Table 7.1. As emphasized already, unlike the user requirements specification, it should be written in a formal notation or notations appropriate to the kind of system described in order to possess an adequate quality level upon which the subsequent design will be based. This is the first step in the life cycle at which **quality is to be purposefully built into the system**, since errors here will feed right through into later stages and become increasingly expensive to remove at an alarming rate. Therefore, effort expended here to maximize the quality of the document will be richly rewarded in terms of lower development and support costs. For this reason, this document and all its successors in the life cycle should be subject to formal document revision control. It is also highly desirable that the users who contributed to drafting and finalizing the user requirements specification should be part of the approval process for this document, in an effort to weed out defects due to accidental lack of consistency one with the other.

This document ought to contain the following sections, for which a debt to the GAMP guide (1996 appendix H) is again acknowledged:

Keep *It*

Simple

Practical Guidance
Create a standard describing how functional requirements are to be expressed, what the document will contain, how it will be controlled, and who will sign it off prior to its use as a basis for subsequent system design work

- **Introduction**: author's name, any contractual aspects, and relationships to other documents.

- **Overview**: key objectives, benefits, high level view of main subsystems, principal interfaces to outside world, assumptions (e.g. specific hardware or operating systems), and any deliberate divergence from the user requirements document.

- **Functionality**: hierarchical top-down decomposition of requirements, both positive (what it should do) and negative (what it should **not** do). Describe the objective of each item of functionality and how it is to be used. Keep the needs of the system designer (the most critical reader of the document) constantly in view. Include critical algorithms or calculations, measures of performance in terms of response times and throughput. Anticipate Murphy's Law (action in case of failure); describe any internal diagnostics; and address access restrictions, time-outs and data recovery. Describe configurable functions and any limits on the possible configuration.

- **Data**: define these in a hierarchical manner, building up the complex objects from simple ones. Highlight critical parameters.

- **Access**: method, speed, update time, reading and writing interlocks (e.g., to preserve database integrity and inhibit simultaneous record update transactions), data capacity, retention time, and archival arrangements.

- **Interfaces**: roles of users, types of workstation and other peripheral devices, formats of displays and reports, interfaces with other systems in terms of data transmission, speed, handshaking, security, and interfaces with any other noncomputer equipment.

- **Availability**: uptime, built-in redundancy (a requirement often satisfied today in the sphere of disc storage with RAID[1] devices), internal diagnostics, standby operation.

- **Maintainability**: potential for enhancement that can reasonably be foreseen, spare capacity, likely environmental changes, expected lifetime.

- **Hardware** and other software specifications (if appropriate).

THE HUMAN–COMPUTER INTERFACE

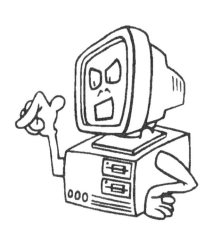

It is vital that adequate attention be given to the human-computer interface, an area which can cripple or break an otherwise successful computer system that complies with its user requirements in every other respect. Its design must be commensurate with the skill level of the humblest of the anticipated users, as mentioned above, and the environment in which he or she will use the system. It must be truly *user-friendly*. For example, in today's ubiquitous Windows™ environment the data entry screens should all be designed with the same look and feel, reducing differences between each screen, and thus the effort required to become competent with the software, to the minimum. In practice, conformity to Windows™ or other platform-specific standards is almost unavoidable nowadays.

Again a system should not be designed where it is possible to execute a lethal command without the command being circumscribed with *third world war* warning messages! Another area generally weak is that of the design of help text, which in some systems borders on the worthless. Developers are generally not the best people to write help text. They are far too familiar with the software and have great difficulty divorcing themselves from their unavoidable presuppositions, which are passed on into the help text as subliminal assumptions. A novice who does not possess this knowledge then finds the help text almost meaningless. Recognizing this, some vendors assign the task to a documentation group (sometimes staffed with those having journalistic skills) independent of the developers, and who are better placed to walk in the footsteps of the novice user most needful of such text. Companies whose raison d'être is the development of graphical user interface software (and this is the vast majority of the industry today) ought to have some or all of the following documents (simple and brief as possible) in their quality management system:

- User interface design standard (what we expect our interfaces to look and feel like, and what evils we will deliberately avoid in design, perhaps based on bitter experience). This will be mentioned again in the next chapter in the context of programming standards.

- User interface design review procedure (making sure we have it right).

- User interface test procedure (how we test how useful it is, and who will be the guinea pigs).

- User interface test report (how we evaluate what users find, in a format that the developers can use to improve the design standard, and so ratchet up the overall quality and performance level in this key area, thus avoiding the unforgivable sin of making the same mistake twice).

THE DESIGN PROCESS

Establishing the system design can be described as the centre of gravity of the entire development life cycle. It rests critically on the functional requirements specification from which it will be constructed, and to a large extent its quality level is determined by it. It resembles the functional requirements specification in the sense that this, too, is a key stage at which *quality is built into the system*, quality whose presence and level will be demonstrated by subsequent system testing but **not significantly changed by it**. The document must possess the traceability characteristic described previously, but in two directions: in a **forward** direction to the structured test plans (sometimes known as qualification protocols), which will be developed as a direct result of this document and, when used, will deliver the evidence to prove the conformity of the design to the user's requirements; and in a **backward** direction to the functional requirements specification.

Without a formal system design document, it is impossible to develop software that meets the requirements of users in a controlled and predictable manner. Yet vendors may still be encountered who claim to be able to develop quality software in a cost-effective manner without any formal design discipline whatsoever. It behoves me (painful duty though it be) to point out the huge, unquantified costs of working chaotically in this way, traceable as it usually is to an unconscious yielding to the seductive allure of the rapid application development tools available today. Introducing a formal design methodology in such an environment has been shown repeatedly to be one of the fastest ways to reduce the cost of software development while at the same time increasing the rate at which it can be developed. Whatever methodology is introduced it should, as far as possible, represent the best of current practice in the firm in order to secure ownership and commitment by everyone—a principle repeated without apology since it is so critical to gaining acceptance of a quality culture. Once the decision is made as to how designs are to be assembled, they should be documented as clearly, simply and concisely as possible.

The design process involves decomposition, the reducing of a complex object into its simpler component objects while analyzing its structure, its interactions and interfaces. Eventually, the process reaches the level of an irreducible object known as the module. This might be defined as a piece of code no longer than 100 lines perhaps, with fixed unambiguous inputs and outputs and which, regardless of invocation context, always behaves in the same way. The process should occur in two distinct phases:

1. **Structural (or architectural) phase:** The entire system is viewed from the top and an overview design document produced describing the overall architecture, data structure, components and interfaces. It relates each component back to the requirements, so achieving traceability, and thus constitutes the key transition point (or centre of gravity) in the life cycle.

Keep It Simple	**Practical Guidance**
	Create a procedure describing how to draft a system design specification, together with individual module specifications where needed, all based on the functional requirements specification and traceable to it.

2. **Detailed phase:** A complete specification of the struc-
    tures, components, interfacing, sizes of modules, database
    layout, algorithms and assumptions about each program
    unit is produced, suitable for programmers to work from.

The second phase critically depends on the successful completion of
the first, though frequently the two phases meld together. However,
from a strictly conceptual viewpoint they are separate; the larger and
more complex the system, the more visible the separation will be.

A detailed description of the wide range of design tools available now is beyond the scope of this book. The reader is referred to
the STARTS Guide for a start! Suffice it to say that the impact of
tools and formal methodologies in the design stage of the life cycle
is extremely cost-effective, as it is with requirements elucidation.
However, the technical difficulties at the design stage and the potential errors are more subtle; thus, the probable payback in terms
of avoidance of later rework is much greater. Tools immeasurably
aid the design process by supporting the method in use, managing
the complexity of the task, making all aspects of the design (and possible flaws in it) much more visible, analyzing it for sufficiency,
recording it, and making it available to others to work from. It is
critical that the tools used are regarded as being subservient to the
structural and detailed designs and not the masters of them. This relationship is shown in figure 7.3, based on a similar illustration in
the STARTS Guide.

At the structural design stage, consideration should be given to
how the software will map onto the hardware, with special reference to networking. Traffic-related issues need addressing at this
stage since they are the source of a particularly elusive type of software defect. This arises from the coincidental attempt of two or
more programs trying to obtain exclusive control to a single resource, such as a database data set, or a peripheral device. Since the
defect is traffic dependent, it is extremely hard to reproduce and repair. In the HP 1000 environment, for example, this problem could
be avoided by the use of *resource numbers*, or by *semaphores* in the
IBM world. General aspects of the user interface may also be considered at this stage, although the detail is usually deferred to the
next stage. Performance requirements should also be carefully considered. There is also a strong link between this stage and the project plan, since it should now be clear whether the projected
timetables and budgets allocated at the outset are accurate or need
revision. The detailed stage which follows is one where tools really

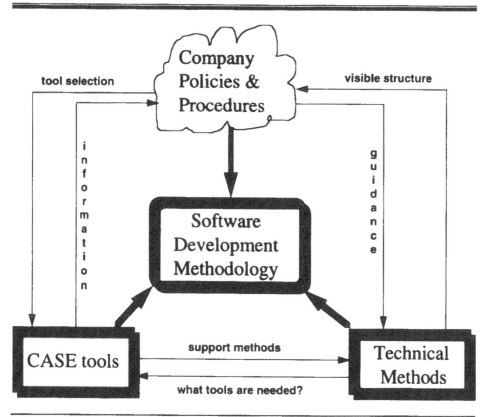

Figure 7.3. The Place of CASE Tools in Software Development

come into their own. Tools can produce the diagrams for the system files and data structures with a fraction of the effort and risk of error inherent in a manual operation.

DESIGN SPECIFICATION

The deliverable from the process is the design specification or set of specifications from which the programmers will work. What should this specification contain? The GAMP guide (1996) suggests the following sections:

- **Introduction**: who produced it, the name of the functional requirements on which it is based, and its relationship to other documents.

- **Overview**: a hierarchical decomposition of the overall system into subsystems usually with the aid of diagrams, as provided by the notation in use.

- **Description**: detailed description of all the subsystems-their purpose and interfacing.

- **Data**: should be shown hierarchically including database data sets, record structure, sizes, and data types. It must contain a description of all the modules or subsystems that are involved and the purpose of each.

- **Modules**: a description for each module should be included, if necessary using pseudo code (see below), unless a separate module design specification is to be created for every module to be built. It should also include details of interfaces to other modules, timing factors (if appropriate), and error handling.

- **Module data**: describing which system data is accessed by each module.

- **Glossary of terms** as dictated by the notation in use.

MODULE DESIGN SPECIFICATION

There should be a *module design specification* for each module defined in the design specification. They may be quite brief, and will be referred to again in the context of testing. The notation(s) used must be appropriate for the system and may include formal grammars, diagrams of data flow and entity relationships, and pseudo code. They should contain introduction and overview sections in line with the design specification followed by:

- **Data**: definition of the data and the data objects, the more complex being composed of the simpler. The notation used should be adequate, including, for example, entity relationship diagrams, and so on.

- **Functionality**: this may be expressed in pseudo code. Pseudo code is a means of using English to demonstrate the basic structure of a module with a superficial eye to the programming language that will be used. For example, a module specification associated with a laboratory information management system to be written in FORTRAN might include the following fragment:

```
DO WHILE (there are more test results to process)
    get the next test result
    IF it complies with the specification THEN
        flag up the test as completed
        pass it into the database
    ELSE
        flag it as a violation
        print up an alarm message on the printer
        in the manager's office
    ENDIF
END DO
```

In this example the CAPITALIZED text represents specific words of the language, whereas that in lowercase *italic* text indicates actions or conditions. Parameters associated with each module should be identified as to input, output or both, and their type (text, integer, real, double precision, etc.) defined.

- **Glossary of terms**

DESIGN REVIEWS

Once the design specification(s) has/have been produced, a formal design review should take place. The purpose of this formal review is to identify and remove defects from the design before the large investment of programming takes place. Since the design is the basis for all of this work, defects allowed to remain are likely to be faithfully incorporated into the code and will be far more expensive to remove either if found in testing or, more likely, discovered in the field after product release. The review (monitored by quality assurance) must assess the design against the functional requirements specification on which it is based to ensure

- That the design is traceable to the functional requirements specification in every respect

- That the design is suitable for the needs of the intended users in every respect

- That the design will enable structured test plans, based upon it, to be assembled so that the system will be testable in every respect.

Keep It
Simple

Practical Guidance
Create a procedure to specify how designs will be reviewed prior to programming, including a formal sign-off of the documents by a second qualified person.

It is vital once again to emphasize the importance of a formal review, since this will abundantly pay for itself in mitigating risk, and in reducing corrective efforts later on. There should be a company standard within the quality management system forbidding the commencement of any programming until this stage has been completed. This review is as important in the small company as in the large, though here it may involve no more than a single meeting especially if the envisaged system is also small. However, the procedure (which may occupy no more than a single side of paper) should state the purpose of the review and those aspects of the design that merit special attention. As time goes on and the value of the review becomes apparent, the standard can be improved in the light of experience.

EXTERNAL STANDARDS

In some system designs algorithms, expressions, calculations or values are derived from external sources. For example, software for controlling an instrument designed to test pharmaceutical tablets and capsules for dissolution characteristics (important to the bioavailability of the drug and, therefore, the effectiveness of the dosage form in the patient) need to carry the limit values from the relevant pharmacopoeia monograph. Again, in an example from an entirely different field, a tax calculation program will need to have access to the latest taxation tables from the Internal Revenue Service. These values may be hard coded into the software, but it is infinitely preferable for them to be held in supplementary files so that they can be changed without rebuilding the executable program and, thereby, generating another version. In any case there must be a formal mechanism for ensuring the validity of any such externally derived data. If this is an issue for the software house, there must be a procedure to ensure the accuracy control of externally derived standards.

Practical Guidance

If appropriate, create a procedure describing how the accuracy of externally derived standards, expressions, algorithms and constants are to be authorized and controlled.

DESIGN CHANGES

In an ideal world, once a design had been initially signed off and approved, and programmers begin to use it as a basis from which to develop code, it would never change. But life is not like that. Invariably, retrospective changes are made to designs after approval, which have the potential to cause havoc with the development process. The danger of thereby introducing error is very high. This danger must be reduced, and the practical way to achieve this is to subject the design specification immediately to strict document change control. Document change control systems will be discussed in more detail in chapter 10; in the meantime, suffice it to say that there must be a formal procedure established for reviewing any suggested change to an approved design so that the implications of that change, both on development work already completed and on that yet to be carried out, are thoroughly explored. If this does not happen (and it usually does not), inconsistencies inevitably creep into the product. Work already carried out is not in accordance with the imposed change, whereas that conducted subsequent to the change is. These effective defects are usually so subtle as to escape immediate detection. It is to achieve this detection that a formal design review is directed.

The procedure should describe exactly what criteria are to be met for the acceptance of changes in design, and how the impact of those changes on the development effort are to be explored. It should describe how such changes are followed through the configuration management system so that all items within the project are brought into line with the change, so that everything once again hangs together (and thus avoiding the programming team being hung separately!).

> ## Practical Guidance
>
> Create a procedure describing how design changes will be assessed for acceptability; how the impact on the entire development effort will be explored; how the configuration management system will be used to avoid inconsistencies creeping in from the change; how the amended design will be re-reviewed, accepted, signed off, and how traceability will be preserved.

The revised design specification should have, like any other document subject to strict control, an audit trail section on its frontispiece documenting all of the changes that have taken place, so that programmers are under no illusions or have any misunderstanding of what they are now required to achieve. The procedure should address this, as well as a review of the project life cycle once again, to make any revisions to timetables and budgets precipitated by the design change.

IMPACT ON OTHER PRODUCTS

Many vendors today have several products in their portfolio, often related in some way both in functionality and in the use of common modules or objects. Therefore it is vital that if changes are made either to the designs of products under development, or to established products in the field, that the question is at least asked as to whether this change affects other products.

> ## Practical Guidance
>
> Create a procedure describing how the impact exerted on other systems in the company's portfolio of changes made to any one system will be evaluated and addressed.

STRUCTURED TEST PLANS

There is one final stage that must take place (and which in my experience rarely does) before programming begins. This is the development of structured test plans derived from and traceable to the design document(s). It is by means of these that the testing intended to follow development can be engineered to be thorough and comprehensive and to address every aspect of the design, both positive and negative. Regrettably what usually happens is that testing becomes, instead, an empirical activity tacked on as an afterthought to programming; therefore it is not surprising that it is so ineffective in detecting in-built defects. These issues will be discussed in more detail in chapter 9.

We are now ready to shift our attention to programming. Are programmers to be left entirely to their own devices and imaginations, to allow their creative talents to flower unrestrained in producing what the design defines? Or should their activities be constrained within standards of good programming practice? It is to these questions that the next chapter is devoted.

Notes

1. Redundant array of inexpensive discs

8

Programming Standards

When a bug appears in our software, we always
blame the programmers. They wrote the code,
so it must be their fault!

A European software vendor

THE EVOLUTION OF PROGRAMMING LANGUAGES

Computer programming involves expressing the task the computer
is intended to perform in the language comprehensible by the particular machine. In the early days of computing, this took place
directly—programmers were obliged to learn the machine's instruction set and write their instructions in terms of this *machine code.*
The difficulties involved were prodigious, requiring an inordinate
amount of effort for even the simplest of tasks. Such *low level pro-*
gramming obliged the programmer to manage even the contents of
individual registers, every movement of a stored value requiring its
own separate instruction or line of code. Although such low level
programs, once written, executed on the machine extremely rapidly,
the rate of program development was painfully slow; thus

programmer productivity was very low by modern standards. The support of such software, in turn, required the same depth of knowledge and intimacy with the machine language on the part of the support programmer; since instruction sets on the different machines were proprietary, cross-fertilization of skills was minimal.

Programming began to be revolutionized by the introduction of languages enabling the expression of instructions at a higher level (i.e., nearer the conceptual level of the *task* and further removed from the detailed mechanics of the *solution*). These cross-platform languages resulted from the development of *compilers* that were able to translate the source code language into the low level code (called *object code*) required by the machine. The programmer forfeited some measure of control over the final code, perhaps sacrificing efficiency, in exchange for a far greater ease of programming and an increase in his or her productivity. This advantage was reinforced by the appearance of libraries of commonly required functions, frequently sold as adjuncts to the compiler, for carrying out common chores. These functions or subroutines were simply callable, with appropriate arguments, from within the source code. Once the source code had been successfully compiled, the program's own object code, together with that of the various external references embedded within it could all be linked together by a *linker* program (normally supplied with the operating system) to form *executable code*, the actual program that would run on the machine.

Each successive evolution of languages, now amounting to several generations, has raised the programming language further above the processing level and nearer to the concept of the functionality required, thus giving rise to the term *high level languages*. Perhaps the most striking innovation was the introduction of a language intended not for professionally trained programmers, but for the new breed of computing novices, anxious to exploit the cheap processing power now placed at their disposal. Developed at Dartmouth College (Pennsylvania, USA) and dubbed *Basic All Symbolic Instruction Code* (and now known universally as BASIC), it brought computer programming to both the scientific and technical community, and the home enthusiast. It coincided with the appearance of the first relatively inexpensive (for the time) microcomputers, of which the PET (Commodore Business Machines), the British BBC computer developed by Acorn, and the ZX81 and Spectrum models, brainchildren of the charismatic Sir Clive Sinclair, are by far the best known. The most prominent characteristic of BASIC was its use of a form of expression extremely close to simple algebra, thus enabling programs for simple numerical tasks to be written almost intuitively by anyone with no more than a rudimentary acquaintance with school level mathematics. No expensive compiler was required, since the language was interpretive—every line being successively translated into machine code as it was executed. Although slow, this was a minor disadvantage since the machine was only performing a single task. The interpreter for the language was usually included in the hardware as firmware, bundled in with the operating system.

Up to this time, computing at all levels had taken place in a character-based, or textual, environment where the screen consisted of a set number of rows and columns and could display only the characters contained within a specific character set. Operating systems were used by means of a textual command language, where commands had to be typed in exactly, using syntax of some complexity and quite unforgiving of errors, thus requiring an aptitude for precision. It was abundantly apparent that computers were quite difficult to use and were really for the serious user or the enthusiast. (As a matter of fact, computers are still difficult to use, despite all the advertising hype to the contrary. The difference today is that they *pretend* to be easy to use. If this fact is doubted, just watch an older person of no more than average intelligence, but totally unacquainted with personal computers, trying to understand and use any of today's well-known packages.)

The appearance of the graphical user environment, of which Windows™ is by far the most ubiquitous example, revolutionized personal computing and brought the possibility of microprocessing to the mass audience of business users, as well as a large caucus of home users and especially children in schools. Programs were now to be executed not by memorizing complex textual commands and typing them in, but by clicking with a pointer device called a mouse on a tiny 32 bit × 32 bit pictorial representation of the program (called an icon). Static pictures, and more recently sound and moving pictures, could be displayed in a multimedia environment, leading to an explosion in applications, fueled by the exponential rise in computing power essential for driving a graphical interface, yet available (seemingly miraculously) at an ever-declining price. Items on the screen, such as icons, window boxes, scroll bars and list boxes, became known as objects, manipulated by software written in object-oriented languages, of which Microsoft Visual Basic® and C++ are among the most common. Such *fourth generation languages* are not process-driven as their third generation forebears, but are *event driven*—the events being the actions the user may take at any time that objects are displayed on the screen.

THE NEED FOR PROGRAMMING STANDARDS

Whilst the changes that have taken place in programming languages have been breathtaking, one thing has not changed: the need for standards by which a programmer must work. Contrary to widespread belief, it is just as possible to create defective and ruinous code, which few can understand and unravel and which is replete with errors, in a fourth generation graphical language as in any earlier one. Indeed, the speed of hardware and the remorseless rise in the complexity of software has intensified rather than diminished the need for supportable coding.

Keep It

Simple

Practical Guidance

Create a programming standards document describing how code is to be described and structured, how variables are to named, how errors are to be trapped, and any language-specific guidance that fosters ease of code support by those other than the original author.

This is a vital issue to all software houses which must, at some time, recruit new programming personnel for replacement or expansion. One important ingredient of an effective induction program for software developers is written programming standards. Many software companies, and especially the smaller ones, have frequently yet to write down the standards used in creating source code. The absence of such written standards is a critical weakness, although this often comes as a surprise to outfits where there have been no new staff arrivals for a long time. In these circumstances, the members of the small programming team have long since agreed to the detailed conventions to be followed in the assembly of code and are deeply familiar with each other's idiosyncrasies. Therefore, it is possible to maintain each other's code without compromising the existing structural integrity.

The chickens come home to roost when a new recruit joins the team. The task before them is now to impart all of the detailed knowledge and unspoken assumptions that everyone has long since absorbed into their bloodstream to the new recruit. The nest has now acquired a large cuckoo, albeit an innocent and enthusiastic one as mentioned in chapter 3 in the context of documentation (see page 86). Total reliance on verbal instruction, dependent on the memory of the trainer and the understanding and retention of the trainee, is disastrous. Many companies still operate like this. Without written standards, it has been shown frequently to be impossible to train a recruit to work safely in a predictable period, or to arrive at any assurance that a safe level of competence has been acquired. Worse than this, the training exercise itself may reveal a lack of consensus over what the prevailing standards actually are!

THE NATURE OF PROGRAMMING STANDARDS

Programming standards define how code is to be written and must be appropriate for the software under development. The standards fulfill the need met by any language—they define the basis for communication. Without such rules, information intended to be conveyed from one mind to another becomes ambiguous and garbled. We examined this issue in the context of notations for documenting functional requirements and design specifications. Programming standards are simply the notation used in the context of programming.

THE PROGRAMMING STANDARDS GUIDE

A written coding manual or programming standards guide is an indispensable essential for any effective programming team. It should be established and maintained even in the smallest organization, since it is not expensive to produce. It should start out by describing what actually happens now; the general conventions that are accepted to apply to program source code files, such as header information, revision code, its nomenclature, and an audit trail of changes. If more than one language is in use, there should be a separate, language-specific standards documents for each (if appropriate). If industry-wide conventions are followed, for example, the Microsoft Windows™ Programming Standards (Microsoft PC28921-0692) for programs designed for the Windows™ environment, these can be referred to with detailed supplementary guidance on additional company-specific conventions. As an aside, it is worth mentioning that the Windows™ Application Design Guide properly emphasizes the importance of an overall design methodology (Microsoft PC28921-0692, p. 5).

THE CONTENT OF PROGRAMMING STANDARDS

What ought to be featured in programming standards? There are certain aspects which are basic and apply to all languages. There must be a clear, overarching programming standard that describes the overall structure of a software product and a top-down approach to coding. This would decompose the required code down to the irreducible level of the module, and specify how uniformity is to be achieved from one module to another. A standard should specify what supporting documents the programmers must expect to have, such as the design specification and the individual module design specifications. The storage location of these documents and their form (paper or electronic) should be mentioned. Any available coding tools and libraries should be described. The objective is to describe everything that is a fixed practice, so as to leave nothing to chance as far as humanly possible.

Beyond this, the remaining standards will, to some extent, vary with the language used. A standards guide related to object-oriented programming in *Visual Basic*® would look very different from one applicable to *FORTRAN 77*, for example. It is beyond the scope of this book to lay down language-specific standards; confining ourselves instead to the essential elements of good programming practice, applicable in a generic manner to all languages, and which the assessment team would expect to find in a well-controlled programming environment. An indication of the defects that these standards are intended to avoid will also be given.

DOCUMENTATION AND CONTROL

The source code is one of the key life cycle documents. This may seem to some readers a mere statement of the obvious, but there is a hidden inference. Many software houses see the source code as the product, which in one sense, of course, it is! However, in another sense, it is *not* the product; it is simply a *document describing the product*. The product is actually the executable code, a sequence of 1s and 0s within the machine that, when executed by the microprocessor, performs a task useful to the customer. This is a vital distinction and conveys a powerful message to the many software houses that have almost no life cycle documentation at all, yet always have the source code! Of course, at one level they must have this, since source code and product are inseparable. But the central point here is that their need of source code arises fundamentally because without it, they cannot debug, maintain, or in any other way control the product. What they also fail to realize is that the measure of control over the product afforded by source code is strictly limited and heavily circumscribed. It is a widely believed fallacy that the product of software development is the source code, the whole source code and nothing but the source code. Rubbish! There are other documents delivered at other points in the life cycle at least as powerful in exercising control over the product for which the source code is no substitute whatsoever. For example, the level of errors in the source code, from which the bulk of support (i.e., non-quality) costs arise, can be controlled to only a very minor extent by the source code alone. Functional requirements documents, a design specification document, structured test plans and test reports are needed individually and together to provide this. The claim, therefore, to be frequently heard along the lines of "we don't place much emphasis on documentation around here" is disingenuous, since every such vendor in reality attributes overwhelming significance to the one piece of documentation the team actually does possess!

Let us, therefore, examine in more detail various generic aspects of programming standards that ought to be featured in any programming standards guide.

Header Information

All source code ought to carry basic header information, including some or all of the following:

- The name of the program

- A brief description of its function and its usage

- When it was developed

- The name of the original author

- Essential input/output information

- The names of any external libraries or databases used

- Any important interfaces required for the program's operation

- A running revision control log and audit trail of changes

There are several source code control packages in widespread successful use, for example, Microsoft's *SourceSafe* and the *Polytron Version Control System* (widely known by its acronym PVCS) produced by Intersolv,[1] that are being used both to implement a basic security policy over code (e.g., that no more than one programmer can secure write access to a given file at any one time), and to enforce the inclusion of some of these items. In these cases, the header information is separated from the program file itself, the defense being that the source file is never accessed outside the environment of the source control package. Whilst the intention of this ought to command respect, this discipline is dependent on compliance with procedure, and that prudence dictates the wisdom of at least including basic header information in every source file, even if this is repeated in the source control package. Source control packages are strongly advocated, since they enforce the discipline of configuration management discussed in chapter 5, which is vital to successful software development. Without such a package, dependence falls back on people and their degree of compliance with procedures.

Keep It
Simple

Practical Guidance

Implement a computerized source code control system to police the allocation of source code files for editing, impose configuration management, and enforce minimum standards of header information and audit trailed change control.

The Audit Trail

The audit trail is of particular importance. As changes are made to a source file, it becomes increasingly difficult to reconcile it to the design documentation, unless careful, concise but comprehensive, notes are kept of who changed which lines, in what way, when, and for what reason. A running log of such changes ought at least to be kept in the source control package (in many of them this is mandatory); in the absence of such facilities, the log should appear in the header of the source file. Additionally, at each point in the code, the commenting out of the old line adjacent to the inclusion of the new has much to commend it. By this means, the evolutionary thought process leading to the code now being the way it is becomes absolutely clear to each successive editor.

Names and Type Definitions of Variables

The intuitive naming of variables in accordance with a scheme or notation that is sensitive to the application or the environment delivers enormous benefits in terms of ease of support and the avoidance of errors. It is so much easier to understand

```
if (data_record_pointer.gt.6) then

    number_of_samples = number_of_samples + 1

    call record_updater (data_record_pointer)

    . . .
```

rather than

```
if (x56.gt.6) then

    y4 = y4 + 1

    call sub1 (x56)

    . . .
```

Failure to exercise discipline in defining the types of variables is a common source of error in many languages. In both FORTRAN and BASIC, for example, variables can be of various types, occupying different amounts of storage space. Integer, double integer, real, double precision, character and Boolean are just a few. Errors commonly occur either when wrongly typed variables are EQUIVALENCED to each other, passed as arguments to subroutines or committed to COMMON storage, leading to chaotic memory arrays. In both of these languages, the IMPLICIT NONE (for FORTRAN) or the OPTION EXPLICIT (for Visual BASIC®) should be absolutely mandatory in the standards, and constitute a hanging offense if disregarded!

The initialization of variables should also be included in the standards. Some languages automatically initialize numeric variables to zero and character strings to nulls. However, there should be specific action taken to initialize all variables, since a common source of error is to attempt to read a variable before it has been assigned a value.

Structure of Code

Many of the fourth generation languages, such as Visual BASIC® and C++, now enforce indentation in source code layout to indicate subroutines, loops and conditional branching. However, if code is being written in a language where good practice of this nature is not built into the tool, there ought to be a specific requirement in the standard.

Labels in the form of a paragraph header comment should be mandatory to show the flow of a program and to identify the exact function of a short piece of code that performs a discrete task. The flow of the program or the processing order for programs of this type should be quite clear. If there is an option menu or other event-driven stimulus determining the flow of code, this should be clearly indicated in the source. Large programs should always be divided into modules, programs of no more than about 100 lines or so of code that perform a discrete task. This limit is important for two reasons:

1. To ensure that the module is amenable to exhaustive structural testing (code review) by the programming group; if it is too large this process will become unwieldy.

2. To ensure it can be exhaustively tested in isolation.

Modular approaches to software development, such as the creation of module libraries, simplify main programs by minimizing the amount of code, and clarifying the intentions of conditional branching. A lack of comprehensiveness in branch design here is another common source of error that can be mitigated by sound programming standards. For example, suppose that the programmer can foresee three possible sets of conditions that might subtend at a particular program point. The code might look like this:

```
If (condition_set.eq.1) then     ! the first set of
                                   conditions that I
                                   can think of applies
                                   here
```

```
        call subroutine_1 (argument_a1, argument_a2)

   else if condition_set.eq.2) then        ! or the second set
                                            of conditions ap-
                                            plies

        call subroutine_2 (argument_b1, argument_b2)

   else if condition_set.eq.3) then        ! or the other set of
                                            conditions applies

        call subroutine_3 (argument_c1, argument_c2)

   endif
```

This might be just fine, providing the programmer had not overlooked some "special circumstance number 4" which complied with none of these conditions. In that event, the branch is skipped completely and the program enters the uncharted waters of the *undefined state* when anything can happen. This kind of fault was a common cause of program aborts, corruption of data, or even system halts in proprietary operating systems of the 1970s and 1980s, and can still today lead to the ubiquitous General Protection Fault with which Windows™ users are so painfully familiar nowadays. The standards ought to demand the inclusion of a catch-all branching clause to cater for any unforeseen circumstances and trigger a graceful termination:

```
   If (condition_set.eq.1) then           ! the first set of
                                            conditions I can
                                            think of applies

        call subroutine_1 (argument_a1, argument_a2)

   else if condition_set.eq.2) then        ! the second set of
                                            conditions applies

        call subroutine_2 (argument_b1, argument_b2)

   else if condition_set.eq.3) then        ! the other set of
                                            conditions applies

        call subroutine_3 (argument_c1, argument_c2)

   else                                     ! any other condi-
                                            tion (should never
                                            be executed)

        call error_handler (argument_a1, argument_a2, ...)
```

```
call (print_report_sys_manager)

stop ("Program Terminated")

endif
```

It is encouraging to see that Windows 95® has attempted to provide the user with some details of the circumstances of a program performing an illegal operation, available by clicking the Details button always displayed on the illegal operation program termination banner. This displays sundry register information which could well provide vital clues to support personnel. It is unfortunate that defective software leads to this display being so familiar to the hapless user of today's desktop.

Unconditional branching exemplified by the use of GO TO statements in BASIC often indicates an ill-considered logical structure for code. Some firms outlaw the use of GO TO in their BASIC programming standards, thereby enforcing a rigid discipline of good logical design on programmers. This factor can have a marked effect on program execution speed or *performance*. Another important standard relevant to defective logical design is that all code should be *reachable*.

Integration of Third Party Library Code

The use of third party code can be extremely cost-effective and is especially common in the object-oriented graphical programming environment. It has the great advantage of speeding up program delivery and avoids the ingress of errors from programmers attempting to construct this code for themselves. However, these weighty advantages are counterbalanced by the need to use these libraries with caution and discretion. Little, if anything, may be known about the QA practices and controls used to supervise its construction. It must be recognized, therefore, that inherent logical errors from the third party may well become deeply embedded into the product, and there may be no practical or systematic way of discovering them. It is most important, therefore, that programming standards underline the need for an overall quality management system that subjects the final product to a thorough, structured test protocol. This is vital, since the code contained within the library module cannot be examined and subjected to independent structural testing. The use of commercial libraries in this way reinforces the need for additional quality assurance rather than abrogating it.

Keep *It*

Simple

Practical Guidance
Include within the quality management system simple, concise procedures covering all aspects of writing code, including compliance with written standards, documenting everything in this regard that is supposed to happen.

Libraries that are supplied with little or no supporting documentation should be studiously avoided.

The use of well-respected, commercially available libraries of prepared code, such as those of *Foundation Classes* (Microsoft Corporation)[2] and *Visual Objects* (Computer Associates)[3] is widespread today. These libraries consist of classes of objects from which the programmer can select prewritten and allegedly tested code in order to construct screen elements (objects) very quickly. If this is the case, it should be described in the written standards. If certain libraries are to be used in-house, procedures to this effect should be included in the standards.

There are already some signs within the industry of a growing awareness of the issue of the quality of third party code. For example, Informix[4] has recently announced plans to vet the quality of all snap-in modules that third party developers create for its enterprise-capable extensible relational database management system, Universal Server™. Informix is committed to ensuring these are of adequate quality and has inaugurated a certification program. Under this, the *datablade*® developer[5] will be obliged to submit the module, *and* its documentation, it should be noted, to the company for QA testing, to ensure that the database's resilience will not be thereby compromised.[6] It is regrettable that this testing appears to be confined to functional testing, rather than to the structural testing of the source code which would deliver a far better degree of quality assurance.

Error Entrapment Strategies

The dreaded undefined state has already been mentioned as an example of a program running into trouble due to defective coding practice. However, programs get into trouble for all sorts of reasons, of which the operator or user is frequently the cause. Programmers ought to take a pessimistic, but nonetheless compassionate, view of users. The policy of one notorious programmer who, in contempt of users who had the audacity to make more than one mistake in running his programs, would print out a large banner message with the telephone number of a prominent Harley Street (London) psychiatrist, is not to be emulated! More seriously, a forgiving attitude in program coding is much to be favoured.

User errors ought to be politely identified and an opportunity to correct them offered with the added option to terminate the program. Internal program errors should lead the program to terminate as follows:

- With a message to the user indicating that the error is internal, and its location

- A diagnostic dump to a file or a printer of key internal variables or other memory values or pointers to assist in subsequent diagnosis

The thrust of this book is directed toward helping to make this an occurrence of increasing rarity.

Use of Examples

Programming standards written as dry prose are unlikely to be as helpful as those replete with examples both of good practice (which may often be seen) and of bad practice (which can be seen only rarely). This is a pity. One or two examples of howlers can focus the minds of programmers wonderfully.[7] The more examples that can be included in the standards, the more persuasive they will be.

As experience highlights frequently repeated programming errors, the standards should be regularly updated to enable successors to benefit from the bitter experience of others (also known as the *school of hard knocks*). Not only will this powerfully endorse the need for compliance with standards, it will also focus attention on the particular needs of the software house and its products.

Dead Code

Dead code is code superseded from earlier versions. Its isolation by commenting rather than its actual removal has already been advocated, since its isolated presence can aid in the understanding of program evolution. Dead code should not be confused with rarely used code, such as that in a large configurable product which might be inactive rather than dead. This distinction is vital, since its premature removal will lead to serious trouble when the need for it arises unexpectedly. A good example of this is rarely used diagnostic routines, or a module for the use of an unusual peripheral device like an obsolete printer.

Ancillary Programming Standards

Code is not the only aspect of programming that requires control in terms of conformity to standards. Many firms operate in-house styles for screen layouts and report formats that new development must abide by and which must be imparted to novices. These are excellent candidates for inclusion in the programming standards guide, which essentially defines how programming is to be conducted in the firm. Many software houses today are constrained to conformity with the Microsoft Windows™ Programming Standards. However, within these there is considerable scope for variations. The programming standards guide, therefore, can well refer to the Microsoft Windows™ Standards where these apply without change, but then emphasize any local features by which the company wishes its software to be characterized. This will clearly be a much more demanding issue for those firms still involved with third generation language tools, but applies to all groups in some measure.

Help Text

Help text is a vital component in product training and successful acceptance in the marketplace. Few users in this day and age are willing to commit themselves to the personal discipline of studying a manual, despite the fact that this is usually the quickest way to use a software product properly.[8] Poorly assembled help text can cripple an otherwise superior quality product that meets the users' needs, but does not aid them in just the way they need. The potential loss

Keep *It* Simple	**Practical Guidance**
	Create a document describing the company's procedure to be followed in the creation, review, and formal "testing" of help text.

of future business from this source is one of the unknowables of poor product quality, but from the general frustration among users is a huge unnecessary burden on software houses. Making the extra effort to get it right is highly cost-effective.

The unsuitability of programmers in general for this task has already been alluded to, as their familiarity with the product at great depth makes it hard for them to appreciate the needs of the novice user. Whoever writes the help text should have the benefit of documented in-house standards describing what is expected of this text in terms of clarity, conciseness, level of detail and style. There ought to be at least one independent review level of the usefulness and relevance of the help text, and a formal procedure describing how this is effected.

THE PROOF OF THE PUDDING IS IN THE EATING

The benefits of the effective adoption of programming standards will be most keenly felt in the support phase of the life cycle after the product has been released, and especially if the original authors have moved on to pastures new. However, there should also be a more immediate benefit, in that there should be far fewer simple programming errors (i.e., errors not related to design or requirements shortcomings) whose correction slows down the project process. The worth, therefore, of the programming standards should become immediately apparent in the testing phase of the life cycle, to which the next chapter is devoted.

Notes

1. Intersolv Inc., 9420 Key West Ave, Rockville, MA 20850. Tel 1-800-547-4000

2. Microsoft Corporation, 1 Microsoft Way, Redmond, WA 98052-6399

3. Computer Associates International Inc., Islandia, NY

4. Informix Software Inc., Menlo Park, CA

5. *Datablade*® is an Informix term used to denote a software module, or plug-in object extension, composed of routines written in accordance with Informix's proprietary programming standard. The datablade's function is to expand the parallel performance and scalability capabilities of the relational database. It does this by supplying the database with its properties, thus enabling the database to store information of a specialized nature.

6. "Modules Face Quality Check", news item in *Computer Weekly*, 18 July 1996.

7. I vividly remember in the mid-1980s spending 2 days and a sleepless night (insomnia is said to be common among programmers) unable to get a FORTRAN program to run successfully. It transpired that I had implicitly "typed" the record number variable for a database as real (4 bytes on this 16-bit machine), because its name began with the letter "r", rather than integer (2 bytes), which it would have been had its name commenced with the letter "i", a feature of the default naming conventions applicable in the language at the time. I never repeated that mistake!

8. When all else fails . . . read the manual!

9

Software Testing

Who can straighten out what he has made crooked? . . .
What is crooked cannot be made straight, and what is lack-
ing cannot be numbered.

Ecclesiastes 7:13; 1:15

The observation has already been made that in the course of visiting vendors, both in North America and in Western Europe, most of them spend an inordinate amount of effort in the functional testing of software. This being the case, therefore, one might be forgiven for wondering whether there was really any need to include a chapter on this subject in a book primarily intended for software developers.

The truth is, of course, that this sobering fact betrays a widespread misunderstanding of the proper place of testing in a well-controlled, standards-conforming, life cycle process methodology. Indeed, the prevalence of testing and its disproportionate importance in the values and activities of so many software firms points to the shameful abuse of testing rather than the proper and praiseworthy application of it.

A TRIO OF DELUSIONS

There are three widespread delusions surrounding software testing among developers today:

1. Functional testing puts quality into the software.

2. Functional testing enables the errors in the software to be found and rectified.

3. The discovery of errors during functional testing phase demonstrates its effectiveness; once these are rectified, the software is evidently fit to be delivered to customers.

All of these arise from a lack of understanding of the realities undergirding the development of soundly engineered software. They are common in the broad mass of software developers still labouring at the first two levels of the Capability Maturity Model that were explored in chapter 1. Before a sound approach to functional software testing will be suggested, a brief recapitulation of the harsh facts behind this trio of misplaced assumptions is in order.

Functional (end product) testing is totally incapable of putting quality into software. All it can do is give a rough and rather unreliable indication of the level of quality already there. Quality has either been incorporated or excluded from the product as a facet of the process by which it has been developed. Testing neither improves nor degrades the fundamental quality level of a finished product.

Functional testing is an extremely blunt instrument for detecting errors in anything larger than the tiniest program. Chapter 5 described how even a quite small program can have trillions of possible pathways; therefore, it is practically impossible to test most software programs to little more than a superficial extent, let alone exhaustively. There is only one way of gaining an insight into the likely level of remaining errors: the method of structural testing or code inspection, which examines the logical structure and technical content of source code in relation to the design specifications from which it is built. Only when this exercise has shown a satisfactory level of innate structural integrity exists does functional testing provide a confirmatory assurance of software quality.

The number of errors found either in structural or functional testing is proportional to the number of errors still remaining but hitherto undetected. If functional testing has found a large number of errors which have since been rectified, this is most definitely NOT a cause for celebration. On the contrary, it is cause for mourning and weeping! It means that the software is replete with defects that will continue to flow in after release to the market, sapping the confidence of existing customers, costing the earth in support arrangements, and, by word of mouth over the ubiquitous grapevine, discouraging potential future business.

Keep *It* **Simple**	**Practical Guidance**
	Include in the quality management system a brief summary of the two different types of testing, where they fit into the life cycle, how they are separate but complementary, and what the limitations of functional testing really are.

TESTING IN ITS RIGHTFUL PLACE

The proper place, therefore, of functional testing is as a late stage in a life cycle process, in which a partnership of structural testing and functional testing, taken together, provide the assurance of innate structural integrity. Within this partnership, the emphasis should be principally on structural testing, since this takes place with a full knowledge of the code and of all the possible pathways resulting from the logical structure under examination. Compliance with good in-house programming standards and practices and the use of a well-reviewed and approved design specification fully traceable to the functional and user requirements avoids the incorporation of many defects in the first place. Since these were never in the product, they do not need to be removed. After all, defects do not arrive in software by accident—they are put there by someone. Is it not, then, sheer lunacy to pay people to put defects into software that others are subsequently paid to try to detect and remove?

How then does testing relate to the other stages of the life cycle? Figure 9.1 answers this question in relation to the V model that was discussed in chapter 1. It attempts to clarify the following:

1. Testing takes place in *phases*, and the relationship between each phase and the corresponding specification documents created at the precoding early stages of the life cycle.

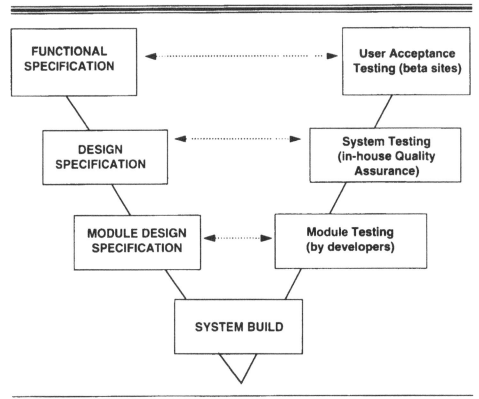

Figure 9.1. Testing Roles Versus Specifications

2. The personnel involved in testing and the location and degree of independence in the testing activities.

The principles, both of testing in phases and of securing independence, are both widely accepted within the software community, although the relationship between each phase and its foundation document is still only appreciated by a few. Figure 9.1 illustrates the minimum arrangements which is common to the majority of vendors today. It will be seen that the need for independence does not apply at every stage. However, the fundamental point of the diagram is to underline the pivotal role played by these documents in ensuring that *quality is being built into the software*, and that this is taking place before a line of code has ever been written. It therefore follows that the testing activity, far from building quality into the software as it is widely believed to do (but which in reality it is totally incapable of doing), simply demonstrates the level of quality that has already been built in (or excluded) by the corresponding early stages.

STRUCTURED TEST PLANS OR SPECIFICATIONS

Testing software is by no means an easy task. For anything but the simplest programs, it is an extremely demanding discipline that must be carefully planned and controlled if it is to stand any chance of giving a reliable guide to the innate quality level of the product in terms of remaining residual defects. Without a structured approach, testing easily degenerates into a haphazard empirical exercise comparable to the use of a blunderbuss to kill flies. Planning the test activities is, therefore, crucial both to ensure its success and to ensure it will be a cost-effective exercise to the organization. It has been hinted already in chapter 7 that structured test plans directly derived from and traceable to the design specification are the essential prerequisite for a satisfactory software testing exercise. The timing of the appearance of the test specifications is important. Since test plans are directly derived from the design specification and traceable to it, they ought to be drawn up at about the same time, and certainly no later than the beginning of development. They must be available before testing commences, thus avoiding the unedifying and somewhat ridiculous spectacle of developers trying to test their modules thoroughly while their minds are preoccupied, quite properly, elsewhere producing the code. Having a test specification ready on which they can rely, and drawn up in an atmosphere where concentration was able to be given fully, comes as an enormous relief to developers.

Test specifications are critical documents on which the effectiveness of testing depends. Even in those firms that draw up test specifications, it is rare that anyone reviews them for accuracy or traceability to the design specification. Each test specification should be subject to formal document control, which will be discussed in more detail in the next chapter. Since it is likely to be updated at least once as a result of test failures, the test specification should come strictly within the configuration management system. Without this, who will know to which version of the design specification the test specification related, or to which test specification the software finally complied? It should be reviewed and signed off by a second competent individual in the interests of finding and removing defects before it is used (i.e., **before testing commences**). Quality assurance should be involved in ensuring this, which is an excellent example of the type of controls which should have been specified in the quality plan.

Keep It *Simple*	# Practical Guidance Create a procedure describing how test specifications will be reviewed by a second qualified person and signed off when approved.

Traceability of test specifications back to design specifications is also critical. It is vital that all aspects of the functionality of the product, both positive and negative, are tested, together with the error routines (often by contriving error conditions in the environment). In more traditional, third generation language development, paragraph numbering was often used to relate each test to its corresponding design feature. In the object-oriented arena, design specifications can often be converted into test specifications with very little effort, sometimes amounting to no more that inserting boxes at the side of each design feature description for recording the pass or fail. However, this does depend on the construction of the design document. There is not always a one-to-one correspondence between a design feature and its test cases—the relationship will frequently be many-to-one. Nevertheless, the design document can often be an excellent template on which to base a structured test plan. If this desirable, labour-saving feature can be anticipated at the outset of projects, or even incorporated into the general standards for design specifications within the organization and documented in the quality management system, so much the better.

What then are these documents and how are they related to the earlier life cycle stages? Figure 9.2 illustrates three testing specifications, each corresponding to a different requirements specification. However, before what each of these specifications ought to contain will be considered, the question of how testing ought to be carried out should be addressed. Are there any general principles essential to successful testing regardless of the testing stage? Yes, there are.

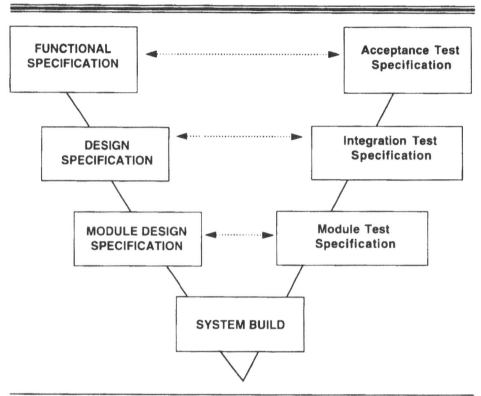

Figure 9.2. Software Testing Specifications

KEYS TO SUCCESSFUL TESTING

The quality plan assembled at the outset of the project should have defined those documents that ought to be available before any testing begins, and by whom they should have been reviewed and approved. At a minimum, this should be the test specification or plan appropriate to that stage, which should have been reviewed and approved as specified, and the procedure for carrying out the tests. If any equipment was involved, such as a computer for running any automated test routines, this should be checked and documented as being in good working order. Accompanying the test specification, or ideally part of it, should be a place where compliance or non-compliance can be entered by a tick or a check mark. This document (and remember it may be electronic, such as a Lotus Notes® page, just as easily as being a paper document) then becomes the *test record* as well as the test specification. The result of each test should then be recorded as pass or fail. Any failures recorded on the document then qualify it to be included in the project post mortem meeting in due course, where a careful analysis of what went wrong on the project can be examined, with a view to improving the process for the future (*kaizen*). If certain raw data were involved, these too should be confirmed as being as specified, since if this is not the case, a defect dependent on the nature of the raw data might slip through unnoticed.

Test failures (and the ensuing finger-pointing) may arise from several causes:

- A fault in the test specification or the test data (*Who approved the test specification?*)

- A fault in the way the test was carried out (*Who did the test?*)

- A fault in the operating system of the machine or some other environmental fault (*Who is giving us operational support?*)

- A fault in the design specification (*Who approved it?*)

- (and yes, this cannot be excluded) A fault in the software itself! (*Who wrote this code?*)

A simple testing flowchart appears in figure 9.3. A running log ought to be kept of test failures, since these raise serious questions over the effectiveness of the disciplines used to control the generation of the code. Of special importance in this regard are any major failures, such as systems halts or crashes, which terminate program execution altogether. Each failure represents a breakdown of control in one respect or another. Although many may be just be a slip of a programmer (we are all fallible), this could either point to a training need (if it indicates a lack of knowledge either technical or procedural), a lack of motivation or concentration (human resource issue), or, more seriously, a fundamental weakness somewhere in the life cycle procedures. Addressing these issues is of supreme value in improving the organization's capability level and, thus, deserves the very best that management can give to it.

Many firms do not retain test records, or even a summary of them. This is more than just a pity; it could become a liability. As the awareness of software engineering and quality issues on the part of purchasers improves, there is likely to be increasing demands to inspect the test records of a released version of code. What other

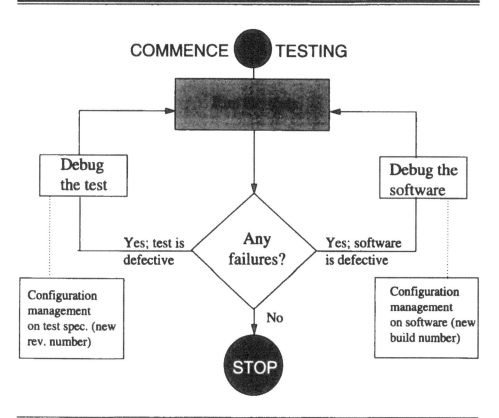

Figure 9.3. The Flow of Testing

impartial evidence can a vendor produce of the quality of the product? We have already seen how market penetration is a very unreliable guide of residual defect levels, since the majority of users may well only be exercising the same minority subset of pathways that constitute a tiny proportion of the total.

Keep *It*

Simple

Practical Guidance

Create a document describing the procedure to be followed in testing software. Include the necessary prerequisites before testing can commence, how testing is to be conducted, and how the results are to be recorded. Give special emphasis to action to be taken on failures.

<table>
<tr><td>Keep *It*

Simple</td><td>

Practical Guidance

Include a procedure for retaining at least a summary of the test results for each released version of product, any failures and the corrective action taken, to be retained for the support lifetime of the product.

</td></tr>
</table>

Therefore, the retention of at least a summary of the test results is to be strongly advocated, including, of course, the failures and the corrective actions arising from their investigation. This may simply be a one- or two-page document, but it provides evidence that the firm is in control of its process and has a mechanism for ensuring continuous improvement. For those who do not summon the structured test plan to perform the dual role of a test log, two simple documents have been been included in the appendices. The first of these is a *Test Results Log* (appendix 7) which can be used to record the results of a series of test cases in the form of a table. In the event of a failure of any level of severity, a *Failure Report* (a specimen appears as appendix 8) can be filled out for investigation by the developers in the first instance and the project team later on. Both of these simple documents, taken together, can form the basis of a simple test recording scheme, though the approach of the structured test plan is more methodical, less labour intensive, and much to be preferred.

MODULE TEST SPECIFICATION

The first stage of testing normally occurs at the module level and can quite properly be carried out by the developers themselves. It aims to demonstrate the achievement in practice of all of the elements described in the *module design specification*. The most successful practice seems to be for each programmer to engage the service of one of his or her programmer peers for this purpose. For each module, a *module test specification*, directly derived from the module design specification, whose place in the life cycle and whose content we examined in chapter 7, should have been drawn up.[1] This document details the individual tests that should be applied, clearly defining what constitutes a pass or a fail, and should mention any areas that will not be tested and why. Tests should be arranged in logical groups and structured to represent each test along the following lines:

- **Test case**: what functionality the test is designed to show to be present or absent; if this test is dependent on any others in the suite or must be run at a certain position in the sequence.

- **Test goal**: how the software ought to behave in this test. What input data is to be used (a script, a command, or a dataset) and how it should be transformed.

- **Test procedure**: the steps involved in carrying out the test and any essential preconditions to be met. This might include setup actions, actions necessary during test execution, what ought to be done to interrupt testing (if need be) and to repeat the test.

- **Test data**: nature and content.

- **Expected test results**: what should happen (or not happen as the case may be) if the software works as intended.

- **Documentation method**: how the actual behaviour will be recorded.

If the test specification can also be used as a test record document (two for the price of one and a permanent piece of documentary evidence of product quality):

- **Test result**: what actually happened (pass or fail).

A common source or errors that is frequently overlooked in software is its behaviour at design *boundaries*. For example, suppose an input is supposed to be less than 100 and provided this is met, the software works as intended, with an error being reported for values greater than this. Error routines are thus designed to catch all entries greater than 100. So everything works correctly for inputs up to 99.99999 and the error routine is invoked correctly at 100.00001 and above. But what happens when the entry is exactly 100.00000? The example may be trivial and almost frivolous, but this principle operates to trip programmers up time after time. Module testing should, therefore, pay very careful attention to policing boundary conditions on passed arguments or other derived data. This issue can assume critical importance in systems designed to control industrial processes. Chapman has described (1984) what he calls the *PAR approach* (proven acceptable range) in the context of process validation to aid the assignment of such values in the software of process control computer-related systems.

INTEGRATION TEST SPECIFICATION

The second phase of software testing (also known as *alpha testing*) is that of the product in its entirety on the basis of satisfactory test results for each of the component modules. It focusses on the interfaces and interplay of the modules together and sets out to demonstrate the achievement of the requirements established in the functional specification. It must be carried out by personnel other than the developers; in many larger firms, dedicated software test groups are led by QA staff; in small firms, this role is often performed by the product support group. Like module testing, it must be conducted on the basis of a written specification, in this case the integration test specification, a structured test plan derived from and directly traceable to the design specification. It should be laid out in the form of test cases along the same lines as the module specification, though, naturally, it is likely to be considerably longer than any of them.

The IEEE (ANSI 829) standard recommends no less than eight different related documents which can be involved in the testing process, and is illustrated in figure 9.4. This is really quite excessive for all but the very largest systems.[2] However, the standard is valuable as a reference guide against which to check in-house specifications to ensure that nothing of importance is overlooked. The control that must be respected is configuration management (e.g., that each successive version of the specification, and each software build, is uniquely numbered and identifiable).

The testing of error message routines is of particular importance at this stage. There is a great temptation to overlook this aspect of software. It arises from a subconscious overestimate of the quality of the software, a desire to assume the best about what is not examined, a reluctance to go looking for trouble, and a hope that error message routines will never be executed. All of these inclinations are, of course, quite fatal but nevertheless widespread. Error message testing addresses not only the actual behaviour of the software in terminating gracefully or taking other controlled action, but

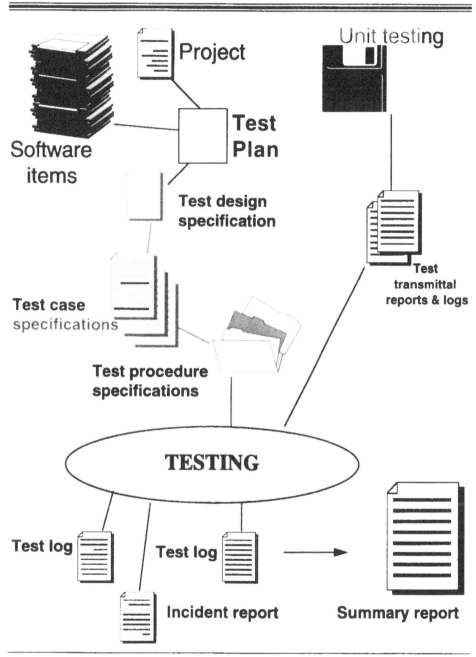

Figure 9.4. The IEEE Approach to Test Documentation

also its interaction with the user. The constant criticism voiced over today's software by users is that the error message text is either ambiguous, unintelligible, or just plain wrong. All error routes designed into the software should be specifically tested at this stage, and the error message text verified by the documentation, support or QA personnel as meeting the criteria of intelligibility, suitability and freedom from ambiguity.

ACCEPTANCE (BETA) TESTING

The last stage of software testing, which almost all vendors seem to be involved in, is that conducted by independent selected customers known as *beta test sites*. Conceptually, this stage is aimed at showing that all of the requirements set forth in the user requirements specification have been met. It should address functionality, performance, any critical parameters and the operating procedures required to use the system. All of the user documentation should also be available now, since product and documentation are inseparable. This includes installation information, since installation is the first task to be performed on product receipt by a customer.

The acceptance test specification should be derived from and traceable to the user requirements specification. For those systems that interface with other systems and equipment at the customer's site, the test specification may need to carry a supplementary (customer site) section addressing behaviour specific to the system's operating environment.

While the document may resemble (and indeed be a revision of) the integrated system specification, it ought to have additional sections, as appropriate, addressing the following:

- Testing of alarms

- Testing of boundary conditions for input, whether manual or instrumental

- Testing of displays and reports

- Testing of critical functions, data and interfaces

- Testing of shutdown and start-up procedures, if applicable

- Testing backup and recovery, if integral or specific to the product

- Testing of security and access restrictions

For vendors of systems in regulated environments, the purchaser will need to qualify (i.e., test and document) the system as outlined in figure 1.9 on page 56. This may, in practice, be very similar to beta testing at selected sites, but with one important difference. The purchaser is obliged to subject the system to the acceptance tests in a very formal manner and document the results as part of the validation plan. For vendors supplying systems of this type, the auditor must ensure that the vendor will afford the purchaser every practical assistance in seeing this activity through to a successful conclusion. This is seldom a problem, since the completion of the sale or contract is usually conditional on it.

AUTOMATED TEST TOOLS

Testing software manually can become an extremely boring task. This is especially true as much or all of the testing will need to be repeated on the entire product as each defect is repaired and a new build operation performed. Bored, demotivated people, with a limited concentration span and level of interest, are quite unsuited to the demands of such an exercise, and are likely to make many mistakes. It is the realization and acknowledgment of this fact, together with the speed and precision of automated tools, that has led to their widespread deployment for testing.

The use of automated tools for software testing appears to be much more common in the United States and Canada than it is in Europe. Quite why this is remains unclear, but the explanation may partly lie in the much larger size of the North American marketplace for software, exacerbating the potential seriousness for the company's future of residual defects. The ability to amortize both the cost of the tool, and the effort necessary to establish the test scripts, over a larger licence base clarifies the value of automation, about which U.S. developers often speak to me in glowing terms. This is seldom the case in the United Kingdom. Where CAST (computer-aided software testing) tools are in operation, they have been very successful and highly cost-effective, and most of these implementations have been in the object-oriented environment. The best groups have built their suites concomitantly with product development, the test engine evolving alongside the product in harmony with the structured test plan. The various commercially available products vary in their strengths and weaknesses. Microsoft's *Test,* for example, includes a library of suites for testing many of the most common objects and controls, thus enabling a product test script to be constructed much more speedily, addressing much of the foundational testing. Another product being used successfully is *AutoTester* (Silvon Software, Westmont, Illinois, USA), applicable to the Windows™ and OS/2® environments, which includes *Test Library Manager* providing change and version control (discussed at greater length in chapter 11) and an audit trail of activity. Yet another product with a good reputation is *QAPlus* (Segworks). As experience with tools grows, a library of company-specific scripts for the more common product functions, and for any coding errors that have crept in, will accumulate, thus enabling the productivity, efficiency and value of testing to rise as time passes.

Automated tools such as these are capable of running the same suite of tests defined in a prepared test script without any human intervention, often overnight, recording the results in a log file with a summary of noncompliances. Every single build can be exhaustively tested overnight, night after night. This is a huge advantage! We have already lamented the failure to retain test records, which deprive the firm of the ability of retrospectively proving the quality of the software by destroying the key evidence of it. For bulky paper records, this action is at least understandable, even if it cannot be condoned. But a compact electronic test log from a sophisticated and comprehensive automated test run can be retained indefinitely at almost no cost whatsoever! *AutoTester,* for example, automatically documents every step of testing, identifying each test by number and requirements identifier; this product is also, incidentally, capable of testing IBM–based character-oriented software through its ability to work with 3270, 5250 (for the ubiquitous AS/400 systems), and Hewlett Packard 2392 terminal emulators.

From an auditor's viewpoint, therefore, the use of such tools is a great credit to a vendor, since it means that functional testing is likely to have been far more thorough and systematic than would be the case otherwise. The major investment required, aside from the initial purchase of the tool itself is, of course, the preparation of the script. This can be very laborious, and many firms have shied away from tools in the belief that these costs outweigh the benefits. Although this was certainly true of the early tools, these costs are probably already being expended in firms still wholly reliant on manual testing. Tools have matured considerably, and their present level of sophistication is making them almost indispensible, especially in view of the fact that the high degree of integration of many of today's products is making residual defects much harder to find. Some tools are even capable of restarting the system should it freeze up or hang during the testing program.

TESTING IN PERSPECTIVE

As the organization matures and improves the performance of the software engineering process, more and more effort will be proportionally devoted to the early parts of the life cycle, thus reducing the level of errors creeping into the code. As this occurs, the presently dominant role of functional testing can be allowed to diminish to that of a minor, final check, since there are now far fewer errors to find. Failures in functional testing, which once demanded an inordinate amount of management effort to deal with, become less common, allowing the staff to claim with some justification that defects have been *designed out*. These savings, coupled with those from reduced needs for support services for better quality products, have been found time and again to more than compensate for the additional effort expended at the early stages. It really is cheaper to do it right the first time!

THE JOB ISN'T FINISHED UNTIL . . .

Throughout the assessment so far, the team has been examining the evidence for quality being built into the software from the earliest stages of the life cycle. Most of this evidence has been in the form of documentation of one form or another, reflecting its centrality within a controlled engineering process. In the next chapter, some practical approaches to handling documentation will be examined, and the minimum documents that should be afforded by every quality assured software development process summarized.

Notes

1. More detailed procedures for drawing up module, integrated and acceptance test specifications can be found in the GAMP guide (1996).

2. A view shared by R. Chamberlain (1994) in which a concise treatment of the IEEE approach to test documentation can be found.

10

Documentation

The spoken word is transient as the wind,
but the written word endures.

Anon

The ANSI (N45:1993) definition of documentation is as follows:

Any written or pictorial information describing, defining, specifying, reporting or certifying activities, requirements, procedures or results.

Throughout this book, the creation of written documents to record the standards and practices of the organization has been emphasized. The thesis undergirding this position has been that the creation of software, being an intensively intellectual activity, depends critically for its success on the control of the information flows in both directions during what must be a stagewise, formalized process. Warnings have been given that if these disciplines are ignored or dismissed, then the process becomes chaotic, however gifted and able the programmers may be, and overhead costs, both those that can be measured and, more importantly, those that cannot, rise steeply and ultimately uncontrollably. The fact has been emphasized that in today's increasingly competitive environment, with customers now becoming less tolerant of defective software, these issues will ultimately determine which software houses will thrive and prosper, and conversely those which in due course will fail. It has also been pointed out that software written for use in a regulated environment must be validatable (i.e., carry documentary evidence that it has been engineered in accordance with a system of quality assurance). This principle is analogous to that applicable to all processes in these environments, a principle defined as

> *establishing documented evidence which provides a high degree of assurance that a specific process will consistently produce a product meeting its pre-determined specifications and quality attributes* (FDA 1987).

However, knowing what ought to be done and knowing exactly how to achieve it are very different. Many companies, in an effort to develop an effective library of standards and procedures, or a *quality management system*, to impose quality disciplines in their process have fallen foul of the dreaded disease of *bureaucracy*. This evil tends to creep into most large organizations at some point in their growth. It consists of documentary procedures and logs outliving their usefulness and being perpetuated beyond their natural life simply for the sake of it. Those that tolerate this situation are either ignorant of the need to challenge institutionalized practice, or reluctant to rock the boat through precipitating and driving forward change, or content to accept wasteful overheads because they themselves are unwilling to take the risk and make the personal effort that effecting change inevitably implies. Bureaucracy is to be deprecated in the strongest terms, but replacement of one evil (that of bureaucracy) with another (that of a chaotic uncontrolled process) cannot be justified. What will be demonstrated in this chapter are the practical approaches to writing procedures that simply and cost-effectively control the information flows and the practices within software development, and by their introduction deliver immediate business benefit to the organization. First to be addressed are the composition and presentation of operational procedures, with attention then being turned to other types of documentation bound up with the development life cycle.

STANDARD OPERATING PROCEDURES

A quality management system should include all of the standard operating procedures (SOPs) that have been written to institutionalize best practice. It is helpful to understand the derivation of the term:

- **Procedure** means a stepwise series of instructions which, if followed verbatim, enable a business process to be executed.

- **Operating** means that this series of steps is a practical, assured way of achieving the objective in view for the process (although there might also be other ways).

- **Standard** implies that this is the only acceptable way of carrying out this process, and that the format of the procedure conforms with an approved set of requirements applicable to all such documents.

SOPs are the essential tool by which the capability of a software development group may be raised from the *creative chaos* or *repeatable* levels to the defined level, as described in chapter 1. Procedures transform such organizations, where highly competent professionals execute business processes from memory and close familiarity but where nothing is documented, to the *managed* model, where everything the organization does to run the enterprise routinely is written down. The main advantages in maturing from creative chaos to managed is that management can control the business more effectively, and that the business is less vulnerable to staff absence or turnover. Once documented, business processes can be scrutinized by consensus to improve productivity and effectiveness, resulting in improved competitive advantage, reduced costs and higher profitability.

SOPs are collectively intended to benefit at least three audiences within the company, however large or small it may be:

1. The **process owners**, those who are responsible at the sharp end for progressing the business process, do not have to rely on their memory, or on verbal instructions which may be incomplete or misunderstood, for knowing how to do a job. If done this way, the job can be completed successfully.

2. The **management** responsible to the owners, or the shareholders, and the customers, for the success of the process.

They may not always be entirely familiar with the fine details of every business process and need a readily available aide-mémoire to be assured that if carried out this way every single time, the process will have the predictable, repeatable outcome. The continued prosperity of the business and the employment of the staff depends on this. Risk is, thereby, significantly reduced.

3. **New recruits** who need to be trained to execute the business properly do not have to depend on the memory, or the eloquence, or the variable training aptitudes, of existing staff to school them in the way things are done. Without SOPs, the success of the business is solely dependent on the culture that prevails. New recruits unfamiliar with this culture and its web of underlying, unspoken, and often unconscious assumptions present a huge risk to a company involved in intellectually demanding work of this type. They cannot possibly be expected to absorb this culture in a fixed time, and there is no reliable way of knowing when they have understood enough to be able to safely work (from the company's point of view) unsupervised to any extent. SOPs mitigate most of these uncertainties.

4. **Quality assurance** personnel or **internal auditors** dedicated to ensuring that established best practice is actually being followed.

The case, therefore, for SOPs is overwhelming. Why do so many software houses then believe that they can operate successfully without them? Very small outfits with perhaps no more than two or three programmers are quite capable of producing good quality software with few or no procedures. Communication is possible within tightly knit groups to an intensive degree, as we have seen, achieving a high measure of control over the information flows inherent in software design and development. However, without SOPs describing their standards and processes, such groups are faced with two serious problems:

1. They are sealed into a prison of their own making in that growth beyond their present small size carries enormous risk. Almost all of the small enterprises in business today aspire to grow. Growth is seen, quite properly, as a sign of life; none of the vendors are willing to admit to a contentment to fossilize and vegetate.

2. They cannot provide impartial evidence that they are capable of building structural integrity into their software. However successful their market penetration, they cannot assure customers that their software is being engineered in a controlled manner and in accordance with standards, and, consequently, cannot assure them either that use of the software does not pose an unknown risk to the purchaser.

How can procedures be written in such a way as to serve the needs of the different audiences while at the same time being cost-effective and nonbureaucratic?

LEVELS OF INFORMATION

One of the most successful approaches is to abandon the attempt to address all of these requirements in a single document, but to divide it into two distinct classes:

Procedures

Procedures are designed to give a brief reminder of the approved method of working. Intended audiences are the process owners themselves, or quality assurance and/or internal auditors.

The process owner readers are assumed to possess all of the requisite background knowledge and practical training to carry out the operation competently and, therefore, require the minimum information only. This should be presented in a crisp, didactic style, with almost no explanation of why things are done the way they are. A procedure should, therefore, appear as a series of steps in the imperative mood, such as the following:

1. Do this first.

2. Then do this.

3. Then do this.

Procedures written by the process owners themselves after this fashion stand the best chance of being followed, since they will be "owned" by those who execute them. They will be full of assumptions and, thus, quite unsuitable for any other audience. The QA or internal audit personnel (usually the same) may not know quite as much about the process, but they should know enough to compare

Keep *It*

Simple

Practical Guidance
Create a document describing how to write simple, concise and brief procedures, where they are to be stored and how the cultural information relating to them (the why and wherefore) is to be recorded and made available.

what is actually happening on the ground with what is described in the document and to recognize noncompliance.

Descriptions

Descriptions are designed to explain to new recruits, and the management, the reasons why things are done the way they are and any other useful background information. This information may be in the form of plain prose, or diagrams of various kinds; it may include specimen forms used in the process, or any other kind of associated data. Authors of such documents may well be the process owners themselves, those with less knowledge of the process, and who are thus less handicapped by intimate familiarity with it usually produce much better results. Many firms have a documentation group, or use the support personnel for this task. Naturally, there must be close liaison between process owners and authors in drafting these standards and explanations, and all must be approved by quality assurance on behalf of the management.

The procedures must contain brief statements of where to find the explanatory standards and descriptions that undergird the form that the process has been agreed to take. These then are the links between the two sets of documents, the procedures being seen as being "in front", while the descriptions lie "behind" them and are generally (though not exclusively) accessible through them. This arrangement is illustrated in figure 10.1.

ELECTRONIC PRESENTATION USING LOTUS NOTES®

Almost everyone now uses word processing and disc media to create and store documents. However, the form in which documents are *presented* has a major bearing on their acceptance, usefulness and the overhead cost of maintaining them. While it is still perfectly

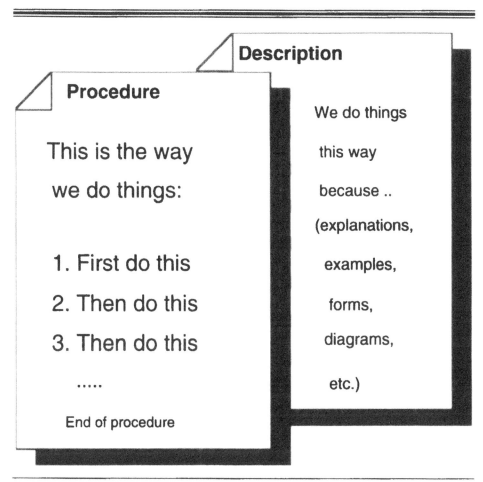

Figure 10.1. Procedures and Descriptions

possible to use paper as the presentation medium (and this is true for most companies which have documented their procedures), there are more elegant methods and, for larger organizations, cheaper ones.

Paper has well-known disadvantages as an information presentation medium, which, although not being much of an issue in the small company, quickly increases in seriousness as the company becomes larger, especially if operating over several sites. Multiple copies of the same document, widely dispersed geographically, make version control and configuration management a nightmare.

Once of the most successful approaches in practice is the use of the groupware product known as Lotus Notes® as the vehicle in

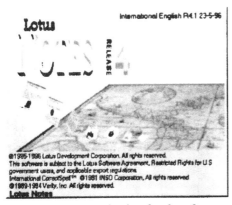

which to retain, maintain and present documents. Notes® is a group information manager that allows users to collect, organize and share information over networks and dial-up lines; it is in this latter sense that Notes® offers enormous advantages over static, single location document management systems. A single database of documents may exist in the form of multiple, replicate copies on individual servers scattered over a number of geographically isolated locations. Changes made to any of these databases are replicated at regular intervals so that all users have access to what is essentially a single repository of information, existing as multiple, dispersed copies, without the inherent disadvantage of an unacceptably long time to access a remote document. Thus, a large company can create a library of standards and procedures that applies everywhere, right across the globe if need be. The architecture has the enormous advantage over a physically unitary database in that users have the added advantage of the performance of a local database, thus obtaining the best of both worlds—one enterprise-wide library but accessible locally. The replication frequency is chosen to balance the need to be up-to-the-minute with the performance penalty on the network inherent in the transmission of the replication traffic. For the kind of application we are considering, overnight replication is usual.

The other major advantage of Notes® is the ability to view documents in a wide variety of different listings, limited only by the number of fields chosen in the documents' form designs. Coupled with this is the ability to link documents together both within and between databases, delivering an elegance in access that paper systems have no hope of matching. The inclusion of a graphical object, such as a screen dump, can be especially effective as a communication tool in procedures.[1] Should hard copies be required, a document can be printed as a walkaway copy, but only on the strict understanding that hard copies are not to regarded as ever having the status of the electronic original.

Figure 10.2 illustrates part of a typical Notes® workspace, where three databases have been created. The Procedures database on the right is the direct repository for the didactic stepwise procedures for daily reference by the process owners, while the descriptions database appears next on the left. There may be several of either type of database, as shown by the "another library" example on the far left.

As the procedures are drafted by the process owners for brevity, simplicity and conciseness they are unavoidably and intentionally shot through with a multitude of assumptions. For this reason, it is vital that quality assurance review them, not of course to remove the embedded assumptions but to *probe* them. Quality assurance needs the opportunity to ask the obvious question, like "why do we do that?" The answer to such an enquiry provides the raw material for supplementary documents which they themselves, or others, should compose in the Descriptions database, and reference from the procedure by means of an interdocument link, as shown in Figure 10.3. Prompt text beginning "For a display of AS400 Tape Labelling Information . . . " written in a different font and color (blue, 12 point bold Times New Roman) from the black 10 point Helvetica procedure text provides the viewer with an immediate opportunity to delve deeper (figure 10.3 is reproduced here only in monochrome). This has proven to be an extremely valuable training aid for novices and a means for management to keep themselves informed of what is really going on.

The document detailing the tape labelling information has been composed in the Descriptions database and a link to it "cut and pasted" into the procedure. It is extremely simple to construct. Descriptive background data accessible in this way does not have to be confined to text. PowerPoint® flow diagrams can be dynamically OLE linked, so that while they are maintainable in their own

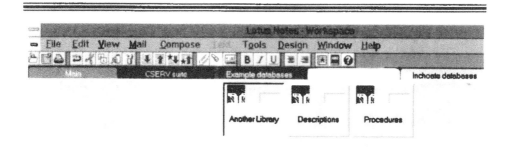

Figure 10.2. A Typical Notes® Desktop Workspace

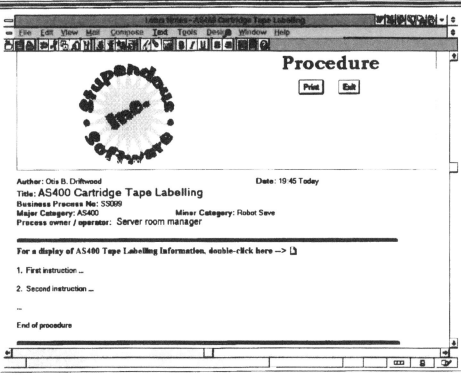

Figure 10.3. Descriptive Information Within a Procedure

application—PowerPoint®—the latest version is always viewable, albeit after pressing the Refresh button, in the Notes® procedure. The possibilities are endless.

Figures 10.4 and 10.5 give examples of procedures for the drafting of SOPs and their supporting information documents in a Notes® environment, applicable to many types of organizations, not only those of software developers but also IT service groups. They are intended for use by the owners of processes to create the procedures for each process, together with the background explanatory material.

Before moving on from the subject of groupware, it would be prudent to sound a note of caution. Despite the well-attested virtues, and the enormous potential of groupware products such as Lotus Notes®, the decision to introduce this technology into a software process must not be taken lightly. It is vital to have a clear and detailed vision of both the strengths and the limitations of an envisaged design, before the commitment to replace paper-based

---

Procedure Documents

1. Write the procedure in a stepwise, didactic style, using the imperative mood, as these instructions are being presented!

2. Use Helvetica 10 point black text.

3. If your procedure uses technical terms and jargon, use a Pop-up to define it on first use. The Pop-up word or phrase will appear inside a green rectangle, on which the reader may click to view your definition. Select the text, press Edit, then Insert, then Pop-up, type the text and then click OK.

4. On completion, select all your text.

5. Use View then Show Ruler to see the ruler, and set the left margin at 1 inch.

6. Press View then Show Page Breaks and set the right hand margin to 7.5 inches. This margin only affects hard copy printout, but ensures a WYSIWYG presentation of the document on paper.

If any explanation is needed, keep it very brief and to the point. An introductory statement at the head of the procedure can often be helpful, especially if the procedure dovetails with others.

Figure 10.4. An Example Procedure for Procedures Using Notes® Release 3.x

---

systems or to formalize communication mechanisms is taken. A number of studies of the effects on user attitudes of introducing information technology into organizations have been undertaken, among which is one by Grudin (1994) specifically concerned with groupware. Although Grudin's work was concerned with the problems of groupware re-engineering in business in general, rather than with software development groups in particular, his conclusions still carry weight. They provide a vital checklist of criteria against which the likelihood of success of a suite of Notes® databases could be judged, and they can be summarized as follows:

- **Tangible benefits:** People are always reluctant to use anything new, especially if it involves extra work, unless they can clearly see the benefit. This, of course, may accrue to

Information Documents

What about all of the assumed knowledge that the procedures themselves do not describe? This is where information documents are involved. When you draft your procedure, ask yourself what knowledge this assumes. Once you have completed your draft, compose any explanatory documents that management and trainees will find useful in understanding the procedure in the Descriptions and Help Library Database. Such a document can then be pasted as an icon into a procedure following a prompt, written in blue Times New Roman bold text to distinguish it from the black Helvetica 10 point text of the procedure itself. Use the following procedure:

1. Compose your document in the Descriptions and Help Library Database.

2. Press Edit, then Make Doclink.

3. Save the document and leave the database, returning to your procedure.

4. Press CNTL E to put the document into edit mode, and type a prompt into the procedure at the appropriate place, such as:

   For more information about the widgets, double-click here →

5. Move the cursor to one or two spaces past the arrowhead and press CNTL V or Edit then Paste. A document icon will appear.

6. Highlight your prompt, press Text, then Font, then select Times New Roman 12 point bold, and blue.

7. Save the revised procedure and leave the database.

Figure 10.5. An Example Procedure for Information Documents Using Notes® Release 3.x

others rather than themselves, rubbing salt into the wound. An example would be the use of a change control database requiring data entry effort from programmers, but where the immediate prime beneficiaries could well be their successors.

- **Getting everyone involved:** Many groupware applications depend critically for their success on everyone participating, so unless this can be achieved, the project will flounder. An example would be a database that records the current state of a project; this would only be useful if everyone on the team uses it.

- **Changing old habits**: The dynamics of relationships within a software engineering team and complex and subtle. People adapt to each other on the basis of shared assumptions and conventions of behavior which may be deeply affected by introducing some aspects of a process technology. Such technology cannot possess this kind of knowledge.

- **Human flexibility**: We have already noted how dumb computers are compared with the almost limitless resourcefulness and flexibility of human mental processes. If the groupware system's lack of flexibility demands the input of an inordinate amount of data to accommodate real life situations on anything more than the rarest of occasions, it will not succeed.

- **Being part of the woodwork**: Some characteristics of a groupware system will be used constantly while others only rarely. In the latter case, if these features require a great deal of learning, which then atrophies through long periods of disuse, these features will never, in fact, be used.

- **Evaluating the system's effectiveness**: There are no reliable systems yet available for measuring the success of process support technology. In-built metrics can sometimes be collected, but their usefulness has yet to be proven. For this reason, it is difficult to generalize about the effectiveness of groupware. Make sure, therefore, that what you develop is exactly tailored to your own organization's needs.

- **Get the requirements clear**: Unlike CASE tools, where the developers of the tools have a clear idea of what the tool must do, and therefore do not need to know the detailed requirements of every potential user, developers of groupware need to understand the requirements of the user organization in great detail, and must not rely solely on intuition.

Grudin has also arrived at many penetrating insights into the effects that the introduction of groupware can have in enterprises, especially those largely characterised by a hierarchical or autocratic structure, and into the human behaviour that can limit or destroy their effectiveness. His comparisons of groupware with both traditional, organisation-wide transactional systems on the one hand, and single user, desktop products on the other, is especially instructive, since groupware shares some common features with both types of computing, while being quite distinct from either. His work will amply repay careful study.

A POSSIBLE ALTERNATIVE APPROACH

Although no examples are to be seen just yet, an *intranet* may offer a more cost-effective medium for documentation in the smaller company. Intranets are created by applying the technology of the Internet World Wide Web to a internal company network. With a web server and web clients connected together, documents and graphics can be posted on the server using hypertext markup language (HTML), providing the essential feature of a centralized documentation repository. It is easy and cheap, and the web browser provides users with a single interface through which all applications may be run. However, the hidden costs of actually developing a central document database subject to the disciplines of configuration management with adequate security may be much greater than is apparent. The tendency of such arrangements to degenerate into anarchy because of the ease with which information can be posted would need to be fiercely resisted through careful network management. The announcement in May 1996 of the *Domino* and *Domino II* products, which turn a Notes® server into an Internet application server and allow web clients to compose, change and delete documents in Notes® databases confirms Lotus' own appreciation of the trend towards web technology.

PROJECT MANAGEMENT DOCUMENTATION

Notes® databases are well suited to facilitating the project management process. For example, in several small companies, the minutes of all project review meetings are recorded in a discussion database, from which comments and suggestions are elicited from the team as a whole. The speed at which this information is disseminated has freed the flow of information and improved the quality of the process. A set of discussion databases can be established for larger projects, each covering a different aspect. These databases can either be very simple, in which case they can be constructed easily and quickly by simply modifying the template examples provided as part of the Notes® package. More complex databases simulating a workflow scenario and linked perhaps with electronic mail obviously take a little longer to develop, but can be highly cost-effective.

SOFTWARE LIFE CYCLE DOCUMENTATION

Throughout this book an attempt has been made to show that documentation ought not to be regarded as an onerous adjunct to the software development process. In a well-controlled engineering environment, life cycle documentation is and should always be thought of as the very lifeblood of the process. It provides the documentary evidence that the process is indeed in control and that there is a realistic chance of the right product emerging with an appropriately low level of residual defects, at a cost which when sold at a price the market will stand and in the projected quantities will leave the organization with a healthy profit.

What documents ought to be generated during the life cycle? Figure 10.6 illustrates those that should be featured in all well-managed software development processes. However, few companies at the low levels of the Capability Maturity Model are capable of migrating to this standard overnight. In the meantime, the creation as an interim step of the following sextet set of documents, which is the absolute minimum for exercising a basic modicum of control, has much to recommend it:

1. User requirements/functional requirements specification

2. System design specification

3. Structured test plan(s)

4. Source code

5. Installation document

6. User manual

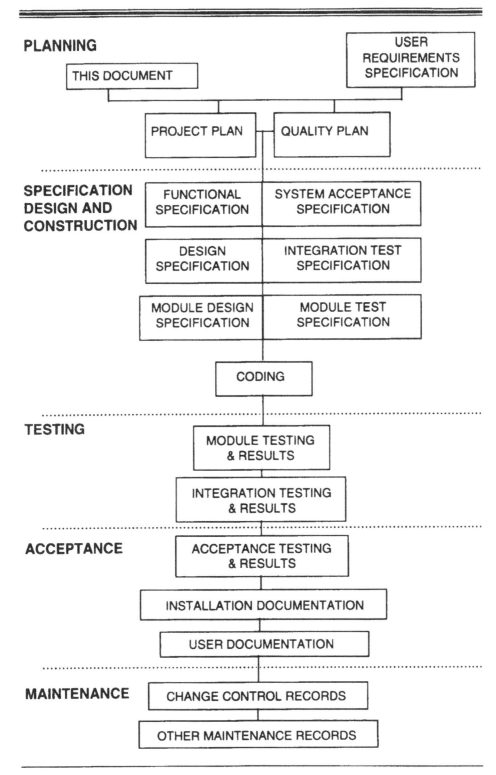

Figure 10.6. Software Life Cycle Documentation

In some companies, the installation document and user manuals are combined; in others, the user requirements and functional requirements may be combined for many projects. The essential point is that these elements should be present in the documentation however it is arranged.

<table>
<tr><td>Keep It

Simple</td><td>**Practical Guidance**

Create a document describing the company's software development life cycle approach (how we develop software around here) and the documents it produces, which prove to us that we really are in control of the process.</td></tr>
</table>

DOCUMENT CONTROL

If documents are to perform their intended role and if the various potential authors are to contribute consistent material, they must all have access to and abide by a defined documentation standard. One such standard in the context of SOPs (i.e., the SOP template in appendix 5) has been alluded to already. However, there should also be a general standard for the layout, style and numbering of all life cycle documents. (The *contents* of each of the life cycle documents themselves have already been addressed in separate standards). The standard should require the inclusion of a contents list or summary, an issue date and a revision code, and a summary of the changes made at each revision. Prior to the formal issue of a document, it ought to be labelled as a draft and identified sequentially (e.g., as A, B, and so on), and then by a new and different nomenclature when issued (say 1.0, 2.0, or some other scheme).

Document issue in a small company may be handled very informally, but in a larger concern, there should be a formal, but simple, document issue procedure which should involve the following five steps:

<table>
<tr><td>Keep It

Simple</td><td>**Practical Guidance**

Create a life cycle documentation standard describing the layout, style, and numbering schemes for both drafts and formal issues of life cycle documents.</td></tr>
</table>

1. Updating the document history.

2. Updating a master index* of documents (lists the reference number, title and issue status of each life cycle document).

3. Opening and updating a document circulation register*.

4. Issuing a document transmittal notice* with each controlled copy (designed to ensure superseded versions are destroyed, an action which the recipient confirms as having taken place by signing and returning the notice).

5. Writing the controlled copy number on the document.

Examples of some of these(*) can be found in the GAMP guide (1996).

Much of this may strike the reader as being appallingly bureaucratic. The truth to which it really testifies is the capability of the medium to obstruct the message—to the drawbacks of paper as an information medium and the cumbersome labour-intensive practices required to address these limitations. The withdrawal of documents and ensuring the destruction of superseded versions is a major headache in big organizations. In several such enterprises, an electronic document presentation medium, either Notes® or perhaps one of the more sophisticated document management packages now on the market (*Documentum*® and *PC DOCS*® are being reviewed by some organizations), is being adopted to avoid much of this effort. In smaller companies, the Notes® approach seems to be more cost-effective in the short term than the document management packages seem to be. Once again, a careful assessment of each of the options for cost-effectiveness, and suitability within the company culture, is absolutely indispensible before any final commitment should be made to any document management package.

DOCUMENT REVIEW

Documents must be formally reviewed to ensure their fitness for use as the basis for the next stage of the life cycle. The review itself might simply be one individual's inspection in a small company. In a larger firm, however, the procedure of inspection outlined in chapter 5 in the context of source code can be easily applied to any life cycle document as was emphasized there. Prior to formal review, the document is entirely the author's responsibility; after review it comes under collective responsibility.

Keep *It*

Simple

> ## Practical Guidance
>
> Create a procedure describing how documents are to be formally reviewed, how these are to be minuted, and how defects are to be reported, corrected and subsequently fed back into process improvement reviews.

There should be a formal review procedure which requires each document to be endorsed by an approval signature, together with a description of the approver's responsibility or qualification to review.[2] Finally, there should be a requirement for quality assurance to approve that the necessary controls set in place to mitigate risk have been observed, and to confirm that the document really is the sure foundation it is intended to be, and on which further work and investment can be securely based.

This is much easier to implement in a Notes® environment than trying to enforce it with paper. It is easy to set up fields to record, say, the last 10 changes to a document, comprising the name of editor (automatic), the date and time of edit (automatic), and a summary of the change (to be entered manually by the author in a text field). A signature field or button can be configured which only certain named individuals (who may be named on the button face) are able to "press" to signify approval. The meanings of the respective signatures should be documented in the quality policy outlined in chapter 5. Once a simple workflow template has been set up, it can be copied, modified and extended. The recent release 4 of Notes® has made many of these tasks easier than was the case in the earlier 3.x releases, though some of the terminology has altered slightly.

In most of the best companies, there is a formal document change control system in place. It need not be complex at all. It is simply a standard that defines who is in charge of technical control of which documents (which may be the same individuals as defined

Keep *It*

Simple

> ## Practical Guidance
>
> Include in the quality policy a definition of the meanings of the respective signatures required on documents (who may approve what and when).

above in the quality policy, and the two pieces of information may be combined). It should also define who checks the quality, and then who implements the changes (which may be someone else entirely for some documents). These needs are clarified as the document control standard is established.

Finally, a common source of error is a lack of coordination between software changes and documentation changes. For example, when a change in functionality is made in the software and a new release is issued, does a revised manual automatically follow? There must be a strict procedure to cover this to avoid users having defective or inconsistent information about the product. Many firms slip up over this, some from a cheese-paring attitude of economy if only a small portion of the manual is now out of date. A number of companies are overcoming this with the use of loose-leaf ring binders for their user manuals, so that individual pages (endorsed with the software revision number and date as footnote text) may be changed and mailed, a practice common with traditional, mainframe vendors for many years.

Keep It *Simple*

Practical Guidance
Institute a document control policy by writing down who is in technical charge of what documents, how the documents are to be composed (templates) and reviewed, who checks the quality, who implements the change, and who maintains the consistency between software changes and document changes.

Other firms are subsuming the document control practices with the overall approach of configuration management, of which it is a part (since each life cycle document is an *item* in configuration management parlance). It has been included here to make it clear what is needed. The name attached to the approach is less important than the reality of the control.

USER MANUALS IN USER EDUCATION

The quality of help text was discussed in chapter 8, wherein a plea was entered for the text to be thoroughly vetted for suitability and comprehensibility in relation to the needs of the novice user before the product is released. Many companies are now acknowledging the fact that many computer users today, like the population in many countries at large, are not in the habit of reading books, having grown up in the television age of visual stimuli. As a result, on-line help text has supplanted the printed user manual and the latter is fast becoming superfluous. While the considerable strength of this point of view is recognized, the history of computing has much to teach us about the value of a good printed manual.

In the 1970s and 1980s, users of large, proprietary systems were accustomed to receiving a large set of well-written manuals along with the system. These frequently amounted to 10–20 volumes, each loose-leafed in a 1-inch binder. The Hewlett Packard manuals of that era, for example, were absolutely superb, being particularly skillfully drafted not only with clear, straightforward, illustrated explanations of what were very complex systems, but in the manner of a stepwise tutorial, which constituted a course in computing in its own right! Such was the quality of these documents that many system managers without any prior experience of the digital computer were able to derive an adequate level of knowledge and competence through the study of these manuals alone. If money was not restricted, this study could be supplemented by residential courses, the two together being capable of providing an in-depth expertise with these systems.

It is regrettable to see how far short of these standards most of the user manuals for today's systems fall, written in poor English on the assumption that if a complex idea is just defined, and no more, then that in itself is a substitute for an explanation. Users who in frustration and contempt consign their manuals of useless and confusing jargon to the trash can/wastepaper bin and reach for the telephone testify to the failure of the software production process, since these calls, like most of those received by the help desk, are in one way or another an indicator of the *absence* of quality. This absence can just as easily arise from the printed manual as the software itself, both of which are part of the product. Why are companies prepared to spend 10 times as much money on support desk overhead than would be required to engage a gifted author to write the user documentation?

It is vital to appreciate that a basic, tutorial primer is totally different from a list of answers to frequently asked questions, as any qualified educator will verify. Computer software is a complex product that cannot be simplified using the vernacular. There are technical terms involved that require a clear and full explanation, enabling the novice to move by *small, incremental steps* from his or her present state of relative ignorance of the subject to that of in-depth, computer-literate competency. To assume that this will some-how happen through a few calls to the help desk is naive and hopelessly unrealistic.

My plea to software houses, therefore, is to re-evaluate the place of the user manual and to invest imaginatively by employing a first-class author to assemble a comprehensive tutorial text that fully explains every aspect of the software. It will require a glossary of terms and call for applied study on the part of the user. The ma-jor advantage for the software house, however, is that once this valuable resource is established, reliance is no longer placed on sup-port personnel who may not have the verbal skills to impart this knowledge through telephone conversation. Understanding a sub-ject oneself and being able to put it across to others are two quite different things, as all of us who can still remember our school days will testify. Instead, callers to the help desk can be given a brief an-swer, and then referred to the full story in the manual that every user will possess. This may sound like an old-fashioned approach, but for learning purposes, the written, printed word that can be studied at the user's own pace at work, or at home, is matchless. Furthermore, the physical presentation of a loose leaf book permits the display of two adjacent pages of text and illustrations simulta-neously with the screen presentation of the product itself; this arrangement is far easier to use than switching between the prod-uct and a single screen's worth of text. It is important to use tech-nology sensitively.

To some readers, the advocacy of paper-based manuals may seem to be a contradiction to what was advocated earlier about the advantages of electronic documentation. In fact, there really is no contradiction whatsoever, in that the circumstances for study and learning are quite distinct from those of record keeping and infor-mation sharing among trained personnel. Let us keep *horses for courses*, selecting the medium, the style and the level of detail of the written word to be appropriate for the needs of the reader.

SOFTWARE REPLICATION

Once the final, released version of the source code and supplemen-tary documentation, such as installation information, licences and user manuals, are ready for distribution, the software replication process comes into play. Replication is just another type of documentation task, but requires careful control since most software products typically consist of a multiplicity of executable files and dynamically linked libraries, all of which may well have existed in a number of developing versions, each contributing to a series of internal builds of which only the final is intended for delivery to the customer as the public release.

The configuration management system must clearly list in detail which version of each of the component items in a release has been issued. This is frequently represented under a software build number which is designated as a particular release. There must be a strict system recording which customers have received which release and when so that support may be effectually provided. There should then be a formal procedure describing how the software suite is to be replicated and how the media (discs or CD-ROM) are to be labelled. This must include virus sweeping of purchased discs, and how the manual version numbers and those of other documentation are to be coordinated with the software release number.

The virus sweeping procedure should include a formal log to record that each disc was clean prior to dispatch. The background to this is explained more fully in chapter 13, but its importance is emphasized here, since these records could be critical in the event of legal action from customers alleging virus-contaminated distribution discs or other media.

If the vendor does not intend to install the software personally, but distribute it through commercial channels, there should be a concession procedure by which the customer can verify that what was received is what was intended to be shipped, and can inform the vendor at once of any nonconformity. The installation procedure should include some simple checks to ensure that installation was achieved successfully, and report this back to the vendor so that support arrangements can be established. This is especially important where hardware requirements are especially demanding and where there is a good chance that software might be installed on unsuitable, unsupportable hardware platforms. There should also

Keep It Simple	# Practical Guidance
	Establish a virus sweeping procedure for software distribution media including the formal logging system.

be instructions (or at least recommendations) on how to back up the software at the customer site. If, on the other hand, the vendor performs the installation, there must be a procedure to establish how access to the customer site and the systems already there is to be obtained, and how successful installation is to be verified. Since every such site will be different, any such procedure ought to be confined to general guidance only of what to check, and what pitfalls to avoid.

Keep It

Simple

Practical Guidance
Create a software replication procedure describing how software and its attendant documentation is to be copied and distributed, including a list of what should be included in the box (if not installed by the vendor), how it is to be identified, and how successful installation at the customer site is to be confirmed.

Attention should also be given to copyright issues and the prevention of illegal copying and piracy. Many firms are now using devices known as *dongles,* a piece of firmware incorporated into a loop-back connector fitted to one of the ports of the computer that the software is designed to read when commencing to execute. Each copy of the software is delivered with its own dongle, each encoded with a unique identifier corresponding in some way to the replication number of the software and hard coded into it. Illegal copying of the software is, thereby, rendered a fruitless exercise. There is clearly an overhead cost involved both in the acquisition and distribution of dongles and in the increased complexity of the replication process, which prevents the strategy from being cost-effective unless the level of piracy becomes especially severe.

While the issues surrounding backups of released software will be discussed in chapter 12, the next chapter will focus on the related areas of software version control, change control and software/record archival.

Notes

1. "A picture is worth a thousand words!"

2. Although the cleaners, who visit the office each evening, are probably quite charming people and would willingly sign any life cycle document if asked, they are probably not *technically* qualified to do so!

11

Change Control and
Archival Policies

Change and decay in all around I see.

H. F. Lyte

THE NEED FOR CHANGE CONTROL

Software products rarely stand still unless they have become senile or retired. They are subject to constant change, both during development and after release into the marketplace. Indeed, a measure of iteration around the various stages of the life cycle is expected, and can arise either from errors in the process or changes in the user's requirements. After release, there is usually pressure to incorporate enhancements arising from users' greater familiarity with the potential of the product. Unfortunately, change is one of the principal causes of risk and loss in software engineering. It entails rework and configuration changes. It threatens to undermine the carefully planned and ordered progress to which all of the engineering disciplines that the evolving international standards in this sphere have been aspiring. It is to mitigate these evils that the principles and practices inherent in configuration management (ISO 10007) (discussed in chapter 5) are directed and of which change control is a part. Both sources of change—those emanating from within the organization and those from the market—should be subjected to the same change control standards.

THE COWBOY CULTURE

The worst offense which formal change control is intended to avoid is the *quick fix* mentality associated with what has become known as the *cowboy culture*. Although almost all software firms today are blessed with staff of exemplary professionalism, the software industry is still saddled with a number of programmers, many self-employed, contract (as they are known in the United Kingdom) or consultant (as in the United States), who remain openly contemptuous of the discipline inherent in software engineering. They make their living by assisting companies (usually the larger ones) on very short-term assignments to make *just job* changes ("we want you *just* to change this small piece of code"), paying lip service to any formal standards and procedures in order to effect required changes in software in the shortest time and for the highest fee. The shorter the shortcut the better; the more lax the controls on documenting what they have done, the better. The financial and commercial sectors are among the worst affected areas in this regard. Managers who employ such individuals share in the guilt of jeopardizing the well-being of their companies, since the most adverse effects of such irresponsibility are unlikely to emerge immediately. If the key thought process underlying a software change has not been documented and defects have crept in, how can the knot be unraveled long after the quick fixer has hurriedly departed to greener pastures? While the short-term thinking implicit in this kind of attitude is thoroughly reprehensible, it is, from another point of view, understandable since the average longevity for data processing managers to remain in their position is only three years. The most careful vetting of all temporary contract/consultant programming staff is to be strongly advocated, with the accompanying suggestion that it is in the long-term interests of every software house to confine its recruitment to permanent employees, committed in the long term to the business and its reputation, as far as possible.

ELEMENTS OF CHANGE CONTROL

Although it would be fair to say that configuration management is a term widely misunderstood (or dare it be said, not understood *at all*) within a large proportion of the software industry, the term *change control* is something most people do understand. Termed configuration control in IEEE parlance (ANSI 828, paragraphs 3.3.2 ff.), change control practice cannot exist in isolation. It depends for its success on the identification and numbering of all of the individual items which make up the complex tapestry of software development. It addresses the actual procedures that use these identifiers to track changes, not only in the item to be immediately changed but in all of the consequential changes that logically follow from it in other items but which, because of the frailty of human nature, frequently get overlooked in a chaotic or unstructured process. It is here that many errors creep in.

Successful change control has five components:

1. A formal way of registering the need for change and so initiating the process

2. Some management approval system for regulating the number of changes

3. A record system to analyze the status of changes and trends

4. Formal procedures that measure the cost and timetables of changes

5. Configuration management controls to track actual changes against the requests that generated them

There are four stages of activity in effecting change in a controlled way:

1. Recording the request for a change

2. Deciding what to do about it (including to reject the request)

3. Making the change(s)

4. Verifying the change has been made as intended and approving it

A typical change control procedure with specimen forms can be found in the GAMP guide (1996).

The reader should notice a parallel between these four steps and the life cycle itself. The steps mirror the life cycle in microcosm and dictate, for example, that the necessary testing that should be deployed to verify the successful implementation of the change be thoroughly defined and documented before the code is touched. For changes that are not trivial (and this decision should not be taken thoughtlessly), there should be a change plan. Like a mini project plan and a mini quality plan, it addresses the costing and timetable estimates (the project part of this micro life cycle) needed to ensure that the change is effected on time and within budget, and the controls to ensure that quality has not been compromised. In accordance with the principles of documentation that have been espoused, the change control procedure should require the initial completion of a form (paper or electronic), an example of which appears in figure 11.1, which now seems to be fairly standard for change control procedures generally.

The form features two sets of numbers that must be tracked if change control is to be achieved. The first of these, the Database Request Number, introduces the need for a *support database* in which all defects and enhancement requests should be logged. All vendors today seem to establish such a database. There are several now on the market from which a choice can be made; *Quetzal* is one widely used successfully, supplemented by one of the commonly available reporting modules such as those produced by *Crystal*. There are many others, though very small software houses seem to favor developing their own, usually using the tools provided by Microsoft Access®. Decisions of this kind seem primarily driven by cost, though one has to wonder whether the *reinvention of the wheel* (figure 11.2) that this effectively represents is really cost-effective.

The important principle at work here is the assignment of a unique reference to every such request. Once the request has been logged, its disposition is decided by management as either approval for progression or rejection. If the latter, a reason should be recorded under Comment and the form then filed for the shelf life of the product. If the request is approved, then in the course of implementation, it should be given a change number. This number should then appear in all source code that is changed under this request, and cross-referenced to the database record that originated it. There will frequently be a one-to-many relationship between the

REQUEST FOR CHANGE

Database Change No: Date: Initiated by:

Product or file(s) to be changed:

Proposed change(s):

Rationale:

Required by:

AUTHORIZATION & DISPOSITION

Disposition: **Approved for Progression / Rejected**

Comment

Signature: Position: Date:

Signature: Position: Date:

Signature: Position: Date:

CHANGE DETAILS

Actual changes required:

Change numbers:

Implemented in build number:

APPROVAL & COMPLETION

Completed by: Position: Date:

Approved by: Position: Date:

Approved by: Position: Date:

Figure 11.1. A Typical Change Control Request Form

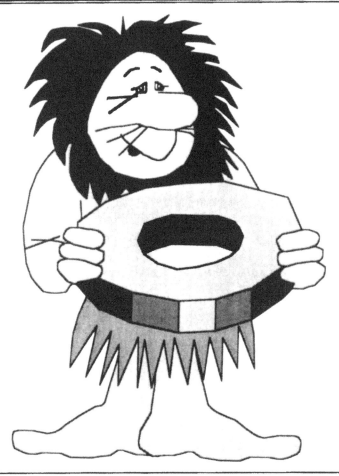

Figure 11.2. Reinventing the Wheel

one database request number (the cause) and a set of change numbers (the effect) arising from it, each number perhaps representing a consequential change on a different file/library or set of these. The auditor should inspect the system to ensure that changes in the source code can be traced back to the originating request in the support database, as a demonstration of a controlled and effective customer-centered approach.

PRIORITIZATION

In most organizations, change requests seem to arise, like the proverbial buses in London, in *convoys*, especially in the early days after initial major releases (dare the suggestion be made that the process is not all that it might be?). There is a pressing need to sort these into a priority order, not only to deal with critical changes in preference to cosmetic ones, but also to combine related changes together to reduce the final number of software changes involved.

Keep It Simple	**Practical Guidance**
	Create a document describing the process and the criteria by which change requests are prioritized in the organization.

The justification for such an aspiration is that every change is not only expensive but risky, and the need should, therefore, be minimized. How much more successful would a software house be if there were no errors to fix, thus releasing 100 percent of the programmers' time from cost-increasing support to profit-generating new development?

Efficient change request systems being operated in a Notes® environment may frequently be seen today. The change requests are typically routed around the managers as a simple workflow application and stored long term in the database. The change requests for each product can then be viewed independently, and sorted in any number of ways, even though they may have originated haphazardly.

DOCUMENTATION CHANGES

There are many software houses where software changes have been meticulously managed and traced back to the source, but where the

Keep It Simple	**Practical Guidance**
	Create a document describing the company's change control procedure including all steps from inception in the support database to final archival of the completed approved change, making sure actual software changes can be unambiguously traced right back to source request, and that all life cycle documents have been updated accordingly.

documentation relating to the product has remained unchanged. First, there is the need to update early life cycle documents, such as functional specifications and design specifications, with traceability features strictly enforced, to reflect the changes. Second, and of more importance to users, is the updating of the user documentation. The result of failure in this department is that unsuspecting novice users are initiated to a product and discover inconsistencies between obsolescent user manuals or help text and current software functionality. The use of loose leaf binders to cut the cost of documentation updates has already been recommended. However, the change control procedure should include or refer to specific steps to review, update and distribute updated documentation together with software changes. This leads naturally to the question of a version control policy.

VERSION CONTROL

However rapidly the functionality of a software product is changing, there must be a documented standard describing the criteria which determines when a new version is to be released.

Keep It Simple	**Practical Guidance** Create a document describing the company's version control policy defining the criteria dictating a major release, a minor release and an emergency release.

In most software houses, a stream of builds is taking place, as one change request after another is processed. After a time, a decision must be made as to when a version release cutoff point has been reached. This version control *policy* document defines what will constitute a major release, what will constitute a minor release, and what circumstances will warrant an emergency release.

Coupled with this will be a version control *procedure*. This will describe the steps needed to ensure that all of the cumulative changes made since the last release are being gathered so that as soon as a version release decision is made, a list of all these cumulative changes can be frozen and recorded for support purposes. It will also describe how document and media revisions are to be disseminated to customers. Version release documentation should include under the version release number a description of the changes made since the previous release, the change release media, any changes in the documentation, any changes to support software, installation instructions, and faults that have not been repaired in this release.

Version control is much easier to achieve if each successive build of the software is regarded as a *baseline*, a central concept of configuration management introduced in chapter 5 and illustrated by figure 5.4 on page 128. Each baseline (build) serves as the basis for further development, with a running systematic record being maintained of all of the changes incorporated into each build from its predecessor. Between each baseline, there may be a number of variants on the previous baseline (i.e., incremental changes to its items [source code files or libraries]). Secure on this foundation, the version release process then sits naturally, rather than precipitating a *frantic fumble* to cobble together all of the change information from a number of uncoordinated sources. A tight tracking system for build numbers is thus implied, showing every file that has changed, a list of its variant change numbers and its new version number, and enabling a report to be generated that details every individual change to each source code file and library from one build to another.

There are many examples of electronic configuration management systems of this type working well, and very cost-effectively, throughout the industry. However, the situation is immensely complicated in some firms who undertake to make changes to released product for the sake of *individual customers*, a situation briefly discussed in chapter 4 in the context of version support. This blurring of the distinction between being a package supplier on the one hand and a bespoke system house on the other bestows many griefs. It results in the actual number of released versions, along with their attendant support costs being hugely increased. It magnifies the complexity of the strict recording mechanisms designed to ensure that the exact version of each item received by each customer is known with certainty. Companies tempted to succumb to these pressures must have a very clear appreciation of the very different business finance models implied by the two contrasting approaches to software development and release. This is not always the case, and is aggravated by the fact that the transition from one model to the other can occur stealthily,[1] each customer's specific demands being conceded incrementally without anyone calling a halt and demanding a rigorous long-term budgetary reassessment and costing. In the pressure of running furiously in order to stand still, management can only begin to recognize the fundamental change that has occurred in the nature of the business when the financial chickens come home to roost. It is much to be regretted that a failure to understand these realities has already led to the demise of several software houses (caricatured by figure 11.3). Package software houses, beset by individual users beseeching them to make specific product changes which do not have a clear place in the strategic vision for the product's future, are well advised to avoid this temptation assiduously at all costs.

Keep It **Simple**

Practical Guidance
Create a document describing the company's version control procedure (what we do when we have decided to issue a new release, and how we coordinate document changes with source code changes).

SOURCE CODE ACCESS CONTROL

Some of the benefits of electronic source code control systems in the context of enforcing the inclusion of header information have already been mentioned in chapter 8. However, the principal benefit afforded by these systems is the security given to source code, both in terms of who can access it and in ensuring that not more than one authorized programmer at a time has write access to it. This assumes considerable importance in the larger organization, where a team of programmers are continually working on the same suite of files. Many companies, however, have yet to implement control systems and are still handling files using only operating system utilities, which do not provide security provisions beyond ordinary network file and directory handling facilities.

Whatever is the case, there is a general recognition that the source code is one of the most precious assets of the company and must be rigorously safeguarded. There should be a simple document within the quality management system which describes the company's approach to source code access and who is authorized to

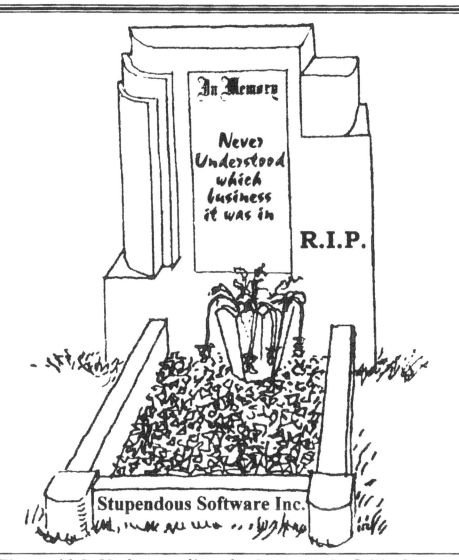

Figure 11.3. Understanding the Business Is Critical
(adapted from an original illustration by John Piper in Church Poems by John Betjeman and published by John Murray, London, © 1981—see acknowledgments)

make changes. In some companies, these provisions are included in the change control documentation, but they must appear in one form or another. The assessment team must try to ascertain whether the documented controls actually work in practice; one of the best ways is to ask the programmers themselves!

<table>
<tr><td>Keep *It*

Simple</td><td>**Practical Guidance**

Create a document describing the source code security measures in place (who may access code, how unauthorized access is inhibited, and how access is systematically controlled and recorded).</td></tr>
</table>

ARCHIVAL POLICIES AND PROCEDURES

Sooner or later in most companies, the need arises for software life cycle and project documents, which are no longer required on the live systems, to be removed permanently. Many companies have been able to postpone the need to do this in recent years because of the precipitate fall in the cost of hard disc storage media. However, the penalty is reaped in the increased capacity required in backup media, and in file systems becoming more cumbersome than they need be.

It is important to clarify at this point the distinction between backup and archiving, which is frequently misunderstood. Archiving is the removal of obsolete information that is unlikely to be required again, but which must be kept for legal or commercial reasons and must be accessible within a reasonable time related to the likelihood of it ever being required. It may need to be readable many years hence. Backup, on the other hand, is the routine copying of current information on disc storage for protection against catastrophe or any other kind of contingency. The media are reused frequently and thus the information is only required to be readable for a very short time.

The first issue that must be raised here is the stability of the media. Many organizations are creating archives on media whose longevity is likely to be less than the expected period of storage. Magnetic tape has a relatively short life, measured in months, during which the integrity of the information can be guaranteed, especially when stored in less than ideal conditions. The alternating magnetic fields on the surface of the tape are vulnerable to degradation, degrading and being in turn degraded by fields on adjacent winding layers, a phenomenon known as *print through*. The problem may be minimized firstly by storage under controlled conditions of temperature and humidity (there are commercial firms who provide this service) and secondly by the periodic respooling of the tapes to alter the relative positioning of each segment. This is not only laborious and expensive; since the media are usually out of sight and, therefore, also out of mind, it is hardly surprising that the chore is often neglected. For these reasons, it is strongly recommend that for archival records, magneto-optical, CD-ROM or WORM[2] devices, which have effectively indefinite lives under ambient storage conditions (as far as is currently known), are used exclusively for this purpose. The recent fall in the price of writeable CD devices has been a welcome development in this connection, alleviating the primary obstacle of expense.

The second issue, of less importance today, is the availability of hardware to read back the archives when required. This problem is especially acute in government circles. In the United Kingdom, the papers of the Cabinet are retained in secrecy for 30 years before being opened for public scrutiny at the Public Records Office in Kew, London. All the while such records were wholly confined to paper, there was never any doubt over subsequent readability. But the advent of computerization has caused archivists some alarm since if nothing is done, software and hardware systems will have been replaced 2 or 3 times over by newer technology by the time the 30 years has expired. This means that some electronic data may be lost forever. A conference to address these issues was convened in Brussels by the European Union at the end of 1996 to explore practical ways of dealing with this. The backward compatibility being designed into hardware and operating systems has ameliorated a problem that caught many companies unaware in the days of proprietary operating systems. It still represents a difficulty for companies holding data from such systems for 10 years or more, who are obliged to retain standby obsolete systems for regulatory or legal reasons. The matter is exacerbated by the diminution of knowledge which inevitably occurs as operators and system managers move

Keep *It* Simple	**Practical Guidance**
	Create a document describing what records and files are to be archived, how this is to be carried out and the media to be used, the expected storage period, and the procedures for periodically confirming accessibility and readability.

on; in-house expertise is lost and must be contracted in with a corresponding rise in maintenance costs. The UK National Radiological Protection Board recently precipitated a crisis by proposing to scrap their database of health records of military veterans because of the costs of maintaining it.

These problems may be expected to diminish with the DOS– and Windows™-based records of today, because of the cheapness and ubiquity of the operating systems, and the tendency to incorporate backward compatibility. However, the possibility of non-readability should not be ignored or dismissed. For companies with archived records in storage, there should be an annual review of the recovery situation and a practical test of the readability of samples of critical data.

MOVING ON

The subject of out-of-date records seems an appropriate note on which to conclude the second part of this book, where issues specifically applicable to the software engineering process have been addressed. An attempt has been made to address all the key aspects of both project management and the software development life cycle. The desire has been to share with the reader those practices and approaches that have been found to be not only consistent with the international standards, but to deliver the financial and quality benefits that attend compliance to them. It is to be hoped that both software vendors, and auditors who visit them, will find value in these insights, to the benefit of developers and purchasers alike.

Having addressed the software process then, the auditor now needs to pay some attention to the environment in which it is conducted. Although separate, the two cannot be totally separated, since the facilities bear testimony to management attitudes in various other ways. It is also important for the auditor to arrive at an assessment of other risks the vendor enterprise may face that could have an impact on the likelihood of its remaining in business to continue to support the product. It is to these issues that attention will be focused in chapter 12.

Notes

1. A principle known as *the inevitability of gradualness,* the most gruesome example of which seems to be that of the frog. Dropped into a bowl of boiling water, it is likely to jump out, quite sensibly, with alacrity. Placed, however, in a bowl of cold water which is then slowly raised to boiling point, the same frog is alleged to remain, accommodating itself to the conditions, until it is too late!

2. Write Once Read Many

Part 3

Environment, Assessment and Future

12

Managing the Development Environment

Computer users are divided into two groups—those that have lost data and those that are about to.

Anon

The core of this book has been devoted to the engineering principles and practical measures involved in creating software fit for its intended purpose. However, this is not the sum total of the purchaser's concern. The issue of software quality is one component of a broader question, the ability of the software supplier to provide a business solution and support it over its intended application lifetime. Some of these issues have already been alluded to in chapter 3. One area not addressed hitherto is the environment in which the software is developed, namely the computer facilities and their management, and it is to this area that the auditor now needs to direct attention.

COMPUTER FACILITIES

The proper management of the computer facilities is not a matter of prime concern to programmers unless there is evidence of mismanagement. This may emerge in a host of ways, from the trivial, such as temporary shortage of disc space, to the catastrophic, such as total loss of a drive. No software development project can continue successfully unless there is complete assurance that the central computers are totally dependable.

There are certain key, routine tasks involved in the running of any computer facility, including the backup of data (which will be considered in detail in a moment), the repair of defective hardware components, and the maintenance of the air conditioning plant. The role of SOPs in ensuring that these routine tasks are performed correctly is just as basic in this area as in the software development arena itself. Yet there are very few sites, other than the most prestigious, where there are any written procedures governing practice here. The pernicious results are just the same, with the service falling down when key people are absent or leave. However, procedures in hardware management tend to be much more straightforward than their counterparts in the intellectual hothouse of software engineering.

Why, then, are written procedures so rarely to be found? The answer appears to be that people do not believe they are necessary or that they deliver any business benefit. Once again, this delusion is difficult to dispel until things go drastically wrong (as they are bound to do sooner or later) in one respect or another. Only then does it become clear (if anyone is prepared to admit it, which they usually aren't) that the ensuing costs could well have been substantially reduced if preventive maintenance or monitoring had been properly carried out on a regular basis. The hidden unknown or unknowable costs of a chaotic operation cannot be avoided.

Facilities managers are strongly urged to document in a simple and concise style the basic steps involved in all routine maintenance and running of the central computer facility. These should include procedures for any regular changing of cards, reboot procedures, system time changes in spring and autumn, changing of filters in air conditioners or emptying of moisture drainage sumps, loading tapes cartridges into drives, generating system management reports on disc or network usage, or whatever other routine tasks are involved in keeping the facility shipshape.

Keep *It* Simple	**Practical Guidance**
	Create a simple procedure for each of the routine tasks involved in running the central computer facility.

Housekeeping and cleanliness are two other aspects of facilities management that ought not to escape the notice of the visiting auditor. Cleanliness is not quite as critical to the health of disc drives as it used to be, and today's sealed units can operate well for years under quite grubby conditions. If, however, a computer facility looks rather like a rubbish tip or broom cupboard, it betrays attitudes not just of the staff but supremely of the management. In one facility, the central computer room was found to be providing hospitality to two bicycles and an upright vacuum cleaner! Whatever extenuating circumstances may be cited to explain situations such as these, the auditor, as representative of the purchasing company, should not hesitate to make a subjective value judgement on the underlying management attitudes which they suggest.

CHANGE CONTROL

Change is as much of a way of life in a hardware facility as it is in software. There is great benefit in maintaining a simple change control log for management and maintenance purposes for the entire central computer kit. Of most concern is the need to associate any unexpected and apparently inexplicable software behaviour to changes in the computers on which it is being developed. This may assist in the early identification of esoteric software *features* (a polite term for defects which we did not know we had, but now that we do, we do not intend to correct!) thought to have no connection whatsoever with the hardware. Isolation of these features might lead either to changes in code, or to a more circumscribed specification of the particular hardware required to run the system successfully. It is vitally important to avoid abortive effort searching for apparently elusive defects that actually do not exist.

Beyond that, change control records in the computer room can help to identify components with a short lifetime, to discriminate between hardware from different suppliers in terms of quality, and to forestall likely failures and interruptions in service.

<table>
<tr><td>Keep It

Simple</td><td>

Practical Guidance

Create a simple procedure to log all hardware changes and maintenance activities.
</td></tr>
</table>

SYSTEM BACKUP

Among the procedures essential to the safe and secure operation of any computer facility, the procedure for ensuring the timely and comprehensive backup of all data is by far the most important. Of all the resources of a software house, the intellectual property represented by the software and its associated documentation are the only ones that are totally irreplaceable if lost. Everything else— buildings, computer hardware and even people (with all due respect) and skill sets—can be eventually replaced in the event of a catastrophe. Software and the thought process that spawned it are, however, quite unique and once totally lost cannot be re-created.

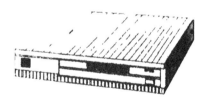

One would have thought that these basic facts of life would be so second nature to everyone in IT today that it would be superfluous, not only to mention them, but also for an auditor to ask pertinent questions about them. The fact is, though, that there are many software houses that take an extremely casual and relaxed attitude to software and documentation backup. Many have no written procedures addressing this activity nor make any managerial effort to ensure backups are being made. In others, backups are made and then left in the same office in a cupboard, ready for the overnight thieves to remove along with all the hardware (though it is usually only microprocessors and memory chips in which burglars are actually interested). Only a small proportion have invested in a fireproof safe which, relatively speaking, is not expensive in relation to the value of the compact items it would actually house and the improved security it would afford to the business.

Even in those companies which do have a backup procedure (seldom documented, regretfully), the protocol being used (the list of files to be saved) is often out of date, not comprehensive, or untimely. Timeliness of the backup is critical to the rate at which files are changing on a system, to enable a systematic restoration from the media in the event of a disaster to recover the latest changes completely.

Backups are normally of two types:

1. Full: where all the files in a directory, a set of directories or folders, or on a physical hard disc or logical drive, are copied

2. Delta or Incremental: where only those files that have changed since the last full backup are copied

The selection between full and incremental backups is dictated not only by which files are changing and how quickly but also by two additional factors. The first is the capacity and data transfer rate of the storage device. The latest devices are becoming so large and fast that many firms are abandoning incremental backups altogether and confining the backup (usually nightly) to a full backup of everything on the server(s). The Hewlett-Packard Colorado T4000S unit, for example, has a capacity of 8 Gb at a recording speed of up to 62 Mbytes per minute on an SCSI-2 interface with 2:1 data compression, or 4 Gb of data on a single uncompressed cartridge. With a typical Pentium® machine, a 1 Gb drive takes about half an hour to back up. This kind of capacity and performance is adequate for most companies. The second factor, intimately related to the first, is the restoration procedure envisaged in the event of a partial or a total loss of the systems from whatever cause. It is of little use having a well-organized backup procedure without a complementary system restoration procedure to accompany it. Each of these procedures will need to concentrate on the files and directories to be restored rather than on the mechanism for carrying each operation out; these are provided by well-documented utilities available with most operating systems and are amply supplemented by stand-alone packages that provide a similar service. Such utilities extend backup provision beyond the desktop to the entire local area network; the best and most widely used of these today appear to be the *ArcServe*® product from Cheyenne Software,[1] and its keen competitor product *Backup Exec*® *for Windows NT* (or *for Netware*) from Seagate Software (formerly Arcada), Lake Mary, Florida. The backing up of documents is just as crucial as source code, but is very often overlooked. Life cycle documents altered under the Change Control procedures should also be included in the backup régime.

Keep It Simple	**Practical Guidance**
	Create a procedure describing how system backups are to be made, the timetable, how the lists of what is to be backed up are to be maintained, and how the media are to be labelled.

Labelling of Media

In most organizations, several sets of backup media (usually high capacity digital audio tapes today) are used for backup. This arises from the fact that a backup is only intended to have a short life, measured in perhaps days or weeks, as opposed to an archive which is intended to be readable for many years. For this reason, metastable media, such as magnetic tape, are quite appropriate for backup operations. Backups and archives are frequently confused in this respect and inappropriate choices of media made—cheap magnetic tape being used for archives or occasionally expensive, writeable CD devices being used for backup. The holding of several sets of media is quite common, so that each set is reused after say three or five backup cycles. A monthly periodicity is to be frequently found, leading to five sets, one for each week or part week of the month.

Keep It Simple	**Practical Guidance**
	Include in the backup procedure detailed instructions as to the unambiguous, clear and robust labelling of backup media.

In these circumstances, it is vital that each and every individual media item be labelled clearly, unambiguously and robustly (since the media is likely to be subjected to considerable handling). The labelling scheme must be devised with the needs of the restoration process very much in mind. It must also be remembered that while most backups are just routine, carried out in a relaxed frame of mind and in the knowledge that the likelihood of the media being needed is low, the reverse is the case with restorations. These often occur in situations of high drama, after the irretrievable loss of data when feelings and sensibilities are running high, and the pressure to recover data is enormous. Calm, reflective, logical thinking is hard for most of us in these situations, where a mistake is capable of compounding the loss. A prepared procedure which addresses every possibility of error in the operation provides an aid to keep one's head when everyone else round about is losing theirs. Testing out the data restoration procedure, perhaps on a loan machine or disc drive, should be part of the periodic disaster recovery drill, as described below.

Quality Control

Quality control in this context is the check to make sure that the backup is being carried out in accordance with the prescribed timetable. This is a business critical activity and should be central to the thinking of any management concerned with the survival of the business. The backup procedure should include the formal signature in a *logbook* (paper or electronic—for example a Notes® form with a simple button recording who did the backup and when) to be entered by the person carrying out the backup. This is caricatured in figure 12.1, intended to demonstrate that meticulous attention to backing up is especially virtuous, since although the job is often viewed as a burdensome chore, it could be the most valuable single action to save the company. This log can be inspected routinely by QA, and failure to conduct the operation, or to record it, should be made a disciplinary offense.

Storage of Media

Media should ideally be taken off the premises as soon as the backup is complete. In some large companies, this is organized by contract with a data storage company, whose van calls at the same time each day to return the oldest set of media and exchange it for the most recent set, hot off the tape drives. These tapes are then

Keep *It*

Simple

Practical Guidance

Include in the backup procedure detailed instructions as to how to log that the backup has just been completed, where the media are to be taken and stored, and who is responsible for this.

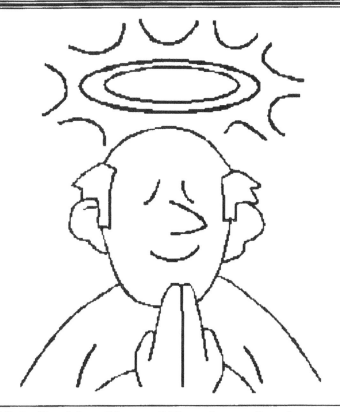

Figure 12.1. Backing Up *and* Keeping a Log!

often stored in a controlled environment, though this is of far more significance for archives than for backups, as we have seen.

The most important principle here is that the media be removed from the site. It is common practice for executives in small companies to take backups home with them. Since the security aspects are not likely to be important, there is no objection in principle to this. However, the location of such off-site backups must be recorded since this is a critical component of our next subject which, like death, is the last subject most software vendors ever talk about but which the auditor must encourage everyone to face full square, and for many this will be for the very first time.

DISASTER RECOVERY OR CONTINGENCY PLANNING

Optimism is a virtue in our fallen world. We all like to believe that tomorrow will be sunny and be free from trouble. It is said that "the sun shines on the righteous", and though this may sometimes be true, the fact is that things can and do go wrong, not just for individuals but for organizations too. One day, sooner or later, trouble will come, and those who have prepared for it are more likely to cope and emerge unscathed (though perhaps chastened) than those who have not. It is within this framework that all organizations, software developers included, should be urged to carry out basic disaster recovery planning.

Contingency planning is by no means confined to large, prestigious companies protecting assets worth hundreds of millions of dollars (or their equivalent). There are some quite small companies that have a neat little *disaster recovery plan*. On the other hand, the situation in a major TickIT-accredited IT organization situated somewhere in Europe, who had excellent procedures, controls, and were exemplary in every respect as a software house, is instructive. After sailing through the team assessment exercise, the delight and pride of everyone involved was conspicuous—until, that is, the question of the disaster recovery plan was raised. An embarrassed silence descended on what up to then had been a convivial and relaxed occasion. Why was there no plan? Why hadn't we ever thought of it? What would we do if *x* happened, or *y*? Within 24 hours, a draft disaster recovery plan had been drawn up, and the company became considerably more secure as a result. It is to be hoped that they will never need it, a sentiment with which they themselves would heartily agree! But they will survive in that event, and now they know exactly *how* they will survive, and why.

What does contingency planning involve? In concept, it is very simple. A small team sits around a table and imagines that the entire company is in ashes around them. Nothing has survived. Situations of differing probability and seriousness are listed. The actions that would then have to be taken to recover business continuity are sketched out. From where would we recover the key files and data (which connects with the backup and restoration procedures mentioned earlier)? From where would we obtain computer hardware? What exactly would be needed? (an up-to-date inventory would be useful for a start!). Where would the disaster recovery plan itself be located? What must be remembered in this context is that while it is easy to think calmly about these issues in the comfortable reassurance that all is well today, when the chips are down, with livelihoods hanging in the balance, and possibly even the bereavement of colleagues to cope with, it is much harder to think strategically. This scenario is not fanciful—it has happened on numerous occasions

Practical Guidance

Create a disaster recovery plan procedure, including regular simulation drills, where the copies of the plan are stored, reports to management of the drills and their outcome.

worldwide, and will happen again. It is this thinking that the disaster recovery plan secures and records.

An excellent aid to disaster recovery planning has been published by Arnold (1988), who has presented a step-by-step guide for a systems or facilities manager to analyse the risks the organization faces, and record the steps that need to be taken in the event of the recognizable and specified contingencies. Use of this book, which is neither long nor expensive, brings the distilled wisdom of a wealth of experience of these issues to the aid of the manager in something approaching a checklist format. Those who have turned to it have found it to be very helpful in handling what is inevitably seen as a chore with pessimistic and dark overtones. It is to be warmly recommended.

The Periodic Drill

Once the plan is in place, it is committed to safe storage in two or more locations and periodically reviewed. How often this occurs varies, though it ought not to be more frequent than at 6 months nor less frequently than at 18 months. The drill simply involves a simulation of the scenario(s) envisaged in the plan. We imagine the catastrophe has occured, and we test out by simulation the procedures we have put in place. Do they still work? Are the media still where we said they were? Can we still obtain *Septium Superfast* desktops and servers from the *Down Your Way Computer Emporium*? If they have since collapsed (like so many hardware suppliers seem to these days, with margins on computer hardware being so wafer thin), what is today's alternative? A simple, roundtable review is conducted, and perhaps a trial restoration of data is made to a temporary server, hired especially for the event. Changes to the plan are made if needed (they usually are), approved under formal revision control, and copies of the revised plan placed in storage while their predecessors are destroyed. A report that the drill was conducted and what the outcome was is passed on to the management.

By this means, the plan is never too obsolete to be credible and the company is far less vulnerable than previously. Thus, the company is more likely to remain in business to support its products, which is one of the prime concerns of users/purchasers, of the vendor and all of the staff, and indeed of the auditor/consultant on behalf of everybody!

Since a hard disc crash is probably the most probable of all disaster scenarios that contingency planning will seek to anticipate, the company would be well advised to at least be aware of the availability of data recovery services should the backup and restoration measures in place finally fail. Such awareness should be very much in the nature of a long stop, since with a disciplined commitment to ensuring the reliability of the established procedures and a professional level of attention to detail, resort to such extremities should never be necessary. The *AuthenTec* company,[2] owned by Alan Solomon of anti-virus fame, is able to recover data from hard discs that have suffered a head crash, where the head has come into contact with the ferric oxide surface spinning a few microns below it, gouging out a section of the disc. The remaining data is likely still to be intact and can be rescued by mounting the platter on a jig, introducing a new head to within the normal tolerance and reading off the data! Another company in this field is *Vogon,* with offices both in the United States, United Kingdom and Germany.

Fire and Flood

Fire protection is essential in any business, and particularly so in the modern office where so much equipment occupies a small area and where the capital funding of the business is often minimal. There should be a periodic inspection by a fire officer and is mandatory in many countries. Notwithstanding, there should be carbon dioxide, Halon or dry powder extinguishers at strategic points in the building, bearing labels showing that they are being inspected at regular intervals under a formal maintenance agreement. The auditor should check and record this.

Flood protection is less critical today unless the company is located in old buildings with overhead services. At one location the central computer room had been drenched on two separate occasions through flange leaks from overhead water pipes! Software development taking place in such environments is, thankfully, increasingly rare today, with software houses generally operating in buildings of relatively recent construction. What cannot be overlooked is the threat of water ingress from a major rainstorm, of which there have been a number of instances in recent years. If the vendor's location is an area where the likelihood of such weather is a reasonable probability, the siting of the company in old buildings, more at risk in these circumstances, should form the subject of adverse comment in the report, especially as so many software houses lease, rather than own, their premises today.

YEAR 2000 COMPLIANCE

This subject, a highly topical potential defect at the time of writing, has been mentioned already in the introduction. All software development houses should incorporate into their programming standards approved approaches to the handling of dates, if such functionality lies within their application area. The auditor should specifically check this item, although the problem will clearly have resolved itself within a few years, since noncompliant software will by then be ostracised within the marketplace.

KEEPING WITHIN THE LAW

Software copyright infringement and outright fraud continues to be a matter of grave concern throughout the entire software industry. The presence of a small minority of pirates marketing bootleg copies of major applications from backstreet outlets, car boots (trunks), through small advertisements, or surreptitiously on the street corner from inside a grubby raincoat sometimes attracts media attention. However, by far the greatest losses of revenue to the industry occur through illicit copying in the commercial and industrial environment. Evidence is mounting of an unwelcome change of attitude in recent months to software piracy on the part of users, with fewer than 1 in 10 now regarding it as theft. Some have alleged that the situation is being exacerbated by the availability of software such as *Netscape* being provided over the Internet free of charge as a *loss leader*, contributing to a dismissive attitude to copyright and the legitimate interests of software authors. Perhaps it is therefore not surprising that the proportion of firms viewing the illegal use of software as theft has fallen to 8 percent, while the number seeing it as just harmless copying has risen to over 50 percent.[3] Nevertheless this is a disgrace, aggravated by the ease with which more copies of a legally purchased application can be installed than the licence agreement authorizes, especially likely under everyday pressures where the licence upgrade process is seen as just another paperwork exercise for which someone else is responsible. The embarrassment suffered by large, prestigious companies inspected for copyright compliance by either internal or external auditors and found to have more copies than their entitlement is hard to overemphasize.

Software vendors find themselves in a unique position in this respect, being vulnerable to the accusation of gross hypocrisy. How hypocritical it is when software companies complaining (rightly) of the infringement and consequential losses from piracy of their own products are found in turn to be committing precisely the same crime with respect to their own suppliers (especially if they support the Federation Against Software Theft)! To avoid this indignity, vendors are recommended take action on two fronts:

1.   Establish a simple procedure to ensure that the installation of packages cannot be carried out until licence upgrade invoices have been obtained and paid for. It is immaterial to whom this task is allocated—quality assurance, support, even finance; the point here is to avoid accidental infringement (much more likely than deliberate piracy) of the law.

2.   The deliberate and illegal internal copying of purchased software should be made a disciplinary offense, as a number of companies have done already. Some have gone so far as to make it a dismissable offense. If there is a clear, effective procedure in place to ensure that licence payments are made, draconian action of this sort should never be necessary. Most people are law abiding by nature in the business environment, and the temptation to behave

---

Keep It

Simple

Practical Guidance
Create a procedure to facilitate the easy upgrading (and payment!) of software licences as a discouragement to staff from making illegal copies of purchased software.

otherwise should be systematically removed as far as possible.

Once such a procedure is in place and an inventory of all packages and users is assembled, a *licence compliance audit* should be carried out periodically by quality assurance. Annually seems to be the most popular frequency. The number of firms across business generally conducting audits of their systems to track pirated software has more than doubled in the past 2 years to 55 percent,[4] driven, no doubt, by the fear of *unlimited* fines, and the derogatory publicity that would surely accompany them. The effort of performing this exercise manually has hitherto been sufficiently onerous to discourage companies from enforcing internal legal compliance. However, there are now a number of products on the market enabling the inventory of executable files on networked desktops to be listed remotely and almost instantly, thus making compliance auditing relatively easy. After an initial data collection sweep into a central database, compliance snoops may be unobtrusively performed either when users log on, or at other times, so enabling suspects or offenders to be brought back to the paths of righteousness earlier rather than later. Internally developed packages can also be included in the inventories in many cases. Products being used successfully in this context and which tend to be components of larger, network management suites are *Saber LAN Workstation* (McAfee Associates Inc.),[5] *LANauditor®* (Horizons Technology Inc.)[6] and *Systems Management Server* (Microsoft Corporation).[7]

Maintenance agreements for products, especially compilers and other tools that critically affect delivered executable code, should also be subject to maintenance agreements, and included in the configuration management system. It is sometimes forgotten that compilers are also programs and prone, like all others, to contain defects. It is by no means unknown for a change in a compiler to cause a previously compilable program to fail to compile, or to alter its executable behaviour in some subtle way. The compiler used is an important configuration item and must be treated as such.

PHYSICAL SECURITY

Burglary is increasingly common in crime-ridden Western society, and software companies are prime targets for the computer equipment on their premises. Computer crime in Britain now affects

90 percent of business according to a recent UK National Computing Centre survey, with viruses and chip theft prominent costing, inclusive of electronic security breaches, £2 billion annually. After a burglary has occurred, the company is even more vulnerable, since the inventory held within becomes known to the criminal fraternity. Premises may be cleaned out repeatedly, and quite probably by the same criminal group. Every effort should be made to comply with the recommendations of the crime prevention team in the local constabulary or police department. One deterrent that appears to be particularly effective against opportunistic theft is continuous video monitoring of premises. Some companies have decided in the face of this problem that relocation of the business to a more public and less vulnerable site has been the only answer. Since the capital plant of most software firms is quite portable, in the very nature of things, opportunistic theft is much easier than in many other industries.

Keep It Simple	**Practical Guidance**
	Create a procedure for the disposal of packaging material of all newly installed equipment, which avoids advertising the new acquisitions to the local criminal fraternity.

The audit assessment team should record the status of external physical security, and also the effectiveness of internal measures, such as numeric entry pads, or card readers, especially to central server rooms, in the interests of assessing the vendor's practical commitment to long-term survival to support the products.

OTHER THREATS

This concludes the team's examination of the hardware environment in which software development takes place, with strong emphasis on the security and continuity of physical resources. However, the team must now turn its attention to a more insidious enemy that is far more difficult to understand and combat, and which has the power to ruin the reputation of any company beyond redemption, while at the same time leaving the physical resources apparently untouched, at least superficially. It is the practical ways to deal with this menace that will be addressed in the next chapter.

Notes

1. Cheyenne is now a division of Computer Associates International Inc., Islandia, NY.

2. Presently at Alton House, Gatehouse Way, Aylesbury, Bucks HP19 3XU, United Kingdom. It should be noted that the company has no connection with the Harris Corporation, Melbourne, Fl, USA, who have the word *AuthenTec* as a trademark.

3. Data from the *Software Theft Survey* conducted by Spikes Cavell for Microsoft and described in a news item in *Computer Weekly,* 10 October 1996.

4. Ibid.

5. McAfee Associates Inc., 2710 Walsh Avenue, Santa Clara, CA 95051

6. Horizons Technology Inc., 3990 Ruffin Road, San Diego, CA 92123-1826

7. Microsoft Corporation, 1 Microsoft Way, Redmond, WA 98052-6399

13

The Virus Menace

There's nothing consistent about human behaviour except its tendency to degenerate towards evil.

Anon

The advent of computer viruses has brought a plague into the heart of Intel-based IT over the course of recent years, which is now costing British business alone more than £100 million annually. According to a recent survey by the UK National Computing Centre, viruses have become the most common problem for British enterprises, affecting 51 percent of firms. Since the whole software industry and, therefore, the vendors are all necessarily at risk, no work devoted to software quality assurance would be complete without a chapter dedicated to exploring the nature of the problem and how it can be combated. Every vendor must be assured that both the software or files he acquires and uses, and the products distributed, are virus-free, since one well-publicized lapse in this respect would be likely to damage the company's reputation terminally.

THE NATURE OF A VIRUS

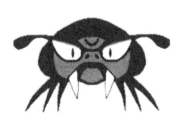

At the outset, it is vital to understand the simple fact that a virus is just a computer program, a piece of software. Like any other software, it can be transferred from computer to computer by floppy disc, or migrate over a communications network between desktops in an office, from one corporation into another and from continent to continent. Like viruses in the biological sphere, it requires a host (a computer's memory) in which to reside and where it can deploy its distinctive characteristic—the ability to replicate itself, behaviour that prompted Cohen (1994) to give it its name. He defined a virus as follows:

> *A program that can infect other programs by modifying them in such a way as to include a (possible evolved) copy of itself.*

To achieve this, it also needs to emulate its biological counterpart in another important respect. It needs to conceal or disguise itself so that it may spread undetected before carrying out its designed action, today referred to generally as *executing its payload*, so that a call to an infected program implies a call to the virus also. Thus, any premature, overt demonstration of its presence will lead to its detection and removal. From the virus's viewpoint, therefore, stealth is the key to success. The generally negative nature of viruses, the wasteful and pointless competition between the digital delinquents that create them and the antivirus scientists who stalk them, and the obligation imposed upon unfortunate computer users to fund these ludicrous cat-and-mouse games through scanners and updates, has led to the awful(!) nouns *malware* and *malicious logic* being coined to describe them.

TYPES OF VIRUSES

There are in the main three types of viruses known at the present time:

1.   Those written in conventional code and capable of infecting a program (.COM or .EXE) file on a hard disc, floppy disc or CD-ROM. There is also one that can infect

C language source code files by contriving code to produce the required functionality when the file is compiled.

2.   Those written in conventional code and capable of infect-
     ing the master boot record of a hard disc or the DOS boot
     record of one of the disc's partitions or the DOS boot
     record of a floppy disc.

3.   Those written in a macro language.

In the first category, a further subdivision can be made into those
that select one or more executables to infect when they are triggered, and those that crouch in a dark corner of memory waiting for
other programs to be executed before pouncing to infect them.
Most viruses in this class are of the latter kind.

  To appreciate the significance of boot sector viruses, it is important to understand the geography of a floppy disc or a hard disc.
In the DOS environment, floppy discs and hard discs are formatted
into a number of circular tracks (called cylinders in the case of hard
discs), which are themselves divided into a number of sectors, as
shown in figure 13.1. The first sector of every disc is assigned by

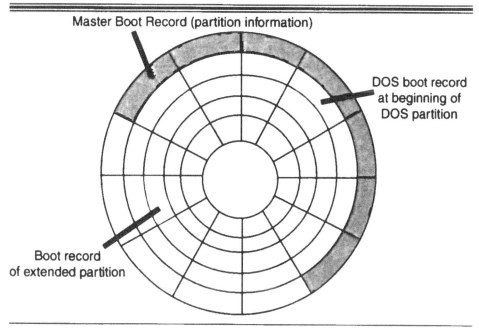

Figure 13.1. Partitions and Boot Sectors

DOS for use solely as the master boot record, and this is still the case even when a floppy disc has been formatted not to be bootable. The master boot record of a hard disc or floppy disc thus commences at cylinder 0, sector 1. This vital area of a hard disc contains information on the *partitions* or physical divisions into which the rest of the disc is divided, and is written on the disc by the FDISK utility before the disc is even formatted. Floppies only have one partition, but the master boot record of a hard disc, which can possess more than one partition, defines where each partition begins and its size. The boot record for each partition, or the boot record for a floppy, describes that partition's characteristics, such as sector size, the number of sectors, and so on. Each partition is viewed as a discrete disc drive. When a computer is booted from the disc, it reads the master boot record to determine which partition has been defined as the *active* partition and where its boot record is located. It then finds this record. The first sector of the boot record contains a small program called a loader that the computer loads into memory first. The sole function of the loader is to load in the rest of the operating system and execute it. In DOS, only the primary partition of a multipartition disc may be used as the partition from which the operating system is booted. However, DOS and its successors are only one of a number of operating systems that can run on the Intel-based PC and its compatibles. Other operating systems, such as OS/2™ or UNIX® may be booted from a second partition, once installed there.

Boot sector viruses can hide either in the DOS boot record at the start of a DOS partition or in the partition sector of the master boot record itself. Once in either of these locations, a virus can be executed undetected every time a PC or server is booted. Such a virus can then infect any floppy disc used subsequently and by this means replicate itself to other computers. A virus installed in the boot sector of a floppy can only become effective if a PC is actually booted from it, the virus thus then residing in the memory (memory resident) alongside the operating system. Some viruses resident on floppy boot sectors immediately copy themselves to the hard disc boot sector, thus executing every time the PC or server is subsequently started from the hard disc. All of the common boot sector viruses, such as Brain, Stoned, Empire, and Michelangelo, are memory resident.

The prevalence of the top 10 viruses, as of June 1996, as well as an indication of their type, is given in table 13.1. Although this

Table 13.1. Virus Prevalence (June 1996) (Reproduced by courtesy of *Virus Bulletin*.)

Position	Name	Type	Incidents	Percentage
1	Concept	Macro	67	19.5
2	Form.A	Boot	34	9.9
3	Parity_Boot	Boot	28	8.1
4	AntiEXE	Boot	25	7.3
5	NYB	Boot	17	4.9
6	Junkie	Boot	14	4.1
7	AntiCmos.A	Boot	12	3.5
8	Ripper	Boot	11	3.2
9	Empire.Monkey.B	Boot	9	2.6
10	Sampo	Boot	9	2.6

material will be well out of date by the time of publication, it is included as an example of the depth and breadth of technical information available from the *Virus Bulletin*.[1] All of these, with the exception of Concept, are boot sector viruses and together account for 80 percent of virus infections. Concept, however, is the most prevalent, accounting for about 20 percent of infections, is an example of a macro virus, a genre which will now be discussed.

Macro Language Viruses

Macro viruses do not exist in the normal executable machine code of a boot sector or in an executable file like most of the file viruses. They are written in the macro language provided by Microsoft Word® or Excel® and, in the case of the former, are designed to infect document files when read. Concept (or Prank as it is otherwise known), once installed, only allows the user to save his or her documents as templates. It is otherwise benign, not causing any other corruption or data loss. However, it replicates through Word documents and is most readily propagated through the transmission of documents as attachments to electronic mail; the infection occurs when the document is opened. Other macro viruses known at present are DMV (very similar to Concept) and Nuclear (causes damage to DOS system files and when printing). The *Laroux* virus affects Excel® spreadsheets when these are opened.

Microsoft has produced a protection macro that can be installed to repair any infected files and to avoid further infections. It can be downloaded from the Microsoft World Wide Web site at http://www.microsoft.com/msoffice or from the MSN™, the Microsoft Network using *go word: macrovirustool,* or other on-line services, such as CompuServe® or America On-Line®.

Polymorphic Viruses

Polymorphism is a term borrowed from the world of crystallography and chemistry. While many chemical compounds exist in a single crystal form (rhombic, monoclinic, etc.), others are capable of existing in more than one crystal form and are thereby said to exhibit polymorphism. In these cases, while the chemical properties of the different polymorphs are identical, the differing crystal shapes themselves may alter some of the physical properties (a fact of special importance in aerosol manufacture, for example). Calcium carbonate, one of the most abundant minerals in nature, exhibits three polymorphs in addition to its amorphous form (common chalk): calcite, aragonite and vaterite. In some polymorphic compounds, the various crystal forms are very stable (e.g., calcite); whereas in other compounds, changes from one crystal form into another occur readily.

The term has been borrowed by the computer industry to describe the type of virus capable of altering its signature (but **not** its payload) when copied, thus making detection harder. However, these changes are not random, but follow a predefined sequence. Thus, by exploring how this encryption is achieved, the best types of scanning software are able to recognise many thousands of different manifestations of the one virus.

Other Types of Viruses

Although a detailed treatment of other types of viruses is beyond the scope of this work, three others will be briefly mentioned:

1. A *stealth* virus makes alterations to information on the disc (usually in the boot sectors) after making a copy of the area prior to infection and copying this to another location. Sitting in memory, it intercepts calls to the sector, returning

the uninfected code and concealing its presence. Being memory resident, however, it is vulnerable to detection.

2. A *cluster* virus changes the address stored in a file allocation table entry for a file, thus redirecting any read transaction on that file to an alternative location. Thus, when the file is read, the virus code is activated, even though the file information remains unchanged.

3. *Mainframe viruses* do exist, but they are far more scarce. To create such a virus requires a detailed knowledge of the operating system involved. Since mainframes operate almost exclusively in closed environments, and those intimately involved in running them are almost always highly motivated and responsible corporate personnel, there has been little activity beyond that of the occasional disgruntled misfit. An additional factor is that mainframe software is exclusively devoted to serious applications; games or other trivial software are not produced for mainframe systems on any significant scale.

VIRUS COMPONENTS

A virus consists of four parts:

1. A **replication** mechanism: the part of the program which copies itself.

2. A **protection** mechanism: the part of the program which conceals it from detection. This might be an encryption process aimed at eluding virus detection software, or a polymorphism algorithm aimed at ensuring that each replication creates a copy differing in signature from the original, in order to elude recognition. Some use stealth techniques to modify the system itself, so that on reading the hard disc the virus remains hidden.

3. A **trigger** mechanism: the part which causes the virus's payload to be executed. It could be the coincidence of a date read from the system clock. Among the most well-known examples of this are the Jerusalem virus, which executes on Fridays falling on the 13th day of the month, and the Michelangelo virus, which runs on the sculptor's

birthday, 6 March. In other situations, the trigger might be the number of times a particular program has run or the number of occasions the system has been booted since infection.

4. A **payload**: the part of the program that makes the presence of the virus evident, initiated by the trigger. It could amount to no more than that (simple announcement of its presence), a so-called *benign* virus. On the other hand, its action could be malevolent, such as the corruption of the hard disc. The most damaging viruses are those that incrementally make small changes to individual files on a hard disc in a random fashion. These changes necessarily become incorporated onto the backup copies of the data. If the virus manages to elude detection for long enough, then all generations of the backup media may have become infected by then, thereby leading to the irretrievable loss of the original, uncorrupted data.

PAYLOAD ACTIVITIES

Six levels of severity have been defined for the activities of computer viruses:

1. **Trivial**: These viruses do nothing beyond replicating and announcing their presence when triggered. They do no intentional damage, are easily removed upon detection and require no subsequent cleanup effort. Unfortunately, the virus code that has actually infected a user's machine may not be beta-tested code, and is most unlikely to have been engineered to any quality standard! It has often been found that so-called benign viruses can acquire a payload beyond the intention of the author, usually after the operating system has been upgraded or new hardware installed. In these circumstances, the virus may crash the computer, causing the loss of work in progress. Viruses intended to be trivial may not always behave in a trivial manner.

2. **Minor**: Alterations to a single file or deletion of one or more executables that were infected are the worst results in this category. A simple restoration from the most frequent backup is usually all that is required here.

3. **Moderate**: The virus may cause wholesale destruction of a hard disc, either by formatting it or by writing garbage all over it. The assignment of the epithet *moderate* to such malevolent action may seem a gross understatement, until it is remembered that regular backups should be both the policy and the practice of all responsible computer users. A restoration from the backup media is all that is required.

4. **Major**: The virus makes undetected changes to a variety of data files over a period of time before it is detected by writing a random bit pattern into them. It may be possible to identify specific files that have been infected and repair them by restoring from backup. This may take a considerable time, but the damage is not irreparable.

5. **Severe**: Now we are getting really serious. If a virus makes subtle incremental changes to a range of files without leaving any trace behind as to what has been done, it becomes impossible to determine exactly which files have been altered. There may have been several generations of backups taken of the files before the virus is discovered. If the period of time between initial infection and discovery exceeds the total cycle time of all of the backup generations, then copies of the files prior to infection may no longer exist. It will be impossible to tell how long the corruption has been occurring.

6. **Catastrophic**: The virus has infected a network and has determined the passwords of the senior players, such as the network supervisor, and communicated this to many others. These individuals have taken advantage of the situation to abuse their newly acquired but illegal privileges. It is impossible to determine with any degree of assurance what has been compromised on the network. There is no way back. The supervisor has lost control and the potential for losses could be devastating.

SPECIFIC ANTIVIRUS DETECTION

The battle with the digital delinquents comes down to the antivirus community keeping one step ahead. Most of the major products have at least a common core set of utilities, which are described below.

Demand-Driven Scanner

A demand-driven scanner seeks for known virus signature bit patterns on the hard disc, using a regularly updated database of signatures. Some of the leading products use heuristic[2] techniques to pick up unknown viruses. Dr. Solomon's *FindVirus* uses advanced heuristic techniques to detect 8 out of 10 unknowns, and also includes instructions on removing and cleaning up the mess, a feature which not all of the products in this category provide. But what of the remaining unknowns? The drawback to all heuristic scanners is that code that might be innocent in one program could be suspect in another. Most heuristic scanners use some sort of points scoring approach to reach their decision, any file exceeding the threshold of suspicion being flagged as *possibly* infected.

The obvious bane, therefore, with this approach is the *generation of false alarms*. If an innocent file is brought under suspicion, how on earth can the user know the truth, or discriminate between a real virus infection and the false witness of a defective antivirus program? A wild goose chase is usually precipitated at this point. The network may need to be shut down, precluding access to the "infected" file. And where does it stop? Have any of our floppies been infected?

The crisis then degenerates into a nightmare when the antivirus software calmly states that no repair is possible. So the backups are then wheeled in from off-site storage, whereupon it transpires that they, too, are infected. At this point, the QA manager quietly has a nervous breakdown, while the chief executive becomes apoplectic! If only the truth that *no virus ever existed* had been known from the start, how much anguish and waste could have been avoided!

This scenario is by no means a flight of fancy. In 1993, an antivirus product mistakenly identified a new version of PKUNZIP.EXE as infected with Maltese Amoeba. Other users were disappointed that their (different) antivirus product reported no such infection. PKWare, the makers of PKUNZIP, protested vigorously that their product was clean and that the antivirus product was flawed, but how could they substantiate their innocence? Since many users reported their antivirus product flagging PKUNZIP as infected *but incapable of cleaning it up*, they were forced to abandon use of PKUNZIP. In another case, a small development company was falsely accused of distributing an infected demonstration disc. The infection arose within the purchaser's operation, but how could the vendor company protect itself? There are serious potential legal questions at stake here, and this is clearly a business-critical issue for all software vendors.

Great care must be exercised in selecting antivirus software on the basis of the sophistication of the heuristic techniques used. Dr. Solomon's product is regarded as one of the best at avoiding false alarms, a finding confirmed by the survey conducted by *Secure Computing* in January 1996. Nearly half of the products tested failed to complete the test without false alarming.

Memory-Resident Scanner

A memory-resident scanner intercepts system calls to enable it to check every program file for known viruses before allowing them to be executed or to be copied. It is similar to the demand-driven scanner, but only checks files as they are used. The best ones of this type are automatic and very fast.

Windows™ Virtual Device Driver

A *Windows™ Virtual Device Driver (V×D) scanner* scans files accessed while Windows™ is running, inhibiting access to any file identified as carrying a known virus. The best product has full 32-bit compatibility and is, therefore, suitable both for Windows™ 3.1 and for Windows 95®.

Fingerprinting Programs

The principle at work in *fingerprinting* is to take a note of the checksum of each boot sector and every executable file, both locally and on the network, and store them in a database. It rests on the assumption that in normal circumstances these checksums should never change from the day they are installed. Any unintended change ought to be regarded with suspicion, since this *might* signal infection by a virus. It includes a utility to replace an infected boot sector. Obvious exceptions are new versions of executables, or intentional changes to a master boot record, perhaps from the installation of a special disc driver like the *Quantum OnTrack Disc*

Manager® software.[3] More recent BIOS chips sport a feature to enable master boot sector writes to be intercepted by the BIOS itself, usually generating a message such as "Boot Sector Write—possible virus!!" It is wise to take advantage of these facilities if they are available.

GENERIC ANTIVIRUS DETECTION

We are left then with a time gap, the period between the propagation of a new virus and its inclusion in the databases of the antivirus community, the window of opportunity when a new virus has a sporting chance of eluding even the most advanced heuristic techniques. What can be done to close this chink in the antivirus armour? A novel approach has been taken by Second Sight, an Australian company which has supplemented the fingerprinting principle with some novel techniques in its *InVircible* product, aimed at being more discriminating in the decision as to whether a change has been legitimate or not. A database is provided consisting of a hidden file held on each directory. These files hold a 66-byte record for each executable recording information such as the header bit pattern, the length of the file, the entry point addresses, the contents, the name and so on. The program's algorithm decides whether the change is legitimate or illegitimate, based on which of these has actually changed. The company aspires to shift the emphasis away from the combat scenario that has characterized the virus scene hitherto, and to develop a generic product capable of detecting all current and future viruses. It seems difficult to understand how any approach to virus detection and removal can be permanent since no software can effectively be designed to protect against something that has not yet been invented! However, this new approach has great value, since it aims to detect all viruses at the point of propagation, rather than when the payload is executed, and offers baits to stealth viruses to precipitate their self-disclosure. At best it should be used to complement, rather than replace, the conventional scanning databases.

Another important innovation available with *InVircible* is the ability to secure distributed software with an integrity signature, providing proof as to whether the software was infected at the factory or at the user's premises. Registered users of InVircible can also process their floppies with *InVircible Armour*, a product which installs a passive protective jacket that prevents file viruses from

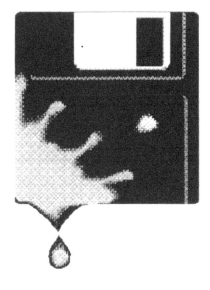

infecting the software, even when the disc is write-enabled (important for registration purposes). The protection for vendors from virus legal liability is clear.

Most of the major antivirus suppliers provide a virus signature update service. Symantec, for example, maker of the *Norton AntiVirus* product, offers a free service via a number of on-line sources, including CompuServe® and America On-Line®, as well as from the Internet and Symantec's Bulletin Board. Software vendors should update their databases at least twice yearly, since new viruses are still appearing at the rate of about 100 a month. The advent of Windows NT® is eagerly awaited by all those concerned with the virus menace, since boot viruses do not work under this operating system.

PRACTICAL ANTIVIRUS MEASURES

Until the problem can be permanently overcome, it is reassuring to realize that with a little care, the risk of virus infection for both the software vendor and the computer user at large can be minimized to a level approaching zero. Indeed, to do so is very cost effective; the UK government has reckoned that the average cost of cleaning up an infected UK business exceeds £4000, so virus protection makes sound financial sense. Here are some suggested actions:

- Implement strict procedures to govern the handling of disc media, to monitor all systems at all times by means of well-established antivirus software, and to ensure through regular surveillance that they are being followed.

- Never use floppy discs or CD-ROMs of unknown provenance without first scanning for viruses.

- When downloading files from the Internet or Bulletin Boards, always scan the files **before** running them.

- Never boot the computer from a floppy disc unless it is certain to be clean. Keep a clean bootable disc, complete with all the important executables on it, in secure storage and intended only for antivirus investigations.

- Use the write-protect tab whenever possible when just reading floppy discs to prevent viruses being copied onto them.

- Confine software acquisitions to licensed copies from reputable vendors.

- Use password security to protect unattended personal computers from unauthorized copying of files.

- Back up regularly, reviewing the strategy frequently to ensure its comprehensiveness.

- Treat unexplained reduction or changes in memory usage at boot up with suspicion (compare with that derived from boot up from a known clean floppy).

- Disable floppy boot up by changing the BIOS boot-up sequence from A,C to C,A.

- Use a recognized, well-known antivirus software product, for example, Dr. Solomon's *Anti-Virus Toolkit*, or *VirusScan* from McAfee, and keep a log of the results of the scans.

- Keep the signature files for your antivirus software up-to-date.

- Use a generic product like *InVircible*, in conjunction with one of the traditional scanning products, for increased depth of surveillance.

Keep It

Simple

Practical Guidance

Create a virus monitoring procedure describing how incoming discs are scrutinized, systems regularly swept, signatures updated, and outgoing distribution discs verified as clean and recorded as such to legal standards.

- Protect distribution floppies with an integrity signature and/or passive protection.

- Maintain current awareness by subscribing to the FAQ sheet,[4] which also contains a fuller bibliography on the subject.

FUTURE TRENDS

How is the virus scene likely to change in the next few years? There are grounds for optimism in some respects and pessimism in others. On the brighter side, it seems that over the last few years there has not been much improvement over the quality of viruses. The major antivirus products, like *Dr. Solomon's Anti-Virus Toolkit*, have become so sophisticated as to be able to detect almost anything, so exhausting most or all of the possible avenues of approach that virus writers might take. Although one virus writer was convicted under the British Computer Misuse Act of 1990 and sentenced to 18 months in prison, this is the only well-publicized case so far of its kind, while the virus situation appears to have settled down to some sort of stalemate. Indeed, over the past few years some virus writers seem to have been behaving positively altruistically in sending their creations directly to antivirus researchers rather than malevolently releasing them.

Unhappily though, the Internet and the World Wide Web will give the real anarchists a fertile breeding ground through which to disseminate the tawdry fruits of their warped imaginations. The macro viruses which can be passed within text documents, and those that encrypt data rather than actually deleting it, are likely to become more widespread. Only time will tell how today's uneasy truce will next be broken.

Notes

1. This international monthly magazine is a first-class technical resource on all aspects of computer virus prevention, recognition and control; it is obtainable by subscription from Virus Bulletin Ltd, The Pentagon, Abingdon, Oxon, OX14 3YP, United Kingdom, Tel +44 1235 555139.

2. Heuristic is defined as learning by investigation. In this context it denotes a rule of thumb approach to problem solving without the exhaustive application of a specific algorithm. Heuristic scanners look for code which *seems* to be suspicious.

3. This is an example of software necessary to enable motherboards with early BIOS chips to accommodate disc drives of more than 1024 cylinders, or about 500 Mbytes, where logical block addressing is used.

4. The reader is referred to the excellent dossier of Frequently Asked Questions (FAQ sheet), available over the Internet on the Virus-L/comp.virus archives, accessible by FTP on corsa.ucr.edu (IP = 138.23.166.133) in the directory pub/virus-1, which is maintained by Nick FitzGerald at n.fitzgerald@csc.canterbury.ac.nz.

14

Assessment and Reporting

*Good sense without vanity, a penetrating judgement with-
out a disposition to satire, good nature and humility.*

Recommendation by
Hannah Godwin
of a prospective wife
to her brother in 1784

Our examination of the software engineering process so far has
been general, in that it has not focussed on any particular product
or version that a vendor is attempting to sell and that a purchaser is
contemplating buying. The consultancy/audit examination that this
book has described, and the practical strategies for improving the
process that it has advocated, have applied to the general process
used by the vendor for all products. However, there can be a huge
distinction between an exemplary, documented quality management system and what actually goes on in practice. Does the quality
management system really work? Are procedures actually being followed? Are they meeting the ultimate test of practical usefulness,
delivering the promised benefits? Or have they fallen into disrepute,
gathering dust in a binder on a shelf while chaos reigns?

One of the best ways of evaluating this, with great relevance to the product purchase being envisaged, is to examine the extent to which the company's practices have been actually applied in the development of this product/version. Even after the most sincere assurances of a well-controlled process, with evidence of effective monitoring by a comprehensive quality management system, we still have no guarantee that for this particular version of this product these procedures have necessarily been followed. Of course, the presumption is that they have. If the purchaser is to confirm that there is no undue risk in purchasing a particular version, and that the quality management system really is effective, the vendor should be able to identify evidence in one or two simple ways that these conditions apply. In this way, the real value of the quality management system can be tested, and the various threads of the team's assessment process can be brought together and summarized.

SOURCE CODE INSPECTION

The source code of the product should conform with the programming standards that have been alleged to apply within the company. The auditor should ask to see the suite of source code files corresponding to the particular version to be purchased and select one at random. Occasionally, a company may refuse the auditor access to source files on the simple principle that these are key intellectual resources of the company and must remain secret. Any inspection by external personnel, whoever they are, therefore represents a real threat that proprietary techniques and information contained within them might be revealed in such a manner as to jeapodize the future of the company.

Such an embargo, while understandable at one level, is entirely misconceived. The auditor normally represents a purchaser whose area of business is totally different from software engineering. Whilst the reservations expressed would be quite appropriate for a visitor from a software *competitor*, they are little short of ridiculous in the context of a software quality audit, where the auditor's interest is entirely confined to compliance with standards. The implied suggestion that the auditor might have an ulterior motive, somehow connected with industrial espionage, is as impertinent as it is fanciful, since in any case the auditor would be most unlikely to possess the technical expertise to decipher anything of commercial value, even if he or she were to be so minded. Regrettably, however, such a position, once taken, tends to be defended with intransigent zeal, and the fact that it is counterproductive both to the vendor and the purchaser cannot be entertained because of the risk of loss of face. This can even be the case when a formal nondisclosure agreement has previously been signed. Happily, however, this scenario, which usually reflects a complete lack of understanding on the part of vendor principals of the nature and purpose of a quality assurance audit, is relatively rare.

The file should be examined in respect of each of the principal categories mentioned under the programming standards. In my experience, compliance or a lack of it becomes clear very quickly indeed. Header information, such as author name, program description, the date and time of creation, and configuration management information, such as revision numbers and an audit trail change summary, should be evident at once. Indentation of conditional branches and iterative loops should be rigorously observed, and is automatic in some languages such as Visual BASIC® and some dialects of C. Each paragraph that represents a discrete function or operation should be separated from previous code by comment lines and text to facilitate readability.

If no changes have been recorded in the first source file, another should be selected for examination. The objective is to inspect how carefully changes are being annotated, not only in the header but also at the particular line of interest. Strict discipline in the numbering of the successive variant (revision) of the file should be evident. If any code has become dead as a result of the change, its isolation by commenting is far preferable to its actual deletion, since the change history of a source file can impart a great level of understanding to a subsequent editor who may never have known the original author.

The auditor should record the name of each file examined, the salient features inspected, and their degree of compliance with the vendor's claimed standards. All of these should be included in the audit report.

Changes in source code after product release usually arise from a request originating in a support database. Each change should, therefore, be traceable back to a record in the support database for a defect repair or an enhancement request. The auditing team should take one of the changes found and attempt to trace it back through the documentation and recording systems. In my experience, this little exercise, which normally takes no more than a few minutes, is extremely revealing of the strengths and weaknesses of the change control, configuration management and tracking systems themselves. Most vendors have expressed profound appreciation of the usefulness of this in identifying practical improvements. The innocent questions of an outsider unfamiliar with the web of internal assumptions can trigger the generation of new ideas and approaches, especially if the auditor can freely share on a totally anonymous basis what other vendors in general have found to be successful without, of course, breaching any confidentiality. This free advice has often proved of enormous value in preventing, once again, the unnecessary reinvention of the proverbial wheel.

TESTING RECORDS

It is relatively rare to find a vendor company which has retained testing records of its products. Most vendors have yet to realize the importance of this key piece of documentary evidence in proving the quality of one's product. The majority seem to believe (with considerable justification at present, it is to be feared) that purchasers will make the optimistic assumption that despite the absence of any supportive evidence, the software somehow *must* be OK. While recording this absence, the vendor should be urged to retain test records in the future; if these are in electronic form, the cost involved is practically negligible.

LIFE CYCLE DOCUMENTS

Regrettably, most vendors still do not effect concomitant revisions to design and requirements specifications when post-release changes are made to source code. This serious omission increases the risk and cost of subsequent support in that maintenance programming personnel not associated with the original work have to guess the design implications of all changes made since release. If, on the other hand, the design and requirements documents have been kept in step with the source code, keeping traceability tight through the process, the chance of adventitious errors subsequently creeping into the product is greatly minimized. It is quite common for 10 errors to be repaired in a release and 5 new, different ones to simultaneously appear. This ought not to be so and can frequently be attributed to a lack of documentation discipline throughout the life cycle. Of course, the majority of source code changes may not require any change in fundamental life cycle documentation; however, the change control record should specifically state this. If a design diagram needs to be revised due to, say, a minor change in a database record, then revise it! It does not take long, but then when the design is later compared with the current release, the one is still consistent with the other.

USER TRAINING PROGRAM

Almost every vendor enterprise, with very few exceptions, organizes some kind of user training in marketing and supporting its product. The auditor should examine course materials and explore whether in the event of any changes occurring as the product is enhanced whether the user training materials are correspondingly revised. All too frequently this does not happen, and new functionality is not covered adequately. Once again, the change control form should state whether any concomitant changes are required in this department.

THE REVIEW MEETING

The examination of the source code concludes the assessment of the state of the software engineering process. It now falls to the visiting auditor/consultant to summarize for the benefit of all involved, and particularly for vendor management, what the team has found and what practical actions have already been agreed to among them as being necessary to improve the process. It is vitally important to re-emphasize that the action points which have emerged are *team recommendations*. They are in no sense whatsoever unilateral attempts by the auditor to *impose* changes, cost and burden on an unconvinced and reluctant vendor. Such would be counterproductive, fruitless and futile. The vendor company operates independently in its own market area, which is usually totally dissimilar to that of the purchaser, who in any event has no sanction whatever over the vendor beyond the sale of a single licence, which on its own could rarely, if ever, justify fundamental changes in software engineering.

The agreed action points *must* be seen by the vendor's staff as being in their own strategic interest irrespective of any purchase that may result from the visit or that has prompted it.

ASSIGNMENT OF VENDOR STATUS

In general, there are three possible outcomes of a vendor assessment, each in terms of a *recommended status* for the vendor; theoretically, at least, there is also a fourth. These are as follows:

1. **Approved:** The vendor's quality management system is sufficiently comprehensive and effective as to ensure the incorporation of an adequate level of structural integrity into the software. The vendor is using a cost-effective and productive engineering process, producing software with a low level of residual defects that does what it purports to do and does not do what it purports not to do. The vendor is, therefore, likely to survive and prosper, and on this basis is accepted as an accredited quality supplier of software to the purchasing business.

2. **Conditional** or **Limited Approval:** The vendor's quality management system is fundamentally sound, but there are important shortcomings. While the level of structural integrity is at least enough for us to use the current version of software in the business without an unacceptably high risk, the inadequacies are serious enough to raise doubts about the level of residual defects and/or the uncontrolled level of cost within the process. Both present questions not only about the quality of future revisions but also over the prospects of the vendor's continuance in business to support the product on a long-term basis in partnership with ourselves. Until the process is improved in the agreed-on respects, further revisions will not be accepted; however, once that happens, the vendor's assigned status is to be elevated to Approved.

3. **Rejected:** The vendor does not have even the basic elements of a life cycle methodology in place, and there is no evidence of the incorporation of any degree of structural integrity into the software. Furthermore, the vendor remains unconvinced of the long-term dangers of working in

a creative, but chaotic, manner and shows no appreciation of the unknown and unknowable costs implicit in working in this way. The vendor's staff cannot demonstrate evidence beyond market penetration that their product has quality built into it. Use of their products, therefore, constitutes an unknown level of risk to any purchaser.

4. **Unapproved**: The vendor has a sound quality management system that has been applied to the development of most of the products, but for some reason not applied to the product of interest. While conceptually possible, this situation arises only on the rarest of occasions.

The vast majority of vendors fall into the category of Conditional or Limited Approval. In larger software houses, this usually means that they have begun to assemble a rudimentary quality management system but have not understood how to develop it. There are some procedures in place, but many parts of the process remain pragmatic. There is little control on the two-way flow of information and little understanding of how costs can be controlled. In most companies, this is clear from a disproportionate emphasis on testing, emanating from a reluctant admission of the belief that testing is the means by which defects are effectively removed and quality put into the software. One of the most pleasing and satisfying aspects of the audit/consultancy process is to witness the appreciation and relief of programmers and managers that someone has, at last, explained the mystery underlying an intractable and long-standing conundrum: despite all their testing efforts, the company is still experiencing a disturbingly high level of errors from customers. At last, the simple steps that can be taken to remedy this are now known and understood.

Great care and discernment is needed on the part of auditors at arriving at a conclusion when very small companies are visited. As has already been explained, it is possible to engineer software to an implied life cycle within a very small, closely knit group of two or three with almost no documentation at all. In these circumstances, the evidence of in-built structural integrity is very hard to assess, being based on a measure of the knowledge and, supremely, the attitudes of the group to quality, followed by the inspection of the source code itself. In most such firms, the case for documentation is easy to make since many appreciate the impediments to safe and secure growth without documented procedures; therefore, it is easy to convince them of the immediate value of making a start on a simple quality management system. This commences by asking them to write down their thought processes and sequence of activities in software development, beginning with a simple description of the life cycle model (usually the Waterfall) that is implicitly in use.

As the effort to produce the agreed-on documentation gets underway, it is satisfying to hear repeated testimonials to the perceived value of having principles written down and agreed to, rather than just being believed, hoped for or assumed. Many subsequently express amazement that they were prepared to forego the benefits of simple, concise documentation for so long, and find themselves going far beyond the specific action points agreed on at the time of the audit visit. The transformation of barely concealed hostility and overt skepticism over standards and documentation into a sober recognition of their indispensability to the future health of the company is one of the most rewarding aspects of the auditor/consultant's job. Furthermore, the willingness of the auditor to be available on a longer-term basis, to afford informal help and advice on request, contributes to the cementing of the long-term partnership that is one of the key objectives of the whole audit/consultancy process. The personal friendships that have blossomed out of the initial contacts made within vendor companies in the course of audit visits are much to be valued.

POST-AUDIT FOLLOW-UP

Conditional or limited approvals should always be accompanied by an agreed-on timetable for their implementation, and the auditor should courteously invite the vendor to define this. Once again, it is the vendor staff's prerogative to state what target they wish to set themselves to achieving the agreed actions, and the auditor should make no attempt to dictate in this regard, since that would amount to impertinence. The response of most vendors seems to be to set an unrealistically *short* timetable to implement these, reflecting a natural enthusiasm to get things done. This reaction is very commendable but it ought to be met with a tactful suggestion from the auditor to reconsider! In most cases three months is a good compromise between addressing both the urgent and the important, a distinction many managers and planners still find very hard to make wisely. The auditor should then offer to contact the vendor, say, within two months to review progress. This is usually warmly welcomed since it offers the gentlest of sanctions on making sure things actually happen—that someone outside the company is going to call us in due course to ask about our performance versus our pledges, pledges we have made supremely to *ourselves*.

Return visits are only made rarely, usually if the auditor happens to be in the vicinity on other business, and even then only by prior appointment. Since the cost of the audit visit has usually been borne by the purchaser, any follow-up visit to the vendor's premises ought to be treated as commercial, professional consultancy, and charged at the going rate. Normally, subsequent contacts with vendor personnel ought to be confined to telephone advice, but happily visits sometimes take place in the reverse direction, where vendor personnel ask to come to review their progress and often bring draft procedures for comment. These visits tend to be especially pleasant occasions, providing tangible evidence of the long-term success of the process and its mutual value to both parties.

COMPOSING THE AUDIT REPORT

Auditors are strongly advised to use a systematic checklist as a aide-mémoire in conducting a consultancy/audit visit; appendix 3 provides an example set of worksheets. It is crucial to point out, however, that the emphasis is very much on the aide-mémoire aspect rather than on the list feature. Asking so-called *closed* questions during an audit, such as "Do you have a life cycle description?" or "Do you draw up structured test plans?", questions which invite a yes/no answer, are of far less value (and require less effort all round) than the request along the lines of "Please show me your life cycle description" or "Can we have a look at some of your structured test plans?" The latter approach reveals far more of what is actually going on than the former. It is for this reason that the worksheets are largely devoted to blank ruled space, upon which the auditor can make copious notes on each aspect of the process, prompted by the reminders of the areas to be examined printed above. With the experience of a dozen or so audits under his or her belt, the accomplished auditor will also recollect many other related questions that can be asked, which are not written down but reflect the benefit of experience of earlier visits elsewhere. He or she will also, of course, be able to share advice over practical guidance of what has been found to work *at the coal face,* so to speak, in other companies.

It is from these first-hand written notes that the *audit report,* usually running to about six pages and structured following exactly the same headings as the worksheets, is composed. The direct relationship between the one and the other optimizes the efficiency of the reporting task, and has been found in practice to work extremely well. As a result, the prime purchaser of the software, by whom the auditor was commissioned in the first instance, receives a detailed, in-depth insight into what lurks beneath the glossy exterior of either the screen display, the brochure or the user manual. Although already mentioned in chapter 2, this warning is eminently worth repeating: it is absolutely essential that the report be written up no later than the next working day. This appears to be a general practice, scrupulously adopted by many auditors employed across industry and commerce in a variety of business areas (financial, for example). Report drafting should **never** be delayed beyond a second audit visit, since the ease with which confusion can arise over what was said in two different companies is a recipe for disaster. Next day reporting is usual for UK visits, since the late afternoon/ evening of that day is usually wholly occupied with travelling home; for audits further afield, the report is best composed back at the hotel immediately after the audit is over, aiming to complete the task no later than mid morning on the next day. In this way, multiple audits may be successfully carried out sequentially and efficiently in a whistle-stop tour, with no possibility of confusion, while minimizing the period of absence from both office and home, and the associated cost. About five hours is usually required for the composition of an audit report, whether handwritten or typed into a laptop computer. If the latter, precautions should be taken to preserve at least two independent copies of the draft in case of loss or corruption during the homeward journey. Auditors are strongly advised always to take two floppy disc copies, retaining one on the person and another in the luggage.

AUDIT REPORT EDITIONS

The flowchart of our reporting process is illustrated in figure 14.1. The audit report appears first in draft stage and is circulated to any other members of the audit team or observers, the purchasing customer who commissioned the audit, and to IT management (for

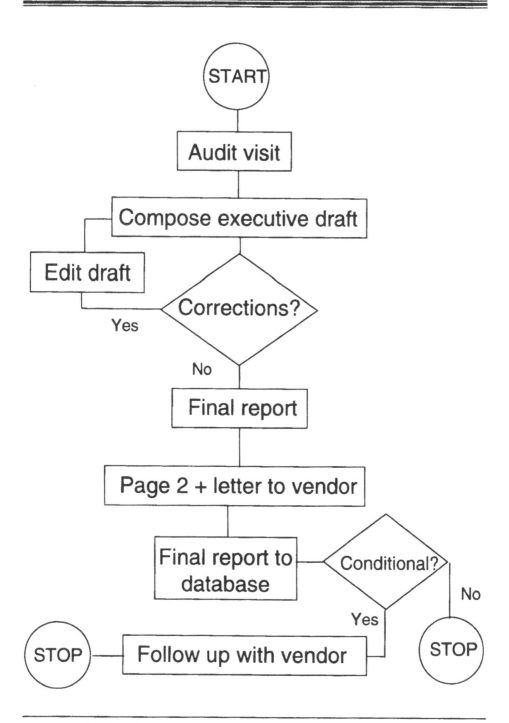

Figure 14.1. The Audit Reporting Process

the wider implications of software installation, reliability and business suitability). The draft gives other audit team members (if any) the opportunity to correct any material inaccuracies, and prompts the customer either to question the auditor on the significance of any of the findings or to question the recommendation. Auditing is not a pure science, being heavily laced with subjective judgement. It is important then to emphasize that the report should not only bear the recommendation but also describe in detail the observations on which the recommendation was based. This is not always the practice of other software auditors. However, the value of this style of presentation is that it exposes the recommendation to wider scrutiny and affords an opportunity to others to *weigh the facts for themselves*. This is a great advantage over other styles of audit report, which simply attribute a numerical score to life cycle or process features and thereby deprive the reader from making any kind of *objective or independent judgement*. Of course, it can make life harder for the auditor in that he or she may have to justify the recommendations under challenge, but this is a healthy incentive to competence and to performing a thorough job, quite regardless of whatever one's own innate sense of professionalism may demand. It is a form of *independent validation* of what may be a key component of an important decision-making process for a purchasing organization.

A specimen audit report, framed like a real report but containing totally fictitious information (since considerations of commercial confidentiality preclude the use of real data), is presented in appendix 4. It is included to illustrate the depth of the type of report the process described in this book delivers and its value to the purchasing company. It should be remembered that a report of this type has been assembled based on about five or six hours of intensive teamwork by the auditor working with, perhaps, the programming manager and/or one or two other senior vendor staff. The actual cost of the audit to the vendor has, therefore, been negligible (though that may not be the case for the corrective actions he identifies as necessary, which should in any case pay for themselves in a relatively short time!).

REPORT APPROVAL AND RETENTION

Once the draft has been examined, comments exhausted, edited as required, and the recommendation approved, the draft is endorsed by the management and evolves into the final report. The second page of the report carries a summary of the findings and any agreed-on actions. This page is intended for transmission to the vendor with a covering letter expressing the auditor's thanks for courtesies and hospitality extended during the audit. The summary provides a permanent record for the vendor aimed at helping him to focus on the actions, if any, that were agreed on, and to which the auditor will refer in subsequent contacts. The report itself is then stored in a central database, from which summary lists are produced periodically and circulated within the purchasing organization. They give potential purchasers of software an indication of the status of vendors in terms of the software product audited, the date of the audit, and the outcome. By this means, an effective software quality procurement policy can be implemented, purchasers being encouraged to refer to the database to identify quality-assured vendors in their own business area when any software purchase is contemplated.

Further emphasis must be made here of the principle that reports are made available for circulation only on the understanding that the implied confidentiality restrictions are respected (i.e., the report is to be confined within the organization and never to be divulged outside it). This can become especially important in two types of circumstances:

1. If sensitive or contentious financial information derived from external credit reference agencies (as mentioned in chapter 3) has been included

2. If the audit assessment has been unfavourable as to merit the recommendation of a Rejected status.

If either of these states of affairs arises, it is quite possible for critical commercial relationships to be affected should the audit findings ever become known *outside* the purchasing company. Clearly, the nondisclosure agreement is intended to demonstrate the good faith of the purchasing company in this regard, since the vendor relationships most vulnerable to such disclosure are unlikely to involve the purchasing company directly. However, the major risk here is not of wilful disclosure, but rather of the *accidental* revelation of such information. The larger the purchasing company and, therefore, the larger the potential readership of audit findings, the greater the risk of such an inadvertent disclosure. The vendor might then be minded to take legal proceedings against the purchasing

company for commercial losses, or damages to the company's reputation; this would then be the unintended but disastrous consequence of an audit assessment, conducted with a vendor by the
purchasing company in the utmost good faith! No purchasing company should entertain such a possibility if evidence that this might
happen arises, regardless of the huge gulf which lies between the
initiation of proceedings, and proving the case to a court's satisfaction. In practice, this would be almost impossible in most circumstances, since the purchasing company plainly had no intention of
harming the vendor by prejudicing the vendor's relationships with
third parties, the fundamental cause of which was the vendor's own
unacceptable process and practice. The purchasing company would
have no case to answer. However, if a purchasing company unwittingly finds itself in these circumstances, it has two further options.
It can either confine the written report to a very tight circle of readers already informed of the legal sensitivity of the contents, or it can
suppress the report altogether, so reducing the risk of accidental
disclosure to a negligible level.

In most cases associated with an outright rejection of a vendor's software development process, the sensitivity of the report is
likely to be short lived. This is because most firms embarrassed to
find themselves in this dilemma are powerfully motivated to initiate
urgent improvement actions, in which the auditor can play a positive or supporting role. Normally, this leads to a radical overhaul of
company practice, and the installation of a credible quality-assured
process, before irreparable commercial damage has been suffered.
Nevertheless, it can land an auditor in a situation of tense drama,
emphasising the need for calm, mature judgement that will withstand the most critical retrospective analysis.

AUDIT/CONSULTANCY PROCEDURE

Great stress has been laid on the need to document each process involved in software development in terms of a procedure to ensure
that it is not only repeatable, but that it is defined for the benefit of
novices, and that management can use the documentation as a
springboard for improving the process. As this chapter concludes,
the reader may be wondering whether what has been preached has
also been practised. Indeed, it would be the height of hypocrisy not
to include in this book the documented procedure for the very

audit/consultancy process that has been described! The reader will find it duly included as appendix 1.

The final chapter will be devoted to considering what the shape of audit consultancy may be in the foreseeable future.

15

Future Trends

Give me chastity and continency, but do not give it yet.

Augustine (354–430)

Software quality procurement has been presented in this book as a means of confining software purchases to those products where evidence can be found of their fitness for their intended purpose. The need for such a policy is a reflection of the lamentable immaturity of much of the software industry today, where most products are not developed fully in accordance with a system of quality assurance. In these circumstances, software purchased without any quality screening, which is the practice of the vast majority of purchasing firms today, assumes the nature of a gamble. There is an optimistic, charitable *assumption* that responsible engineering must undergird the production of all software. The less questions that are asked about it the better. After all *ignorance*, which can always be offered as a plausible defense when things go wrong, is much to be preferred to *knowledge*, coupled with subsequent *inaction* and consequent *guilt*, when it becomes hard to make a credible defense against a charge of irresponsibility or negligence. The software industry relies on this prevalent ostrich-like attitude to continue to produce software riddled with defects at a level that would precipitate legal action in many other commodities or spheres of business and commerce. Indeed, we are now beginning to see the first straws in the wind, especially in the context of the millennium bomb, to indicate that the music is about to stop and the party is about to end. The time for the industry to put its house in order is already long overdue, but until it does, the need for the audit/consultancy process that has been described will remain. Therefore, the final chapter is devoted to the possible shape that this activity might assume across industry and commerce in general in connection with software of all types, not just that where regulatory compliance makes the exercise mandatory.

PURCHASER COST

For a single auditor conducting an audit/consultancy visit along the lines explored here, the total cost including salary and expenses averages about £600 at home, and about £1000 overseas. These costs are often criticized as being excessive in relation to the low purchase cost of some software packages. However, to make such a comparison is to misconceive the business case for the exercise. The objective for the audit assessment is to decrease the likelihood of business losses in terms of time, data or continuity from software failures. Such losses bear no relation to the original cost of the software, be it £100 or £10,000. The cost of the audit, therefore, ought to be viewed as an insurance premium. Expenses of this type tend to be regarded in retrospect as an excellent investment should a claim need to be made during the period of coverage; if no claim needs to be made, the cost of the premium must be seen as reasonable in relation to the risk mitigated.

The advantage of a one-to-one purchaser/vendor audit is that the purchasing firm obtains a detailed insight into the operation of the vendor and the quality of the product, and can concentrate on the vendor's areas of particular interest. However, there are disadvantages in single company auditing/consultancy over and above the purchaser's expense. As quality awareness grows, vendors might become subject to multiple audits, as has already happened in some sectors; if the purchaser standards are not uniform, confusion could result, which could discourage vendors from making the necessary improvements. Some auditors may not emphasize or explain to the vendor the business benefits which he can reap from specific improvement activities as this book has tried to stress, and the audit may then degenerate into the sterile standoff that is the death-knell of progress. Regrettably, it will take many years for quality awareness to develop across the broad swathe of industry and commerce to a level where this is likely to become an important issue.

JOINT AUDITS

Another means of reducing the cost of auditing in the absence of vendor certification would be if two or three purchasing firms interested in the same product cooperated to assess a single vendor. Not only would this save time and cost all round, it would ensure a consistent standard being advocated by the group of purchaser firms. Unfortunately, where this has been suggested, serious barriers have been erected which question the practicality of the approach, and I see no immediate prospect of removing them. To be specific, vendor firms are understandably reluctant to reveal their process weaknesses to more than one purchaser firm, since the potential loss of business from being found irredeemably wanting is much greater. The establishment of the team approach to audit/consultancy that is indispensable to the exercise is far more difficult to achieve outside the one-to-one relationship between purchaser and vendor.

Secondly, purchasing firms have been markedly reluctant to share audit information with each other, on the assumption of vendor consent, despite pledges of intent at lower corporate levels to do so. When the purchaser firms are in the same market such as in the pharmaceutical industry, for example, the competition is so intense that stiff resistance to divulging vendor information (with vendor permission) emerges from management from the fear that this may then contribute to a competitor's business advantage. The strength of this resistance was abundantly evident at a meeting held in 1995 attended by about 20 companies where these issues were exhaustively explored.[1] No evidence of a significant change in the climate in our industry is yet discernible in this respect, and similar competitive restrictions can be expected to be as forcefully applied in other industries.

This issue has received attention within the UK Pharmaceutical Industry GAMP Forum in recent months in the context of the narrower field of suppliers of software for purposes associated with regulated drug manufacture. Resistance to combined audits can be expected to arise from either the software vendor or purchaser communities. In the case of the pharmaceutical industry, there is already a strong consensus of the standards required. As a result, there is little resistance now from most of the vendors to sharing audit information, since many of them recognize that compliance with accepted standards is business critical. In these circumstances, the difficulties that have arisen so far have come not from vendor companies fearful of disclosure of proprietary technical information or process weaknesses, but from purchaser companies unwilling to share vendor information with each other. This reflects the intense competition in the pharmaceutical industry, its rapid rate of change and its feverish pace of global rationalization. It is expected that within the next few years, the number of major players will reduce to single figures, mainly from the pressure to achieve the minimum critical mass essential to making scientific research, drug discovery and dosage form development truly cost-effective.

However, in the wider world, where there is no consensus yet over standards within the various purchaser communities, the resistance to combined audits arises from vendors. Divulging the unfavourable contents of an audit from one purchaser may jeopardize the business from a second purchaser whose currently lower standards might readily be met.

Therefore, future combined audits are likely to be extremely infrequent for the foreseeable future. However, in the longer term, the TickIT accreditation scheme, or something very like it, must represent the best way forward both within the pharmaceutical-regulated software area, and in the wider software world.

INDEPENDENT AUDITS

A third approach which has already shown promising signs of alleviating this problem has been the engagement of a qualified independent auditor/consultant who can act on behalf of one or more purchasing firms. It would be vital for the consultant in these circumstances to adopt the positive, supportive attitude toward the vendor that this book has exemplified if the process is to be of benefit in the long term. Enlightened self-interest is far more likely to deliver the motivation to institute cultural change than externally imposed sanctions. By acting as an honest broker in this way, the auditor's advice is likely to be given more weight since he or she would be viewed as representing the interests of purchasers in general rather than just the immediate interests of one company.

TICKIT CERTIFICATION

The reduction of the costs inherent in purchaser auditing was the intention behind the TickIT accreditation scheme, where certification provides purchasers with an assurance of a sound engineering process being in place subject to regular surveillance monitoring, thus avoiding the expense of an individual audit. However, although after 5 years in operation, over 800 firms have now been accredited in the United Kingdom and 200 abroad, this remains a small minority of the industry. It seems that the vast majority of software houses, while being aware of the TickIT standards, have yet to take the first steps toward implementing the basic tenets of compliance. Many cite the cost of the TickIT assessment, accreditation and surveillance costs as the reason for this. In fairness to the British Standards Institution, the TickIT Guide pulls no punches in clearly setting out what these costs are. There is no doubt that the TickIT scheme has enormous value, and it is much to be regretted that it has not enjoyed even greater success. The appearance of similar schemes in other countries is much to be welcomed, imitation being, of course, the sincerest form of flattery! Harmonization of these schemes is widely recognized as being an important objective, and rightly so.

In the light of this, vendors should be encouraged to distinguish between the practices that TickIT advocates, and the business benefits that stem from them on the one hand, and the certification process on the other. It is quite possible to aspire to the former without proceeding to the latter. Vendors are keen to discover the simple, practical measures that they can adopt to implement the ISO 9000-3 (TickIT) principles, and see an early financial return for their investment, without shouldering the burden of the entire TickIT accreditation process. This conception seems to command wide acceptance, and its clarification has been one of the aims of this book.

Certification, however, offers the prospect to purchasers of avoiding the costs of individual audits which, if totaled, would dwarf the cost of the TickIT scheme. It may take some years for sufficient quality awareness among purchasers to accumulate enough momentum to encourage vendors at large to seek certification, which will only happen when they perceive that their market demands it. This is certainly not yet the case.

OTHER CERTIFICATION INITIATIVES

TickIT is by no means the only quality scheme in existence for software. I have already drawn from the GAMP Guide at several points in my journey and used the Capability Maturity Model from the Software Engineering Institute as a staircase showing where improvement initiatives are directed. I feel one other, very recent scheme merits a mention, that of the Software Conformity Assessment Scheme from Lloyd's Register.

Lloyd's Register is an international society which was formed in the 18th century for the classification of merchant shipping, providing rules for the construction and maintenance of ships. It came into being as a reaction to the poor standards of safety in the building and operation of ships at that time, and the huge consequential losses both of life and of treasure resulting from defective and shoddy construction. It is supervised by a committee comprising shipping owners, marine engineers and insurance underwriters. The name Lloyd originates from Edward Lloyd, the owner of a coffee house in London which was a popular meeting place for merchants, ship owners and insurance people. Lloyd's was incorporated as a recognized body for the regulation of marine insurance by an Act of Parliament in 1871, which was extended to all other forms of insurance (except life insurance) by the 1911 Lloyd's Act.

The long and successful track record of the society in the marine safety field suggests that the pattern might just as readily be applied to the regulation of software, since software is as crucial to the economy of the civilized world in the late 20th and 21st centuries as shipping was in the 18th. Furthermore, the concerns over quality and loss that gave rise to the inception of Lloyd's in the shipping sphere are analogous to those for software today.

The Lloyd's Software Conformity Assessment is a certification system based on the assessment of software products against published criteria. It involves the inspection of requirements, design, testing, verification, configuration, management, maintenance procedures and practices. Its foundational philosophies are to all intents and purposes identical to those on which this book is based. For example, it stresses that testing alone cannot deliver the required assurances of innate quality, and that the quality management system is important but secondary to the key factor of managerial attitudes. It does not attempt to constrain excessively the methodology used, providing that complies with basic principles of good software engineering. The interests of the customer or user are paramount, and the methodology should be responsive to changing technology. All of the deliverables of the development process are assessed for their degree of conformity with standards, which once again exemplifies the principle of documentary evidence that I have stressed is essential for a purchaser and which is produced naturally by a well-defined life cycle methodology. Once again, the very presence itself of the deliverables is vital evidence of the integrity of the process. The Lloyd's approach is illustrated in figure 15.1.

Within the GAMP Forum in the UK pharmaceutical industry, there have already been some signs of interest in a Lloyd's Register approach to the certification of vendors. I very much hope that a

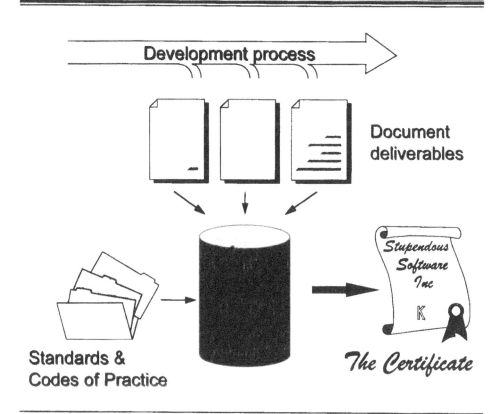

Figure 15.1. The Software Conformity Assessment Scheme

certification scheme along these lines, but across the entire spectrum of business applications, will be established in the not too distant future, so that standards can be lifted throughout the software industry, while at the same time reducing the overall cost of software engineering.

Notes

1. The meeting referred to was a special interest group meeting, held as part of an event entitled *Validation of Computerized Systems—Guidance for Suppliers,* sponsored by the International Society for Pharmaceutical Engineering and held in at the Golden Tulip Barbizon Palace Hotel, Amsterdam, on 12–14 March 1995. The principal purpose of the event, attended by representatives of most of the major European pharmaceutical manufacturers, as well as a large number of software vendors, was to launch the GAMP Guide in mainland Europe.

The Epilogue: Living Out
the Values

Values are caught, not taught.

Anon

This book has concentrated on the practical methods and procedures inherent in developing software that meets the customer's expectations, and ensures as far as possible his or her custom in the future. While one chapter has been devoted to the human relationships aspect of corporate management, the issues have been addressed in largely functional terms (i.e., those actions that will directly promote the process).

In concentrating on *what people do*, it would be very easy to stop there and ignore a wider, deeper and potentially much more powerful determinant of company fortune, that of *what people are*. This is closely related to the values that a company assumes to itself. These issues have been hinted at in the context of changing the company's culture, and the way people respond to change. Leadership has also been explored, particularly as it affects those on the purchasing side of the fence, by whom the auditor is commissioned to initiate the consultancy/audit visit. Let me then close this book with a few reflections on what I believe are the best values on which to base a software house (or any other kind of enterprise for that matter).

VALUES

Values and convictions fundamentally determine how we behave. Our attitudes to other people are driven by our perception of their value as people in relation to our own self-image. None of us in the Western world are able to insulate ourselves from the general decline in moral standards of ethics and behaviour that has characterized society in many countries in recent decades. The abandonment of what are called old-fashioned conventions of decency, consideration and good manners is bemoaned universally. The decline in the moral values of society has become a major political issue in Britain in recent months after a series of notorious atrocities,[1] which have prompted much public speculation as to what is now wrong with society. The rise in militant feminism is widely recognized as being to some degree a reflection of the awareness among women of a decline in respect and care afforded to them by men, and a desire to assert their equality (with which all would agree) rather than their complementarity (which few have the courage to defend). All of these societal influences radically affect us all, not only as individuals at work, but also in the fortunes of our companies. Codes of altruistic behaviour and good manners that could safely be taken for granted among staff and management 50 years ago can no longer be assumed. Companies are, therefore, being compelled to spell out and reinforce by peer pressure, often bordering on coercion, standards of ethical behavior that company personnel can no longer be assumed to abide by, either voluntarily or instinctively.

THE SERVANT MODEL OF MANAGEMENT

All of these values have a common thread running through them. It is the recognition that others should be regarded as at least as important as ourselves, and that success and well-being in the business world are promoted by an attitude of service (not servility) towards them, rather than the self-assertive pride, the sense of self-importance and the lust for power and prestige which are so destructive to interpersonal relationships. Although most would agree with these sentiments at a superficial level, their deeper implications for managers, when fully expounded, are disturbing, and strike some as both revolutionary and unrealistic. A moment's thought about the question *"Who are the most important people in our company?"* quickly illustrates how radical this thinking is. In many companies, the managers see themselves, and behave as though they are, the most important people, there to be served by those *beneath* them and in turn serving the chairman or chief executive who is the head of the company. The language we use to express these relationships, and the hierarchical organizational diagrams we produce to depict them (one of the first documents, the reader may remember that the auditor requests), betrays our values.

The critical importance of not only asking this question, but of arriving at the right answer, should be apparent to everyone caught up in the unprecedented changes now sweeping the industrialized societies of the world, which were touched on in the introduction. These nature of these changes, and their implications for interpersonal relationships at all levels of society, including their impact on mental health, were explored with deep prescience many years ago by Toffler (1970). His book was evocatively titled *Future Shock* to describe the malaise, mass neurosis, irrationality and disfunctional antisocial behaviour (the latter being most acutely expressed in mindless violence), that would characterize a society subjected to a great and unprecedented accelerative thrust of change. The era in which such a society would appear (at which we have already arrived) was poignantly dubbed the *800th lifetime*. This term arises from dividing the estimated 50,000 year existence of *homo sapiens*, self-conscious man as we know him, into 800 lifetimes of about 62 years each. Now of these 800, fully 650 were spent in caves; he then continues:

> *Only during the last 70 lifetimes has it been possible to communicate effectively from one lifetime to another—as writing emerged. Only during the last 6 did the masses ever see a printed word. Only during the last 4 has it been possible to measure time with any precision. Only in the last two has anyone anywhere used an electric motor. And the overwhelming majority of all the material goods we use in daily life have been developed within the present, 800th lifetime which marks a sharp discontinuity with all*

*past human experience. Man's relationship with resources
has reversed itself, evident in economic development.
Within a single lifetime agriculture, the original basis for
civilization has lost its dominance in nation after nation . . .
Moreover, if agriculture is the first stage of economic development and industrialism the second we can see now
that still another stage—the third—has suddenly been
reached. In about 1956 the US became the first major
power in which more than 50% of the non-farm labor
force ceased to wear the blue-collar of factory or manual
labor . . . outnumbered by white collar occupations of retail trade, administration, communications, research, education . . . the world's first service economy had been
born.*

He goes on to describe today's *super-industrial* society as being
characterized by a whirlwind of change occurring at an exponential
rate, causing a breakdown not only in the presuppositions upon
which many have built their lives, but also in mankind's capacity to
cope in such an unstable environment. In the light of this present reality, it seems therefore vital for all of us to rediscover those permanent and unchanging values essential to enable us to establish and
sustain harmonious relationships. Such values would aid us in
restoring some measure of stability in life, at both the individual and
the corporate level, for which so many now crave.

With that background, therefore, the question from which we
digressed re-presents itself with greater urgency: who really are the
most important people in a company? In the service economy of today, nothing less than the health and prosperity of the business depends on our getting the answer to this fundamental question right.
While it is clear that everyone in a company is providing a service,
who is really serving whom? Toffler exposes[2] the inability of the obsolescent hierarchical bureaucracy of yesterday, caricatured in
chapter 6, as sclerotic, and today unable to respond quickly enough
to the need for rapid decision making by those at the sharp end of
the business. It seems evident, then, that at one level at least, those
in direct contact with the customers or the process should be regarded as the most important, and that their managers' function is
to provide (serve) them with the environment in which their efforts
can be optimized, for the good of both company and customer alike.

It is this underlying, altruistic philosophy that is promoting the
modern emphasis on *team work*; although it is not often expressed

in these terms, it is the attitude that characterizes the most successful organizations in almost every business sector. The management in any enterprise can be thought of from this perspective as the *backroom office*, supporting the primary service providers, the staff. Shut down the backroom office and the service continues (at least for a time), while shutting the front office causes trading to cease at once. A football team is often quoted as another example—dismiss the manager, but the team will still play on Saturday (though it might not get paid!).

Now, of course, these are caricatures and grossly oversimplistic, but they serve not only to highlight the mutual interdependence of management and staff, but more importantly to demonstrate the absurdity of management believing itself *more important* than those who are managed. It also emphasizes how counterproductive, and out of place, the managerial outlook of self-assertive exertion of power and authority is in today's competitive environment.

Once this is recognized and **lived out** day-by-day in healthy personal relationships, then, and only then, will management acquire the *moral* authority (which is far more effective in influencing the behaviour of others than compulsion) to stamp on the company the values, without which, the full potential of its staff (the most precious, and expensive, corporate resource) can be developed.

Here, then, is a set of values in six categories which, if adopted and promulgated by life as well as lips, will foster business success in any enterprise. The reader may have noticed that running through them is a golden theme of *altruism, humility* and *self-sacrifice*, as opposed to *self-aggrandizement* and *self-preservation*. Without shared values such as these, even the finest and most cost-effective software development methodology will not ensure the survival and prosperity of the company, the aim to which this book has been devoted.

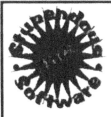 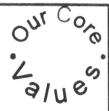

Customer Focus

Our customers are at the heart of everything we do

We strive to understand what our customers need and deliver the solutions to meet those needs.

When a customer brings a service problem to our attention, we assume responsibility for resolving it.

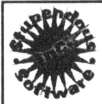 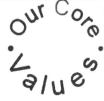

Mutual Respect

We respect our colleagues, just as we do our customers.

We treat each other with fairness, courtesy, candor and sensitivity.

We encourage diversity.

We are respectful of our colleagues' personal lives.

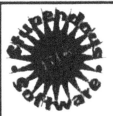

Teamwork

We put the company interest before that of our department or group.

We are all accountable for our company's success or failure.

We build on each others' strengths.

We look for ways to help each other.

Initiative

Our Core Values

We act with a sense of urgency.

We are innovative and creative.

We are continually on the lookout to add value.

We value leadership.

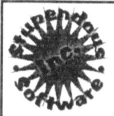

Professionalism

Our Core Values

We set ourselves exacting standards.

We act in a disciplined way in accordance with company standards and procedures to achieve our goals.

We continually develop our skills and competencies and broaden our knowledge.

We take pride in the company.

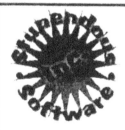

Quality

Our Core Values

We must earn our reputation every day.

We strive for operational excellence

We are determined to make our product the best in its market sector.

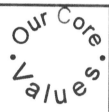

Notes

1. Three of the most appalling were the gunning down by one Thomas Hamilton of 16 schoolchildren and their teacher in Dunblane, Scotland, on 13 March 1996, for no apparent reason; the sadistic torture and murder of the young boy James Bulger by two lads of school age; and the stabbing to death of the headmaster Philip Lawrence by a youth outside his school while trying to stop a disturbance.

2. "The Collapse of Hierarchy" (Toffler 1970), page 123 ff.

References

ACARD (1986) *Software, A Vital Key to UK Competitiveness.* UK Government Advisory Council on Applied Research and Development, H.M. Stationery Office, London. Crown copyright and is reproduced with the permission of the Controller of the H.M.S.O.

ANSI/IEEE standard 1016-1987. *IEEE Recommended Practice for Software Design Descriptions.*

ANSI/IEEE standard 610.12-1990. *Standard Glossary of Software Engineering Technology.*

ANSI/IEEE standard 730-1984. *Software Quality Assurance Plans.*

ANSI/IEEE standard 828-1983. *IEEE Standard for Software Configuration Management Plans.*

ANSI/IEEE standard 829-1983. *IEEE Standard for Software Test Documentation.*

ANSI/IEEE standard 830-1984. *IEEE Guide to Software Requirements Specifications.*

ANSI/IEEE standard 983-1986. *Software Quality Assurance Planning.*

ANSI Standard N45.2.10-1993.

Arnold, R. (1988) *Disaster Recovery Plan.* Wiley, New York (ISBN 0-471-556963).

Benington, H. (1956) *Production of Large Computer Programs* In *Proceedings, Symposium on Advanced Programming Methods for Digital Computers* by U.S. Office of Naval Research (Report ACR-15).

Boar, B. (1984) *Application Prototyping—A Requirements Definition Strategy for the 1980s.* Wiley, New York.

Boehm, B. W. (1981) *Software Engineering Economics.* Prentice Hall, Englewood Cliffs, NJ.

Boehm, B. W., McClean, R. K., Urfrig, D. B. (1975) Some Experience with Automated Aids to the Design of Large Scale Reliable Software. *IEEE Trans. Software Eng.* (March).

BS 4778 Part 2 (1991) *Quality Vocabulary.* British Standards Institution, London.

Chamberlain, R. (1994) *Computer Systems Validation for the Pharmaceutical and Medical Device Industries,* 2nd ed. Alaren Press.

Chapman, K. G. (1984) The PAR Approach to Process Validation. *Pharmaceutical Technology* (December).

Chapman, K. G. (1991a) A History of Validation in the United States, Part I. *Pharmaceutical Technology* 15 (10): 82–86.

Chapman, K. G. (1991b) A History of Validation in the United States, Part II Validation of Computer Systems. *Pharmaceutical Technology* 15 (11): 54–70.

Cohen, F. B. (1994) *A Short Course on Computer Viruses,* 2nd ed. Wiley, New York.

Crosby, P. B. (1979) *Quality Is Free—The Art of Making Quality Certain.* McGraw-Hill, New York.

De Marco, T. (1982) *Controlling Software Projects.* Yourdon Inc., New York.

Deming, W. E. (1986) *Out of the Crisis.* Massachusetts Institute of Technology Center for Advanced Educational Services, Cambridge, MA. Reprinted from *Out of the Crisis* by W. Edwards Deming by permission of MIT and the W. Edwards Deming

Institute. Published by MIT, Center for Advanced Educational Services, Cambridge, MA 02139. Copyright by The W. Edwards Deming Institute.

Dijkstra, E. W. (1976) *A Discipline of Programming.* Prentice-Hall Inc., Englewood Cliffs, NJ.

Dorling, A. (1993) SPICE: Software Process Improvement and Capability Determination. *Software Quality Journal* 2: 209–224.

Fagan, M. E. (1976) Design and Code Inspections to Reduce Errors in Program Development. *IBM Systems Journal* 15 (3): 182–211.

FDA (1987) *Guideline on General Principles of Process Validation.* Food and Drug Administration, Rockville, MD.

Fowler, P. and Rifkin, S. (1990) *Software Engineering Process Group Guide, Appendix D: An Introduction to Technological Change.* Technical Report CMU/SEI-90-TR-24. Software Engineering Institute, Carnegie Mellon University, Pittsburgh, PA.

The GAMP Supplier Guide on the Validation of Automated Systems (1996). Available from the International Society for Pharmaceutical Engineering, Nieuwe Uitleg 21, 2514 JB, The Hague, The Netherlands (for Europe) or from ISPE in North America at 3816 West Linebaugh Ave., Suite 412, Tampa, FL 33624. Tel: 1-813-960-2105; Fax: 1-813-264-2816.

Gilb, T. and Graham, D. (1993) *Software Inspection.* Addison-Wesley Publishing Company, London.

Grudin, J. (1994) Groupware and Social Dynamics: Eight Challenges for Developers. *Communications of the ACM* 37 (1): 92–105.

Humphrey, W. S. (1988) Characterizing the Software Process: A Maturity Framework. *IEEE Software* (March): 73–79.

Humphrey, W. S. (1994) *The Personal Process in Software Engineering* appearing in *Proceedings of Third International Conference on the Software Process,* Reston, VA, (October); 69–78. Published by the International Software Process Association and the IEEE Computer Society Press.

Humphrey, W. S. (1995) *A Discipline for Software Engineering.* Addison-Wesley Publishing Company, London.

ISO 10007 (1995) *Quality Management—Guidelines for Configuration.* International Organization for Standardization, Geneva, Switzerland.

ISO 10011-1:1990. *Guidelines for Auditing Quality Systems.* International Organization for Standardization, Geneva, Switzerland.

ISO 8402:1994. *Quality Management and Quality Assurance—Vocabulary.* International Organization for Standardization, Geneva, Switzerland.

ISO 9000-3. *Guide to the Application of ISO 9001 to the Development, Supply and Maintenance of Software.* International Organization for Standardization, Geneva, Switzerland.

ISPE (1996) *A Comparison of Existing Guides.* Proceedings from the ISPE/PDA sponsored conference, Computer-Related Systems Validation—An International Perspective for Users and Suppliers, January, in Baltimore. Available from International Society for Pharmaceutical Engineering, Tampa, FL. (For address, see above under GAMP Guide.)

Korteweg, M. (1993) Computer Validation in Clinical Research: Regulatory Requirements in the European Community. *Drug Information Journal* 27: 315–319.

Lientz, B. and Swanson, E. (1980) *Software Maintenance Management.* Addison-Wesley Publishing Company, London.

Lucas, E. G. (1987) Psychological Aspects of Travel. *Travel Medicine International* pp. 99–104.

Martin, J. (1987) *Recommended Diagramming Standards for Analysts and Programmers.* Prentice Hall Inc., Englewood Cliffs, NJ.

The Windows™ Interface: An Application Design Guide (Microsoft Windows Software Development Kit). Microsoft document No. PC28921-0692.

Myers, G. J. (1979) *The Art of Software Testing.* Wiley, New York.

Ould, M. A. (1990) *Strategies for Software Engineering.* Wiley, New York.

Perry, D. E., Staudenmayer, N. A., and Votta, L. G., Jr. (1996) Understanding and Improving Time Usage in Software Development. In: *Software Process,* edited by F. Alfonso and A. Wolf. Wiley, New York.

PDA (1995) Validation of Computer-Related Systems (Technical Report 18). *PDA J. Pharm. Sci. and Technol.* 49 (suppl. S1).

PMA Computer Systems Validation Committee (1986) Validation Concepts for Computer Systems Used in the Manufacture of Drug Products. *Pharm. Technol.* 10 (5): 24–34.

PMA Computer System Validation Committee (1993a) Computer System Validation—Staying Current: Vendor—User Relationships. *Pharm. Technol. Intnl.* (September).

PMA Computer System Validation Committee (1993b) Computer System Validation—Staying Current: Security in Computerized Systems. *Pharm. Technol. Intnl.* (June).

Price Waterhouse & Co. (1988) *Software Quality Standards: The Costs and Benefits—A Review for the Department of Trade and Industry.* Price Waterhouse & Co., Chartered Accountants, 32 London Bridge St., London SE11 1XX; tel: 0171 939 3000; fax: 0171 378 0647. Crown copyright and quoted by permission.

Royce, W. W. (1970) Managing the Development of Large Software Systems: Concepts and Techniques. Published in *Proceedings of WESCON.*

Sakamoto K., Kishida, K., and Nakakoji, K. (1996) Cultural Adaptation of the CMM: A Case Study of a Software Engineering Process Group in a Japanese Manufacturing Factory. In: *Software Process,* edited by F. Alfonso and A. Wolf. Wiley, New York.

The STARTS Guide, 2nd edition (1987) National Computing Centre, Oxford Road, Manchester M1 7ED. Crown copyright is reproduced with the permission of the Controller of the H.M.S.O.

The TickIT Guide (A Guide to Software Quality Management System Construction and Certification to ISO 9001) Issue 3.0 (1995). BSI/DISC TickIT Office, London. Extracts from the TickIT Guide Issue 3.0 are reproduced with the permission of BSI Customer Services, 389 Chiswick High Road, London W4 4AL, UK.

Toffler, A. (1970) *Future Shock.* The Bodley Head, London (now part of The Curtis Brown Group, New York).

Trill, A. J. (1993a) Computerized Systems and GMP—A UK Perspective Part I: Background, Standards and Methods. *Pharm. Technol. Intnl.* (February): 12ff.

Trill, A. J. (1993b) Computerized Systems and GMP—A UK Perspective Part III: Best Practices and Topical Issues. *Pharm. Technol. Intnl.* (May): 17ff.

Glossary

*Let every man say what he meaneth,
and mean what he sayeth.*

Anon

This glossary includes the definitions of many of the technical terms
that are referred to directly or indirectly in this book; these are believed to be the most generally acceptable meanings of the terms defined. It has been assembled from a number of sources, including
the ANSI/IEEE standard 610.12-1990, and is intended to be of general help to all software developers and auditors. It makes no attempt to be comprehensive, but definitions have been selected
either on the basis of our estimate of the scope for misunderstanding, or of their widespread usefulness to the software development
and user communities as a whole. Definitions for network-related
terms have been included to reflect their increasing inclusion in the
everyday jargon of IT, and which, therefore, may be helpful to the
auditor/consultant encountering them in the course of vendor site
visits.

Where there are multiple contexts in which a term is used, the
entry has been confined to those definition(s) with the greatest
relevance to the context of software development and quality

357

assessment. Where a particular term is widely used in more than one context, a number of common definitions may be provided.

Acceptance criteria: The criteria a software product must meet to complete a test phase or meet delivery requirements successfully.

Access control mechanism: Features of the product in hardware or software, or operating procedures, designed to allow only authorized access to a computer system.

Accuracy: A quality feature of something that is free from error.

Address: A unique number identifying a particular network or network workstation (network address), or identifying a location in computer memory (memory address).

Algorithm: A finite set of well-defined rules for the solution of a problem in a finite number of steps.

Alpha testing: Initial testing of software by a person not directly associated with the development process.

Application programs: Programs specifically written to fulfil an identifiable technical or business need.

Application software: Software specifically produced for the functional use of a computer system.

Architectural design: The process of defining a collection of hardware and software components and their interfaces to establish a framework for the development of a computer system.

Architecture: The description of a system in terms of the components, interfaces, and protocols that it utilizes and the way in which they fit together.

Assemble: To translate a program expressed in an assembly language into machine code and perhaps linking it to invoked subroutines.

Assembler: A computer program used to assemble.

Assembly language: A computer-oriented language whose instructions usually correspond on a one-to-one basis with computer instructions.

Audit: An independent review for assessing compliance with software requirements, specifications, baselines, standards, or procedures.

Automated design tool: A software tool that aids in the synthesis, analysis, modelling, or documentation of a software design.

Availability: The probability that software will be able to perform its designated system function when required for use.

Backup: Provisions made for the recovery of data files or software or for the use of alternative computer equipment after a system failure of disaster.

Backbone: The primary connectivity mechanism of a hierarchical-distributed system. All systems which have connectivity to an intermediate system on the backbone are assured of connectivity to each other (e.g., a network backbone is one that interconnects to other networks).

Baseline: A configuration identification document, note, or record formally designated at a specific time in a configuration item's life cycle which serves as the basis for the further development of the item, which can then only be changed further through formalized change control.

Beta testing: Final testing of software immediately prior to release by a selected group of independent end users.

Bit: The simplest unit of data in a digital computer capable of two values only, on or off, 1 or 0.

Boolean: An algebraic system formulated by George Boole for formal operations in logic in terms of true and false entities.

Bootup: The execution of a short computer program (the "boot" program) which is permanently resident or easily loaded, that when executed loads a much larger program, usually an operating system, into memory and executes it.

Bottom-up: Pertaining to an approach that begins with the lowest level software components of a hierarchy and proceeds via progressively higher levels to the top level component.

Boundary value: A minimum or maximum input, output or internal data value applicable to a system or process.

Bridge: A device that connects two or more physical networks and forwards packets between them. It can usually be set to take care of filtering packets (to forward only certain traffic). It can be used to connect LANs by forwarding packets addressed to other similar networks. Possessing no intelligence, it passes on all data, even if garbled.

Bug: An accidental condition in software that causes it to behave in an unintended manner.

Build: An operational version of a software product that incorporates a specified subset of the capabilities of the final product.

Byte: A collection of eight bits.

Canned configurable: A commercial off-the-shelf software package with which the user can create application programs by filling in the blanks or writing macros in the language provided, without any change to the executable code.

CASE tools: Computer-aided software engineering development tools enabling developers to ensure that software of sound structure is being created.

Certification: The procedure and action by a duly authorized body of determining, verifying, and attesting in writing to the qualifications of personnel, processes, procedures, or items in accordance with applicable requirements.

Change control: The procedure by which a change is proposed, evaluated, approved or rejected, scheduled and tracked.

Client-Server: A network system design in which a processor or computer is designated as a server to provide services to other network-connected processors and/or computers. The computer (usually a workstation) that makes the service requests is called the client. The network devices (file servers, disk servers, print servers, database servers, etc.) that provide the services to client workstations are called servers.

Code: The representation of a computer program in a symbolic form that can be accepted by a processor.

Code walk-through: A review process in which a designer or programmer leads one or other members of the development team through a segment of design or code that he or she has written, while the other members ask questions and make comments about style, possible errors, violation of development standards and other problems.

Command language: A set of procedural operators with a related syntax, used to indicate the functions to be performed by an operating system.

Comment: Information embedded within a computer program, command language, or set of data intended to provide clarification to human readers without in any way affecting machine interpretation. May also be descriptive, reference, or explanatory information interspersed among source language statements, but having no effect on the target language.

Commercial off-the-shelf (COTS) configurable: A commercial off-the-shelf software package configurable to the user's needs by filling in the blanks provided for this purpose without any change to the executable code.

Compile: To translate a higher order language program into its relocatable code or absolute machine code equivalent.

Compiler: A computer program that compiles source code.

Computer: A functional programmable unit that consists of one or more associated processing units and peripheral equipment, that is controlled by internally stored programs, and that can perform substantial computation, including numerous arithmetic and logic operations without human intervention.

Computer system: Computer hardware components assembled with software to collectively perform a specified function.

Computer-related system: One or more computerized systems in its relevant operating environment.

Computer-related system validation: Establishing documented evidence which provides a high degree of assurance that a specific computer-related system will consistently operate in accordance with predetermined specifications.

Computerized system: A computer system plus the controlled function with which it operates.

Conditional control structure: A programming control structure that allows alternative flow of control in a program depending on the fulfillment of specified conditions (e.g., if . . . then . . . else).

Configuration: The requirements, design and implementation that define a particular version of a system or system component.

Configuration audit: The process of verifying that all required configuration items have been produced, that the current version agrees with specified requirements, that the technical documentation completely and accurately describes the configuration items, and that all change requests have been resolved.

Configuration control: The process of evaluating, approving or disapproving, and coordinating changes to configuration items after formal establishment of their configuration identification.

Configuration identification: (1) The process of designating the configuration items in a system and recording their characteristics. (2) The approved documentation that defines a configuration item. (3) The current approved technical documentation for a configuration item as set forth in specifications, drawings and associated lists, and documents referred to therein.

Configuration item: (1) A collection of hardware or software elements treated as a unit for the purpose of configuration management. (2) An aggregation of hardware/software or any of its discrete portions that satisfies an end-use function, and is designated for configuration management.

Configuration management: (1) The process of identifying and defining the configuration items in a system, controlling the release and change of those items throughout the life cycle, reporting and recording the status of configuration items and change requests, and verifying the completeness and correctness of configuration items. (2) A discipline applying technical and administrative direction and surveillance to identify and document the functional characteristics of a configuration item, to control changes to those characteristics and to record and report change processing and implementation.

Control structure: A construct that determines the flow of control through a computer program.

Controlled function: A process and any related equipment controlled by a computer system.

Correctness: (1) The extent to which software is free from design and coding defects. (2) The extent to which it meets its requirements. (3) The extent to which it meets user expectations.

Critical section: A piece of code to be executed mutually exclusively with any other critical section of code (these are code segments that make competing use of a particular resource or data item).

Criticality: A classification of a software error or fault based on an assessment of the degree of impact that the fault will have on the development or operation of the system.

Data: The representation of facts, concepts or instructions in a formalized manner suitable for communication, interpretation or processing by human or automatic means.

Data dictionary: A collection of the names of all data items used in a software system together with their properties.

Data flow diagram: A graphical representation of a system showing data sources, data sinks, data storage and the logical flow of data between nodes.

Database: A file or collection of files containing data and structural information relating to the data.

Dead code: (1) Superseded code from earlier versions. (2) A residue of a system modification.

Debugging: The process of locating, analyzing and correcting software faults.

Design: The process of defining the software architecture, components, modules, interfaces, test approach and data for a software system to satisfy specified requirements.

Design language: A formal notation with special constructs used to develop, analyze and document a design.

Design review: The formal review of an existing or proposed design for the purpose of detecting and correcting defects that could impair the fitness for use or degrade the performance, safety or economic viability of the envisaged system.

Design specification: A specification that documents a design of a system or component.

Document: (1) A human readable data item. (2) To record information in human readable form.

Documentation: Technical data in human readable form that describe or specify the system at any stage in the life cycle.

Driver: A program that exercises a system or system component by simulating the activity of a higher level component. (Drivers are principally used for the control of peripheral devices. One piece of high-level system code is translated into many peripheral-specific low-level instructions to implement the function represented by the high level system code).

Dynamic path analysis: The process of evaluating a program based on its execution pathway.

Efficiency: The extent to which software consumes the available computing resources in performing its intended function.

Embedded system: A computer system integral to a larger system whose purpose is not computational (e.g., fly by wire aircraft control system).

Emulation: The imitation of all or part of one computer system by another, so that the imitating computer behaves in exactly the same manner as the imitated system (e.g., terminal emulation software for personal computers to mimic mainframe terminals).

Emulator: Hardware, software or firmware that performs emulation.

Error: (1) A discrepancy between a computed, observed or measured value and the truth. (2) A human action that results in software containing a fault.

Executable code: (1) Code directly executable on a computer. (2) Code produced by passing object code through a linker.

Failure: The termination of the ability of a functional unit to perform its required function.

Firmware: Computer programs and data loaded in a type of memory that is nonvolatile and cannot be modified by the computer during processing.

Flowchart: A graphical representation of the definition, analysis or solution of a problem in which symbols are used to represent operations, data, flow and equipment.

Formal language: A language whose rules are explicitly established prior to its use.

Formal notation: A means of recording information about a system to avoid ambiguity, to facilitate automated processing, to prove logical consistency and to promote reasoning.

Formal procedure: A procedure that has been documented, approved, carries official endorsement, and is the accepted means of executing the process.

Frame relay: A recently developed switching interface, operating in packet mode, that constitutes the cloud into which each location can connect, thereby requiring only one router. This eliminates the need for every location to lease lines to connect to every other location (requiring a router on each side of the line), and therefore greatly reduces the expense of the network.

Function: (1) A specific purpose of an entity or its characteristic action. (2) A subroutine invoked during the evaluation of an expression, in which its name appears, that returns a value to its point of invocation.

Functional requirements specification: User requirements for a computer system or configuration item expressed in a formal notation suitable as the basis for defining a system or item design.

Gateway: The original Internet term for what is now called a router. In current usage, the terms *gateway* and *application gateway* refer to systems which do translation from one native format to another (e.g., X.400 to/from that of the RFC822 electronic gateways).

Hardware: Physical equipment used in data processing.

Hierarchy: A structure whose components are reranked into levels of subordination according to a specific set of rules.

High level language: A programming language that includes features closely related to intended functionality, and that does not reflect the structure of any one type of computer, thus enabling it to be used to compose machine-independent programs.

Hub: A LAN device which is used in certain network topologies to allow the network to be lengthened, or to be expanded, with additional workstations.

Implementation: The realization of an abstraction in the more concrete terms of hardware and/or software.

Implementation phase: The period in the system development life cycle during which a software product is created from requirements and design specifications.

Incremental development: A development methodology in which the life cycle phases overlap and are pursued iteratively rather than sequentially, resulting in the incremental completion of the software product.

Independent testing: Testing of software by an organization or individuals who are technically and managerially separate from code development personnel.

Inspection: A formal evaluation technique in which life cycle documents or code are examined in relation to their source documents and standing rules for the purpose of detecting bugs.

Installation and checkout phase: The period in the system development life cycle during which the product is integrated into its operating environment and tested there to ensure conformity with requirements.

Installation qualification: Documented verification that all key aspects of hardware installation adhere both to appropriate requirements and to the computer system design specification.

Instruction: A program statement that causes a computer to perform a particular operation or group of operations.

Instruction set: The set of instructions of a computer or programming language from which all the instructions used must be drawn.

Integration: The process of combining software and/or hardware elements into an overall system.

Integration testing: An orderly progression of testing in which hardware and/or software elements are combined to form an integrated system.

Interactive: The characteristic of a system in which each user entry triggers a response from the system.

Interface: A shared boundary between one system component and another.

Interoperability: The ability of two or more systems to exchange information and to mutually use the exchanged information.

Interpret: To translate into machine code and to execute each source language statement of a computer program in a sequential manner.

Interpreter: Computer program that interprets computer programs.

Interrupt: The suspension of the execution of a computer program by an event external to the process, in such a way that the suspended execution may then be resumed.

Iteration: (1) The cyclic repetition of a sequence of programming language statements until a given condition is met or while a given condition is true. (2) A single execution of a loop.

Kernel: The nucleus or core (e.g., of an operating system).

Key item: An item within a set of data that contains information about the set, including its identification.

LAN: Acronym for local area network capable of linking computers, terminals and other equipment for the purposes of exchanging information.

Level: (1) The degree of subordination of an item in a hierarchical arrangement. (2) A rank within a hierarchy.

Life cycle: A process which can be viewed as a set of discrete stepwise stages.

Linker: A computer program used to create an executable program file from one or more independently translated object code modules by resolving cross-references between them, and by combining them with externally referenced executable code (often held in software libraries).

Load map: A computer-generated list that identifies the location and size of all or parts of a memory-resident program.

Loader: A program that reads object code into main storage prior to execution.

Logical file/record: A file/record independent of its physical environment.

Loop: A set of instructions that can be executed repeatedly while a certain condition prevails.

Machine code: A computer program that can be directly executed by a computer.

Mail gateway: A computer or device that connects two or more electronic mail systems (usually dissimilar systems on different networks), and transfers messages between them. (Sometimes the mapping and translation can be quite complex, generally requiring a store-and-forward scheme, whereby a message is completely held for translation prior to being re-transmitted. Normally messages are passed though as they are being received, without holding).

Maintainability: The ease with which the maintenance of a program can be performed in accordance with its requirements.

Message packet: The unit of information by which a network communicates, each containing a request for services, information on how to handle the request, and the date to be transferred. A message unit that can be individually routed over a LAN is called a data packet and contains a predefined limited amount of data. Messages exceeding the limit must be broken into multiple packets before being sent across the LAN.

Multiserver network: A network having two or more servers operating on it.

Network: A complex system consisting of two or more interconnected computers.

Network station: Any computer or other device connected to a network. It can be a workstation, bridge or server.

Nonvolatile: A characteristic of memory that preserves the stored information indefinitely even if the power supply is interrupted.

Object code: Program code resulting from compiling source code.

Object-oriented programming: Program development by expressing functionality in terms of objects (encapsulated data and services that manipulate it) and the information flows between them.

Operating environment: Those conditions and activities interfacing directly or indirectly with the system whose control is central to maintaining the computerized system's validated status.

Operating system: A set of programs provided with a computer to manage its resources for the successful execution of programs or application software.

Operational qualification: Documented verification that the system or subsystem operates as specified in the functional requirements specification throughout representative or anticipated operating ranges.

Packet: see Message packet.

Parameter: (1) A variable that is given a constant value for a given application. (2) A variable that is used to pass values between program routines.

Patch: A change made directly to object code without re-assembly or re-compilation from source code.

Path analysis: A process aimed at identifying all possible pathways through a program to detect incomplete paths or identify unreachable code (code that is not on any path).

Performance: The ability of a computer system to perform its functions in relation to time, throughput or number of transactions (i.e., its capacity to do its intended job).

Performance qualification: Documented verification that the integrated system performs as defined in the functional requirements specification in its normal operating environment (i.e., the computer-related system does what it purports to do).

Peripheral device: A device, other than the computer itself, used in data processing.

Platform: A computer and its operating system viewed as a basis for loading and executing programs or application software.

Policy: A directive specifying the objective to be accomplished.

Portability: The ease with which software can be transferred from one platform to another.

Precision: (1) A measure of the ability to distinguish between nearly equal values. (2) The degree of discrimination with which a quantity is stated.

Privileged instruction: An instruction that can only be executed by a supervisory program.

Procedure: The stepwise description of the sequence of actions necessary to execute a business or technical process.

Process: A unique, finite ordered sequence of events defined by its purpose and necessary to create a specific condition or state of affairs that does not yet exist.

Program: (1) A sequence of instructions suitable for processing by a computer. (2) To create a sequence of instructions.

Program library: An organized collection of programs with their associated documentation.

Programming language: An artificial language designed to generate or express programs.

Programming standards: A documented set of rules defining how source code is to be developed.

Project plan: A management document describing the approach that will be taken for a project. It describes the work to be done, the resources to be allocated, the methods to be used, the configuration management and quality assurance procedures to be followed, schedules to be met, and organization details.

Prompt: A message informing a user that the system is ready for the next piece of information.

Protocol: (1) A formal description of message format and associated rules that have been established to allow two or more systems to exchange information. (2) The rules that control the formatting and transmission of data. (3) A set of conventions or rules that govern the interactions of processes or applications within a computer system or network.

Pseudo code: A combination of programming language and natural language used to facilitate program design.

Quality: The totality of features and characteristics of a product or service that bears on its ability to satisfy given needs.

Quality assurance: A planned and systematic pattern of the organized arrangements necessary to provide adequate confidence that an item or product conforms to established requirements.

Quality metric: A quantitative measure of the degree to which software possesses a given attribute that affects its quality.

Quality plan: A management document describing the deliverables to be expected during a project, the quality metrics of each, and the controls which must be evident to demonstrate the incorporation of defined characteristics.

RAM (Random Access Memory): Volatile memory in which programs execute and whose contents may be altered by any time.

Real time: (1) Pertaining to the processing of data by a computer in connection with another external process according to time requirements imposed by the external process. (2) Pertaining to the actual time during which a physical process takes place and to which the system is inextricably bound.

Record: A collection of data treated as a unit.

Redundancy: The inclusion of duplicate system elements to improve operational reliability by ensuring continued operation if a primary element fails.

Regression testing: Selective retesting to detect faults introduced after a system change to verify that the change has not caused unintended adverse effects, or to show that the system still meets its functional requirements.

Relocatable code: Machine code possessing relative addresses needing to be translated into absolute addresses prior to execution.

Repeater: A device that disseminates electrical signals from one cable to another without making routing decisions or providing packet filtering.

Requirement: (1) A condition or capability needed by a user to solve a problem or meet an objective. (2) A condition or capability that must be met by a system or system component to satisfy a business or technical need.

Requirements notation: A formal notation with special constructs and verification protocols used to specify, verify and document requirements.

Requirements phase: The period of time within the system development life cycle during which the requirements (user and functional) are defined and documented in written specifications.

Resource number: A shared variable used to synchronize shared processes and coordinate the simultaneous attempts by two or more programs to lock a single resource (Hewlett Packard computers).

Retirement phase: The period of time within the system development life cycle during which support for a software product is terminated permanently.

Ring topology: A closed loop topology in which data passes in one direction from workstation to workstation on a LAN, with each acting as a repeater, passing data to the next workstation on the ring.

Robustness: The extent to which software can continue to operate correctly despite erroneous inputs from whatever source.

Router: (1) A system responsible for making decisions about which of several paths a network's (or Internet's) traffic will follow, utilizing its routing protocol (to gain information about the network and algorithms) to choose the best route. (2) A network layer intermediate system, a bridge operating at a protocol level involving hardware and software (therefore classified as intelligent) to route data between networks, whether similar or dissimilar.

Routine: (1) A program segment that performs a specific task. (2) A program that is frequently used or invoked.

Routing: The path a message must follow to reach its destination, or the procedure used to decide the best path for the data to take in order to reach its destination.

Run time: (1) The time taken for a program to execute. (2) The instant at which a program begins to execute.

Semaphore: A shared variable used to synchronize shared processes by indicating whether an action has been completed or an event has occurred (IBM and other computers).

Senility: The characteristic of software in its retirement phase.

Software: Programs, procedures and documentation pertaining to the operation of a computer system.

Software development life cycle: The process from conception of a software product to its retirement, expressed as a sequence of discrete stages pursued in a controlled, stepwise manner.

Software engineering: The systematic and documented approach to the development, operation, maintenance and retirement of software.

Software library: An organized collection of programs, functions or subroutines with their associated documentation.

Software quality: (1) The totality of features of a software product that bear on its ability to satisfy given needs as expressed in its specifications. (2) The composite characteristics of software that determine the degree to which the software will meet the expectations of the customer.

Source code: The primary, documented, set of instructions, expressed in human readable form, for use in creating a computer program.

Spiral methodology: A software development methodology in which the sequential phases of the life cycle are repeated iteratively until the development is complete.

Structural integrity: An attribute reflecting the degree to which a program or application software satisfies functional requirements and whose development methodology conforms to the generally accepted international standards of good software engineering practice.

Structural testing: The examination of the internal structure of source code including high and low level code review and path analysis to gauge compliance with programming standards and procedures.

Structured design: A disciplined approach to software design that adheres to a specified set of rules based on principles such as top-down design and data flow analysis.

Structured programming: Any approach to organizing and coding programs that reduces complexity, improves clarity and facilitates debugging and modification.

Structured test plan: A document describing the tests to be applied during the test phase, traceable to the design specification and including for each test the case, goal, procedure, required data, execution method, expected result, and documentation method.

Subprogram: A program unit that may be invoked by one or more other program units.

Subroutine: A sequenced set of statements that may be invoked at one or more points in a program that receives and returns information by means of passed arguments or other mechanism, other than that of the subroutine name itself.

Supervisory program: A computer program that controls the execution of other computer programs and regulates the flow of work.

Syntax: (1) The relationship among characters or groups of characters, independent of their meanings or the manner of their interpretation or use. (2) The structure of expressions in a language. (3) The rules governing the structure of a language.

System: An assemblage of people, machines and methods organized to accomplish a set of specific functions.

System design: The process of defining the hardware and software architectures, components, modules, interfaces and data for a system to satisfy specified requirements.

System documentation: Documentation conveying the requirements, design philosophy, design details, capabilities, limitations and other characteristics of a system.

System software: Software designed for a particular type, make or family of computers to enable them to execute application software (e.g., operating systems, utility programs and compilers).

Test phase: The period of time in the life cycle during which the components of a software product are evaluated and integrated, determining whether the requirements have been satisfied.

Test plan: A document describing the approach to be taken for the test activities, including the testing to be performed, the test schedules, personnel requirements, reporting requirements and any risks requiring contingency planning.

Test report: A document traceable to the structured test plan describing the results of the tests defined in the latter.

Testability: (1) The extent to which software facilitates both the establishment of test criteria and the evaluation of the software with respect to those criteria. (2) The extent to which the definition of requirements facilitates analysis of the requirements to establish test criteria.

Throughput: A measure of the amount of work performed by a computer system over a period of time.

Time sharing: (1) An operating technique of a computer system that provides for the interleaving in time of two or more processes within one processor. (2) The ability of a system to allow two or more users to execute programs or application software simultaneously.

Token Bus: A network using a logical token-passing access method. Unlike a token-passing ring, permission to transmit is usually based on node address rather than the calling workstation's position in the network. It uses a common cable set, with all signals broadcast across the entire LAN.

Token-passing ring topology: A LAN design in which each workstation is connected to an upstream and a downstream workstation. An electronic signal called the token, a unique combination of bits whose possession constitutes permission to transmit across the network, is passed from workstation to workstation around the ring. One workstation may not send a transmission to another unless it has possession of a free token (i.e., one not currently in use). Since only one token is allowed per network it follows therefore that only one workstation can broadcast at a time.

Top-down: Pertaining to an approach that starts with the highest level component of a hierarchy and proceeds through progressively lower levels.

Topology: The physical layout of network cabling.

User documentation: Documentation conveying to the end user of a system instructions for using the system to exploit its intended function.

User requirements specification: Requirements for a computer system or configuration item defined by users and expressed in language fully comprehensible by them.

Utility programs: Programs or routines designed to perform some general function required by all application software regardless of functionality.

Validation: The process of evaluating software at the end of the development process to ensure compliance with requirements.

Variable: (1) A quantity that can assume any assigned value according to its type. (2) A character or group of characters that refers to a value which within a program corresponds to an address.

Verification: (1) The process of determining whether or not the products of a given phase of the life cycle fulfil the requirements established during the previous phase. (2) Formal proof of program correctness. (3) The act of reviewing, inspecting, testing, checking, auditing, or otherwise establishing and documenting whether or not items, processes or documents conform to specified requirements.

Virtual storage: The storage space that may be regarded as addressable main storage by the user of a computer system in which virtual memory addresses are mapped on to real memory addresses.

Virus: Executable code designed to attach itself secretly to files or programs in order to foster its self propagation and execute its intended function.

Volatile: A characteristic of memory that results in total loss (amnesia) on the interruption of the power supply.

VPN: Acronym for virtual private network.

WAN: Acronym for wide area network. When a LAN connects to public lines (because it must link over a large geographical area), it becomes a WAN.

Workstation: A desktop computer that performs local processing and accesses one or more LANs.

Part 4

Appendices

Appendix 1

The Audit Process
Operational Procedure

In any organization, regardless of the nature of its business, processes can only be executed repeatably if the manner in which the process is to be operated is documented in an *operational procedure*. Even then, this document must possess the level of detail required by the trained staff member responsible for following it. The process of carrying out team-based consultancy audits is no exception.

The audit procedure presented here is endorsed with the logo of the fictitious company Prudent Purchasing Inc. for two reasons:

1. To emphasise that this is a process of the purchasing company as opposed to the software vendor enterprise.

2. Like all well-presented and credible procedures, it needs to conform both to the letter, and to the spirit, of the company's culture.

The presentation of this document is, therefore, similar to the standard operating procedure template presented in appendix 5 in the context of the vendor company's own quality management system. The document would normally be issued complete with the auditor's worksheets, provided here in appendix 3. The displayed page numbering, however, does not include these. Because the procedure properly belongs within the quality management system of a purchasing company, the example is endorsed with the corporate logo of the imaginary enterprise, Prudent Purchasing Inc., to emphasize this.

PRUDENT INC PURCHASING	Prudent Purchasing Inc. **OPERATIONAL PROCEDURE**	ISSUED BY NAME: H. Garston Smith DEPT: Information Services PROCESS OWNER: Software Quality Assurance Auditor	PAGE 1 OF 4
SUBJECT **AUDITING OF SOFTWARE VENDORS**	CIRCULATED TO:	CHECKED BY: (A. Manager)	REF.NO. SOP001
		APPROVED BY: (A. Senior-Manager)	DATE ISSUED January 1997
		CANCELS ISSUE OF July 1996	

1. Document Control

File reference: d:\office Documents\standards and procedures\AUDIVEND.DOC

Security: No special restrictions

Distribution:

Acknowledgments:

1.1 Document History

Issue	Date	Author(s)	Comments
1st version	11 April 1995	H. Garston Smith	Superseded
2nd version	24 July 1996	H. Garston Smith	Superseded
3rd version	1 January 1997	H. Garston Smith	Current

Related Procedures

1.2 Changes History

2nd version: Re-definition of responsibilities; clarification of implications of Conditional status; clarification of scope; addition of creditworthiness enquiries; updating of logo.
3rd version: addition of specific check for Year 2000 compliance

1.3 Changes Forecast

None

	Prudent Purchasing Inc	PAGE 2 of 4
PRUDENT INC PURCHASING	**OPERATIONAL PROCEDURE:** **AUDITING OF SOFTWARE** **VENDORS**	SOP001

Principle

The assurance of quality in software of whatever origin is an essential activity in ensuring fitness for its intended use. The absence of the required quality constitutes an unacceptable risk to today's I.T-centred businesses. In regulated environments the assurance of software quality is also a legal requirement. This procedure describes the steps of the auditing process, owned and executed by the auditor and directed to fulfil this key business need. The standard against which the software engineering process is assessed is that defined by ISO 9000-3, known as the TickIT standard. Useful supplementary guidance is also available in the GAMP 96 Supplier Guide for Validation of Automated Systems in Pharmaceutical Manufacture, published by UK Pharmaceutical Industry Computer Systems Validation Forum under the auspices of the ISPE, ABPI and IQA, second edition, May 1996.

Scope

This procedure is applicable to all software, regardless of intended area of use, in the following categories:

    (i)   custom-built or bespoke software (GAMP guide 1996, category 5)

    (ii) configurable software packages (GAMP guide 1996, category 4)

    (iii) Standard software packages (GAMP guide 1996, category 3) that are not sufficiently ubiquitous to enable their innate quality to be safely inferred from their extent of market penetration alone.

Qualification

This procedure is intended to be used only by a qualified/certified Software Quality Assurance Auditor.

Responsibilities

The purchaser (sometimes a project manager) of software in any of the above categories is responsible for requesting the audit in the first instance before a final commitment to purchase is made. The auditor is responsible for ensuring the conduct of this procedure, and thus provides a service to the purchaser.

Outcomes

On completion of this procedure the supplier will be accorded one of the following ratings:

1.   Approved: all software developed by this supplier may be purchased.

2.   Conditional or Limited Approval: the existing version of the software product as audited may be purchased although no further versions will be accepted until the remedial activities specified are completed.

3.   Unapproved: the software product forming the focus of the audit may not be purchased

4 . Rejected: no software whatsoever developed by this supplier may be purchased.

	Prudent Purchasing Inc. **OPERATIONAL PROCEDURE:** **AUDITING OF SOFTWARE** **VENDORS**	PAGE 3 of 4 SOP001

Procedure

1. The process is initiated by a purchaser providing you (the auditor) with full details of the vendor, including a named contact, as well as details of the software product whose purchase is envisaged.

2. Make contact with the vendor Explain carefully the purpose of an audit, its consultancy and team-assessment nature and seek to show the vendor the mutual benefit to both organisations of the proposed exercise. This is vital. Conclude by sending to the named contact at the vendor site a summary list of the areas to be examined (*detailed in appendix 3*) to avoid any surprise, and enable the vendor site both to share any concerns in advance and to prepare themselves for a full one day visit. Arrange the visit as soon as is practicable

3. Prepare a set of worksheets to facilitate the gathering of information during the audit, from which the audit report will ultimately be compiled. (These are simply one page per section, headed with the checkpoints and with ruled space beneath for making notes.)

4. Meanwhile make discrete enquiries regarding the financial health of the company to be audited, to ensure its creditworthiness and financial viability, factors which must be mentioned in the audit report.

5. Conduct the audit in a courteous and positive manner, making every effort to inculcate a team approach with the vendor site management, with a view to establishing a long-term business partnership through the purchase of software. Any tendency for the audit process to degenerate into a 'police action' constitutes a major failure in this respect. The assignment of the rating rests on the production of demonstrable evidence of the structural integrity of the software product and its fitness for use, rather than absolute perfection, together with the general software engineering standards and disciplines adopted at the site.

6. Use the worksheets during the audit to ensure that all the points detailed that are relevant for the particular location are addressed, and that all the details are recorded.

7. At the completion of the audit, conduct a review meeting with audited site management, summarising the team's findings, any defects found and the agreed improvement actions, the recommendation (approved, conditional, unapproved or rejected) that will be made to purchasing company management.

8. If it has proved impossible to reach this stage within one working day, arrange a second day without delay to complete the process This, however, should be extremely rare

	Prudent Purchasing Inc. **OPERATIONAL PROCEDURE:** **AUDITING OF SOFTWARE VENDORS**	PAGE 4 of 4 SOP001

9. On return to base, assemble the site draft audit report on the basis of the notes accumulated on the worksheets. The report consists of three parts:

I.   A supplier abstract summary page intended for return to the vendor, that summarises the overall assessment, agreed action points, if any, and the recommendation (no more than one paragraph each)

II. A summary page, which summarises the main findings and recommendations (no more than one page).

III. The detailed findings, assessment, agreed action points and recommended status.

10. Distribute (manually or electronically) the site draft report to other member(s) of the audit team, if any, and to the purchaser, to serve as a preliminary notice of the audit findings, to facilitate any factual or textual corrections, and to explore the possible implications of the report.

11. After any corrections have been made, issue an executive draft report (manually or electronically-this is the final version but without the assignment of the Official Status) to the Senior Manager charged within the organisation with the responsibility of assigning official status to audit recommendations (normally the head of the organisation). On confirmation of acceptance of the recommendation, endorse the executive draft, so converting it into the final report.

12. Distribute (manually or electronically) the final report, carrying the Official Status, to everyone with an interest in the software purchase, including the individual responsible for maintaining the library of software quality assurance reports.

13. Finally send a copy of the supplier abstract page to the audited site, under cover of a courteous letter of thanks.

14. Follow up with the vendor any agreed actions endorsed by the Official Status within the agreed timetable

15. Management will withhold approval of any software purchase contravening the terms and conditions endorsed in the relevant audit report, and reserve the right to specify conditions as to its use (e.g., confinement to a local, non-network PC).

(End of procedure)

Appendix 2

A Vendor
Screening Checklist

The following list of closed questions may be submitted to a vendor in the early days of market research by a purchasing company. It requires only a minimum of effort on the part of a vendor to complete the document. Its usefulness to a prospective purchaser is limited by the closed nature of the questions and amounts only to the roughest of guides as to whether the vendor has any life cycle methodology or not. It can be used to superficially discriminate between possible vendors on quality grounds, but on no account should it be used as a substitute for a full, in-depth team-based assessment.

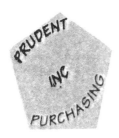

Quality Questionnaire for Software Vendors

Please answer Yes or No by a tick (✓) in the boxes provided.

		Yes	No
1.	Does your company have certification to any recognized international standards?	☐	☐
2.	Do you have a written project management system, including the definition of responsibilities within projects?	☐	☐
3.	Do you have a separate and independent quality assurance individual or group?	☐	☐
4.	Do you have a written quality management system describing the controls on the software engineering process?	☐	☐
5.	Is a written software development life cycle methodology in use?	☐	☐
6.	Is a written functional specification or design document a mandatory prerequisite for software development?	☐	☐
7.	Does a written programming standards guide or coding manual exist to define standards for programming?	☐	☐
8.	Is a written user requirements document a mandatory prerequisite for all projects?	☐	☐
9.	Are structured test plans produced in advance of testing?	☐	☐
10.	Are the testing personnel independent of the development personnel?	☐	☐

11. Are test results recorded and retained?   ☐   ☐

12. Is a written formal change control system for
    software and documents in operation?   ☐   ☐

13. Are formal written backup and contingency
    procedures in place?   ☐   ☐

Signed: _____ Date: _____

For: _____ (Name of Vendor)

Appendix 3

Software Quality Assurance Auditor's Worksheets

The attached set of worksheets comprise an example of the documentation which an auditor might use in leading a team-based audit assessment with representatives of the vendor's development team, and on which the results may be recorded. The headings of the sections correspond exactly both to those of the audit scope document sent by the auditor to the vendor in advance of the audit, and to the headings of the final report, the deliverable from the process. Once again, the frontispiece is endorsed with the purchaser's corporate logo, which I have represented as Prudent Purchasing Inc., to emphasise the auditor's function as a representative of the ultimate customer in whose interests the assessment was initiated.

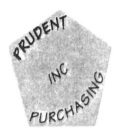

Software Quality Assurance Audit

AUDITOR'S WORKSHEETS

Assigned Audit Reference Number: _____

Vendor's name: _____

Vendor's location address: _____

_____

Date of audit: _____

Prudent Purchasing Inc. assessment team representatives:

_____

_____

_____

_____

Vendor's assessment team representatives:

_____

_____

_____

_____

Product and version to be audited: _____

SECTION 1: COMPANY ORGANIZATION AND PROJECT MANAGEMENT

- History

- Size

- Financial background

- Future

- Organizational structure (organigram, division of tasks and responsibilities in relation to products and their life cycle)

- Separation and independence of QA unit

- Project management and definition of responsibilities

- Project plans with assigned responsibilities; time schedules

- Is there a recognizable project life cycle in existence?

- Project development protected by change control and security measures?

_____

_____

_____

_____

_____

_____

_____

_____

_____

_____

_____

_____

SECTION 2: PRODUCTS AND THEIR SUPPORT

- Product portfolio

- For the specific product of interest:

  - number of staff working on it

  - longevity in marketplace

  - approximate number of users (relevant to likelihood of emergence of defects

  - frequency of revision (not retired, not bug-ridden or exploding, but acceptably stable, say 1–2 annually)

  - reference list of major customers

  - active user community

  - escrow agreement for source code and development tools

  - support for at least one older version

- Support mechanisms (telephone hot line, etc.)

- Licence vendor or long-term support partner?

_____

_____

_____

_____

_____

_____

_____

_____

_____

_____

_____

SECTION 3: QUALITY ASSURANCE

- What value does quality have here?

- Is quality one of the principal aims of the business?

- Does a quality culture exist?

- Written quality management system?

- Certification status, if any?

- Is quality built-in or attempts made to test it in retrospectively?

- Are formal inspection techniques with metrics (Fagan, Gilb) used as an aid to measuring and ensuring quality in the engineering process?

- Internal audits (periodicity, documentation, corrective action)

- Handling of complaints, prioritization of defect repairs, enhancements versus defect repairs (change control)

_____

_____

_____

_____

_____

_____

_____

_____

_____

_____

_____

_____

_____

SECTION 4: SOFTWARE DEVELOPMENT—STAFF

- Programmers' training (records, effectiveness, internal and external)

- Investors in People or similar program?

- Average longevity of stay

- Is there a coding manual or programming standards guide, code dictionary or style manual?

_____

_____

_____

_____

_____

_____

_____

_____

_____

_____

_____

_____

_____

_____

_____

_____

_____

_____

_____

SECTION 5: SOFTWARE DEVELOPMENT—DESIGN

- Details of the software development life cycle being used

- Development tools (CASE, Rapid Application Development, etc.) in use?

- Is the need for traceability throughout the development process recognized?

- Is the design reviewed against the functional requirements for suitability, traceability and testability?

- Do records of such a review exist, and were the acceptance criteria predefined?

- Evidence of accuracy control of all system comparison standards, formulae, decision rules and assignment criteria (recognised published source information; authority review for all decision rules; regular management review of documentation of all source code accuracy standards)

- Is there a sign-off for design reparations, re-review and acceptance?

- Is the approved design subject to change control and audit trail?

- Is the impact of proposed changes on other systems assessed?

_____

_____

_____

_____

_____

_____

_____

_____

_____

SECTION 6: SOFTWARE DEVELOPMENT—PRACTICES

- Programming standards:

    - header information (program name, description, when developed, by whom, input/output, use of library calls, interfaces, revision control, etc.)

    - how variables and registers are named

    - how the code is optimally structured (use of indentation to indicate loops & subs; use of labels; use of matching "if . . . then . . . else" or equivalent, chronological, process order, option menu or alternative logical sequencing; separation into modules; well-controlled integration of standardized or third party code)

    - secure error entrapment strategies (internal syntax error detection; internal audit trail procedure; internal logical error detection; avoidance of program termination in undefined states; noncritical error correction procedure through revisions & updates; critical error correction through immediate user notification)

    - how function keys are assigned uniformly

    - how menus, screen masks, and reports are structured

    - how HELP texts are structured

    - which program libraries are used

- Do SOPs exist defining all of these?

_____

_____

_____

_____

_____

_____

_____

SECTION 7: SOFTWARE DEVELOPMENT—TESTING

- Does a structured test plan exist (test case 1, test goal 1, test procedure 1, test data 1, test execution 1, expected results 1, documentation method 1, . . . test case 2 . . . test case n)

- Is there a formal test plan review by a second person?

- Is the test plan traceable back to the functional requirements?

- Are the tests structured in phases (module, interfaces between modules, the overall system in terms of cooperation between modules, the tests of the application limits by proven acceptable range)?

- Have the error message routines been tested, and are they informative and unambiguous?

- Are (automated) test tools used?

- Are the testers independent from the developers?

- Does the vendor provide validation support to purchasers?

_____

_____

_____

_____

_____

_____

_____

_____

_____

_____

_____

_____

SECTION 8: DOCUMENTATION PRACTICES

- Is there a clear description of how the individual documents from the different development phases link together and of what they contain?

- Does the assembled documentation cover the entire SDLC? It should at the very least include the following:

    - user requirements specification

    - system design

    - source code

    - installation document

    - user's documentation

- Does each document

    - have a contents list or summary?

    - have a revision code and issue date?

    - have an approval signature and a description of the approver's responsibility (e.g., qualified to review)?

    - have a QA review and signature?

- Are the meanings of the respective signatures defined in the QA policy?

- Is there a document change control system in operation in terms of

    - who is authorized to make changes to which documents

    - who is in charge of technical control of such changes

    - who checks the quality

    - who implements the changes

    - who coordinates document changes and software changes

- Is there a standard for SOPs (itself an SOP, defining for what processes SOPs should be written, and how an SOP should be formatted)?

_____

_____

_____

_____

_____

_____

_____

_____

_____

_____

_____

_____

_____

_____

_____

_____

_____

_____

_____

_____

_____

_____

_____

_____

_____

_____

_____

_____

SECTION 9: CHANGE CONTROL AND ARCHIVAL PRACTICES

- Does a written change control policy exist?

- Does a software version control policy exist? It should define the following:

    - what constitutes a major release

    - what constitutes a minor release

    - what constitutes an emergency release

    - how coordination of all documentation changes is achieved and how traceability is maintained

- Does a security policy exist regarding unauthorized access or changes to source code? Does it actually work in practice?

- Have archival policies been defined? Are they being followed? Where are obsolete records retained? For how long? On stable media?

_____

_____

_____

_____

_____

_____

_____

_____

_____

_____

_____

_____

SECTION 10: THE DEVELOPMENT ENVIRONMENT

- Hardware standard operating procedures

- Hardware environment (cleanliness, housekeeping, change control records, etc.)

- Backup and contingency policies and practices:
    - disaster recovery plan
    - regular drills, with records
    - fire and flood protection
    - maintenance agreements in effect

- Virus protection measures; signature updates

- Year 2000 compliance

- Purchased software:
    - Licence agreements in effect
    - Maintenance agreements in effect

- Physical security is adequate and under regular review

_____

_____

_____

_____

_____

_____

_____

_____

_____

_____

SECTION 11: VERSION–SPECIFIC CHECKLIST

• Make sure that the following inspection points have examined records appertaining to the specific version of the software about to be purchased:

- that its source code complies with the general standards and practices relating to programming

- that its change control is being managed in accordance with the generally applied standards

- that its testing records exist and meet the generally applied standards

- that traceability back through design to user requirements has been duly maintained through adequate application of change control disciplines

- that a user training program exists and has been maintained under overall change control

_____

_____

_____

_____

_____

_____

_____

_____

_____

_____

_____

_____

SECTION 12: POST–AUDIT FOLLOW–UP

- Vendor's commitment to address outstanding issues:
  - detail the issues
  - agree on a timetable
  - agree on the nature of the follow-up arrangements to review progress

_____

_____

_____

_____

_____

_____

_____

_____

_____

_____

_____

_____

_____

_____

_____

_____

_____

_____

_____

_____

Appendix 4

A Specimen Vendor Assessment (Audit) Report

In this appendix, the reader will find a specimen report included to illustrate the scope and depth of the final deliverable that the process described in this book is capable of generating. The report is, of course, totally fictitious, emphasized by the use of our familiar vendor name Stupendous Software Inc., but has been assembled to simulate the kind of data which should have been gleaned through working with members of the vendor's programming staff in a team context. It illustrates the depth of insight into what lies beneath the seductive allure of the glossy brochure which a prospective purchaser of a software product can obtain through commissioning an audit assessment along these lines.

This example report also demonstrates the value of the process to the vendor. The strengths and weaknesses identified in the process, with the help of a visitor experienced in exploring quality management systems in a number of other organizations, offer a springboard for a raft of cost-effective improvements. These, if implemented fully, make possible better cost and budget control in most companies, as well as a lower level of residual defects in released product. These gains more than recompense the additional cost of the extra QA controls or other improvement actions within a relatively short time.

The overview and summary section of the report, together with the summary list of any conditional actions, is usually formatted to occupy no more than one page. It is this page that is returned to the vendor under cover of the letter of thanks, as described in the text. Any conditional actions are also mentioned within the body of the report, on subsequent pages, in the context of their origin, thus accounting for their appearance twice in the report. Such an approach has been found to work well in practice.

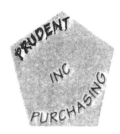

Software Quality Assurance Audit Report No. SQAA 001

FINAL REPORT

Vendor: Stupendous Software Inc.

Audited location address:

Date of audit:

Audited on behalf of:

PPI audit team:

Audit site management:

SUMMARY OF FINDINGS

Software reviewed: X-FILES Version 1.3

Overall assessment: This product has been engineered in accordance with a system of quality assur-
ance which has ensured the incorporation
of an adequate level of structural integrity.
However, there is need for improved documentation and control of cost in a number of key areas which are essential if the
vendor is to maintain software quality, improve control of the project process and
ensure continued business success.

Recommendations: A status of *Conditional* is recommended.

Distribution list

Name or Recipient	Department	PPI Location

*Note: This report contains confidential information and requires per-
sonal discretion regarding security. Inadvertent disclosure to third
parties could expose the company to legal proceedings. However,
within this framework, recipients are encouraged to share this report
with others.*

Officially Assigned Status: _____

By: _____

Date: _____

SQAA Report Author: _____

SOFTWARE QUALITY ASSURANCE AUDIT

Stupendous Software Inc.

(date)

Conducted on behalf of the
(*name of purchasing department*)

OVERVIEW AND SUMMARY

Stupendous Software Inc. (SSI) has been developing its own software for about three years, using a written quality management system (QMS) which provides the major disciplines of a formal life cycle. The QMS is surprisingly good for a company so young. This is rather unusual and is a great credit to the organization. As a result, there is evidence of the incorporation of an adequate level of structural integrity within the software already produced.

There are, however, a number of aspects of the company's procedures which are poorly documented. These have reflected and perhaps exacerbated a lack of clarity of the company's identity as a software developer (between bespoke and package developments which rest on different financial models). An unacceptable level of cost and a lack of focus on the company's strategic interests have already been evident. Remedy of these shortcomings through improvements to the QMS and elsewhere will immediately strengthen the company's ability to produce and maintain high quality software on time and within budget, contribute to customer satisfaction on the basis of realistic customer expectations, and improve the prospects for the company's prosperity in the medium term. Meeting these conditions will also go a long way toward achieving ISO 9000-3 compliance in practice and pave the way to eventual certification if and when required.

The recommendation is being made, therefore, to accord this vendor a status of Conditional, the 10 conditions being as follows:

Condition #1:   A written project life cycle document appropriate for both traditional and object-oriented software projects, clearly defining the point of release and distinguishing development practices from maintenance practices, is required.

Condition #2:   The Design Standards procedure requires amendment to specify an independent review of designs, including approval or quality assurance signature and date.

Condition #3:   A written procedure for the formal assessment of the impact of changes in one product on others is required.

Condition #4:   Programming standards require modification to include a definition of specific strategies to avoid logical errors.

Condition #5:   A Quality Procedure defining SSI's approach to software testing, including test plan traceability, the testing of error routines by contrivance and verification of error message text clarity and freedom from ambiguity, is required.

Condition #6:   A written description of the software development life cycle, the documents it delivers and how they link together is required.

Condition #7:   The chief executive should endorse the company's quality-oriented Mission Statement and Quality Policy by formally assigning responsibility for quality assurance to a competent named individual.

Condition #8:   The Quality Assurance Policy should mandate a Quality Assurance Review, signature and date for all life cycle documents.

Condition #9:   A written software version control policy is required.

Condition #10:   A written disaster recovery plan specifying regular drills is required.

COMPANY ORGANIZATION AND PROJECT MANAGEMENT

SSI was founded in late 1992 as Tremendous Software (the name being changed in 1993) by Otis B. Driftwood to support and maintain the W-Files Laboratory Information Management System (LIMS). The company has developed this product into the X-FILES LIMS System, a mid-range laboratory system applicable to any analytical laboratory.

In 1994, the company extended its activities to become the exclusive distributor in the United Kingdom and Eire for the Y-Files software products of Y-Files Software (based in the United States) of interest primarily in the pharmaceutical business sector. Its experience in first-hand software development has, therefore, been quite limited until relatively recently, when it has produced its own product, X-FILES, designed to log and track enquiries in a medical quality control context and to generate standard reports.

The company has enjoyed a successful track record selling the software on behalf of other companies, becoming the leading distributor of Y-Files and dedicating itself to a number of the leading companies in the Fortune 500 league table. The applications for its products has widened to include forensic and other specialized laboratories. Its guiding principle has been only to market those systems which can be supported in-house. Turnover reached £10 million in 1995 and staff complement has now increased by 4 on the 1995 figure to 28.

The company has established partnership arrangements with other companies and also Stretchford University, employing postgraduate staff in software development. Growth has now outpaced the available space at its premises, which it owns, and new offices are being sought to accommodate a total of up to 40 staff, expected within the next year or two. The company's policy is now to recruit only graduates for all positions except secretarial support. The company has taken steps to join the Investors in People scheme.

The company sees its future as a integrator of LIMS and data acquisition systems rather than just a bespoke software house, licensing software products from other suppliers. The range of industries needing this type of products is huge.

Independent financial references indicate that the company is likely to be trading at a profit of about £150,000 (the company is exempt from being obliged to file a profit and loss account) on its stated turnover of £10 million. Its risk category is low normal, and there is no record of any public information of an uncomplimentary nature.

An organizational structure diagram was presented for inspection. All seven software development staff have job descriptions detailing their responsibilities in the context of software development projects.

The company has not officially designated anyone as responsible for quality assurance, a shortcoming that must be rectified at once. This responsibility is actually carried out at present by the head of Software Development. Independent software testing is carried out by a member of the Technical Support Unit.

Project plans are drawn up for each software engineer using *Prestige Project* version 4, showing activities against time and the deliverables expected. The progress review procedure is documented in the Quality Management System Standards, version 1.00 dated 20 May 1996. A progress form stipulated by the procedure is used to record the results of this review.

GANTT charts are used to assign responsibilities and plot time schedules as part of the project management process. Although a project life cycle could be discerned, it has not been documented. This failure has contributed to the difficulties already mentioned regarding the cutoff point between release and maintenance stages. This requires rectification at once. The project life cycle needs to accommodate the special aspects of object-oriented design.

> *Condition #1: A written project life cycle document appropriate for both traditional and object-oriented software projects, clearly defining the point of release and distinguishing development practices from maintenance practices, is required.*

PRODUCTS AND THEIR SUPPORT

The company sells four products in addition to X-FILES:

- Y-Files, a top-end laboratory information management system

- A-Files, a laboratory data acquisition system

Within these products, two third-party components are used:

- C-Files, a generic database

- D-Files, an object-oriented text retrieval software for indexing a relational database system

X-FILES has three people actively maintaining it and was originally conceived in 1994. The first prototype was delivered in March 1994. The following year, the product was overhauled completely with a much more open and flexible architecture, resulting in the release of version 1.0 in September 1995. No less than four further versions have been released since then.

Closer examination of this worrying scenario of exploding functionality revealed that most of the changes triggering the release of each version have been enhancements rather than defect repairs, indicating a lack of clarity in definition of the requirements early in the life cycle. Indeed, it has revealed some confusion of identity within SSI over whether it sees itself as a bespoke software house or a supplier of packages. While the company's efforts to meet the requirements of customers is laudable, the company has only recently begun to understand the financial implications of this confused thinking. There is an urgent need to clarify the cutoff point between development and release and to define and distinguish the policies and practices in the **development** phase from those in the **maintenance** phase, especially in relation to customer-initiated enhancement requests. The life cycle requires strengthening in this respect.

X-FILES has only 35 users spread over 4 or 5 pharmaceutical houses and a welding institute. This is far too small for an active user community to form. Because of the unsatisfactory requirements explosion situation, the company is seeking to migrate every user to the current version and cease support for its predecessors, and is wise to do so. The company is anxious to be seen as a long-term support partner to its customers.

QUALITY ASSURANCE

Although SSI has only been developing its own software for two years, it has done so from the start in accordance with a written QMS established by the head of development at the outset. This is a great strength and is supported by the company's Mission Statement which is totally customer-focussed. The QMS is continually being enhanced under a vigorous quality culture supported from the top. Each procedure within the QMS is version numbered, dated with the author's name and storage filename. It contains a written Quality Policy (version 1.00 dated 20 March 1995). The company recognizes the value of ISO 9000-3 (TickIT) compliance immediately and hopes one day to apply for certification when market conditions demand it.

The QMS ensures quality is built into software by means of the project process charts and a Quality Plan drawn up at the commencement of a project, detailing exactly how the software will be quality assured during development. Peer reviews of code are conducted in accordance with Code Review procedure version 1.00 dated 20 May 1996, with a form being used to record the results. An annual review of the working of the QMS takes place.

The Configuration Management Procedure version 2.00 dated 7 April 1995 describes the use of the Software Performance Report, which is filled in by customers needing to log defects or request enhancements. Following this, a Software Modification Notice is drawn up detailing the corrective action to be taken. Each series of forms is uniquely numbered and cross-referenced with traceability logs on each. Furthermore, a Future Release form is kept describing in full the defect repairs and enhancements incorporated into each release.

A standard for Standard Operating Procedures has been issued (Document Standards version 2.00 dated 7 April 1995).

SOFTWARE DEVELOPMENT: STAFF

Detailed records are kept of the training both on-the-job by experience and via formal courses both internal and external. Pretraining briefing forms are used to define and clarify training needs. Post-training briefing forms are used to evaluate training and ensure that the company is receiving the financial benefits in terms of skills and competencies that the training was intended to deliver.

The head of development and the senior programmer have been with the company 1.5 years and 2.5 years, respectively. The remaining 3 staff have joined more recently, and 2 are students whom the company hopes to recruit permanently in the foreseeable future.

Programmers' Style Guides have been drawn up for each of the three languages used at SSI: Visual Basic (version 1.00 dated 5 June 1995), C++ (version d.01 dated 1 November 1995) and C (draft.01

dated 18 April 1995). These latter documents which purport to be drafts are now well established and should be reissued as final documents within the QMS.

SOFTWARE DEVELOPMENT: DESIGN

SSADM is in use as a CASE tool, although the company is beginning to make use of the Rational Rose tool in object-oriented software development.

The need for traceability has only been partially understood. A single Test Specification and User Requirements document was drawn up for X-FILES, which effectively achieved traceability but did not serve the purpose of a test record with boxes to confirm compliance and noncompliance, as was used in other software testing.

Designs are reviewed against the functional requirements for suitability and testability. The design specification for X-FILES (version 1.0 dated 14 February 1995) was inspected. It had been reviewed by the senior programmer, but this was not recorded. There should be a formal procedure with sign-offs for the critical stage of design review on which so much cost and risk hang.

> *Condition #2: The Design Standards procedure requires amendment to specify an independent review of designs, including approval or quality assurance signature and date.*

Designs are subject to change control and an audit trail record of changes is maintained. Although the importance of assessing the impact of changes in one product on others in SSI's portfolio was acknowledged, there was no formal procedure for ensuring this was done.

> *Condition #3: a written procedure for the formal assessment of the impact of changes in one product on others is required.*

SOFTWARE DEVELOPMENT: PRACTICES

The C programming standards were reviewed in detail. They specified the inclusion of header information (program name, description, when developed, by whom, and revision control), how variables were to be named (the Hungarian notation for Windows™ Programs), and guidance on the structuring of code and the use of indentation. The standards were deficient in not defining any error entrapment strategies, or precautions for ensuring programs do not enter undefined states.

> *Condition #4: Programming standards require modification to include a definition of specific strategies to avoid logical errors.*

Windows™ standards are used for ancillary program features, such as how function keys are assigned and how menus and screen layouts are structured. The *Expert* text authoring tool is used to assemble help text. The *Really Useful Objects* Library is used extensively.

SOFTWARE DEVELOPMENT: TESTING

Structured test plans are created for software, though more formal methods to ensure traceability back to design and requirements are needed. Test plans are reviewed by a second person, though this is not recorded. In fact, there is no formal procedure within the QMS defining SSI's approach to testing. This must be provided and should include the testing of the clarity and freedom from ambiguity of error message text.

> *Condition #5: A Quality Procedure defining SSI's approach to software testing, including test plan traceability, the testing of error routines by contrivance and verification of error message text clarity and freedom from ambiguity is required.*

Automated test tools have not been used, though their use in the future is not precluded. Independent testing is carried out by Technical Support Group personnel.

DOCUMENTATION PRACTICES

Although the QMS is quite comprehensive, it carries no description of the software life cycle model in use and how the documents from the different phases link together.

Condition #6: A written description of the software development life cycle, the documents it delivers and how they link together is required.

The assembled documentation covers the development life cycle and includes a combined requirements and test plan document, a design document, source code, an installation document and a user's manual. Each document carries a contents list or summary, a revision code and an issue date. However, there is no approver's signature, or a quality assurance signature. In fact, although the head of development has assumed responsibility for quality assurance, the company has not substantiated its customer-focussed mission statement by officially assigning the quality assurance responsibility to anyone!

Condition #7: The chief executive should endorse the company's quality-oriented Mission Statement and Quality Policy by formally assigning responsibility for Quality Assurance to a competent named individual.

Condition #8: The Quality Assurance Policy should mandate a Quality Assurance Review, signature and date for all life cycle documents.

The document change control system defines who is authorized to make changes to which documents and who is in charge of their technical content. There is no definition of who checks the quality, but this will be met by condition #8.

CHANGE CONTROL AND ARCHIVAL PRACTICES

The Change Control Procedure is featured in the Configuration Management document mentioned earlier, and plenty of evidence was available to demonstrate its effectual working. However, when software version numbering was reviewed, there was no document describing SSI's approach to version control, defining what is meant by a major release, a minor release, an emergency release, or the meaning of the numbering nomenclature in use.

Condition #9: A written software version control policy is required.

Unauthorized access to source code has been prevented hitherto by the use of the security provisions of Netware. However,

Source Files VerySafe is now to be used, affording a greater level of protection and ensuring good standards of source code documentation and allocation are imposed.

No archival policies have yet evolved at SSI since the company has not yet had to address this issue. It is not likely to arise in the immediate future.

THE DEVELOPMENT ENVIRONMENT

A tour was made of the building which, though well kept and clean, was now patently too small for the business and is up for sale. As a result of a recent burglary quite a lot of vandalized equipment was being retained for insurance disposal. However, in the main, it was clear that the hardware on which software development is conducted was being maintained, and was now mostly brand new.

The servers are backed up nightly. The written procedure (version 1.03 dated October 1994) defining this was inspected, but did not make clear exactly what was being backed up and when; this information is held in the *Tape Backup System* definition files. Tapes are removed off-site daily for storage. The logbook indicating that backup is being done was inspected, and was found to be up-to-date, with records going back many months.

A risk assessment team meets regularly, a pertinent precaution since in recent months the premises suffered burglary and is thought likely to suffer again. However, more serious contingencies, such as total loss of all data, do not appear to have been imagined in detail, and a disaster recovery plan covering what will happen in major imaginable contingencies, with regular drills, is required.

Condition #10: A written disaster recovery plan specifying regular drills is required.

All disks arriving on site are checked for virus infection using *SuperVirus Software* with up-to-date virus signatures.

Physical security is as good as can be expected. Windows are double glazed and locked, and the front door is double deadlocked, with alarm lines to the police station. The isolated location of the building is a disadvantage, which will only be overcome by a move.

Licences are held for all purchased software. Illegal piracy inhouse is a dismissable offense defined in the Personnel Handbook.

VERSION–SPECIFIC CHECKS

The X-FILES version 1.3 suite of source files was reviewed, and a sample file XFLDLL.C was selected by the auditor at random from the list to ensure conformity of source code to inspected standards. This file, a definition source file for the XFLAYER.DLL dynamic link library, was well laid out. It carried comprehensive header information of author, date, description and version number. There was also a full audit list of about a dozen previous changes, each annotated with version number. The same number appeared in comment at the point in the file where the change has occurred. These changes could be traced back to the software modification notes incorporated in the Change Control System. Each paragraph was preceded by comment and a small subheader. Indentation conformed with standards.

No test records have been retained for X-FILES, though consideration will be given to their retention in the future for retrospective audit purposes. A comprehensive user training program is available either at SSI headquarters or at client sites. It includes training material and course notes.

POST–AUDIT FOLLOW–UP

The vendor has undertaken to implement the improvement actions within three months.

Appendix 5

Standard Operating Procedure Template

If standard operating procedures are to be instantly recognizable as such, and to conform with internal standards regarding layout, content and document control, they must be written in accordance with an approved format. The following example, identified with the company logo (Stupendous Software Inc.), emphasizes once more that the layout and content must spring from within the company's culture and must express it, rather than being the imposition of an external format, foreign to the assumptions and conventions accepted generally by the members of the company team.

	Stupendous Software Incorporated **OPERATIONAL PROCEDURE**		ISSUED BY	PAGE
			NAME	OF
			DEPARTMENT	
SUBJECT		CIRCULATED TO:	CHECKED BY	REF.NO.
			APPROVED BY	DATE ISSUED
			CANCELS ISSUE OF	

1. Document Control

File reference:

Security:

Distribution:

Acknowledgments:

1.1 Document History

Issue	Date	Author(s)	Comments

Related Procedures

1.2 Changes History

1.3 Changes Forecast

	Stupendous Software Incorporated **OPERATIONAL PROCEDURE:**	PAGE of

Principle

Scope

Procedure

1.

2.

3.

4.

5.

Appendix 6

Specimen Implied Structural Integrity Certificate

Certificate No:

Implied Structural Integrity Certificate

Microsoft Access® Version 2.0

Access® is a Windows™-based relational database management software package developed by Microsoft. Version 2.0 was released into the market in April 1994. Prior versions included 1.0, which was released in December 1992, and 1.1, released in April 1993. Over one million copies of all versions of Access® have been sold. No serious defects have been reported to date on version 2.0. Based, therefore, on its successful market history, and the large user base, the Structural Integrity of Microsoft Access® version 2.0 is considered acceptable.

CAUTION

Only limited information is available on software packages when a software quality assurance audit has not been conducted. Information such as development standards, procedures, and change control cannot be determined without such audits. As a quality assurance audit was not conducted on this software, the acceptability of the Implied Structural Integrity applies only to the version specified. Those wishing to use successive versions should contact Central Quality Assurance Audit for further information.

Issued by: _____

Approved by: _____

Date: _____

Appendix 7

Test Results Log

Test Log Identification:

Source code, file, or module under test:

Version number:

Other configuration management information:

Test environment:	Hardware:

Procedure	Result	Other Observations	Failure Report #	Tested By	Date

Appendix 8

Test Failure Report

Failure Report Number:

Source code, file, or module under test:
Version number:
Other configuration management information:
Tested by: Date:

Test environment:	Hardware:

Expected results:	Actual results:

Other anomalous observations:

Follow-up action (process improvement implications, if any):

Appendix 9

Skill Needs Profile

SKILL NEEDS PROFILE

Page 1 of 3
Document Reference:
Revision:
Date:
Supersedes:

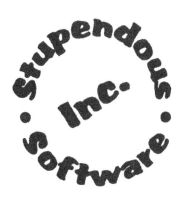

Job Title:
Management Group:
Location:
Main Purpose of the Job: (A concise single-sentence statement of the achievement the incumbent is paid to deliver).

SKILL NEEDS PROFILE (page 2 of 3)

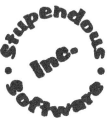

Academic, Technical and Professional Qualifications:

Essential:

Desirable:

Work Experience and Skills:

Essential:

Desirable:

Personal Qualities: (e.g., communication, teamwork, assertiveness, perfectionism, calmness, maturity, decisiveness).

SKILL NEEDS PROFILE (page 3 of 3)

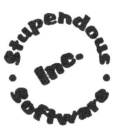

Health Considerations:

Training To Be Offered:

Interview and Other Details:

Issued by:

_____   _____
Name   Date

Appendix 10

Vendor Quality Assurance/Life Cycle Enquiries

In appendix 2, a vendor screening checklist for the initial and rather superficial assessment of the quality of a vendor's process was provided. In this document, a much deeper and more searching set of enquiries is set out, avoiding the closed questions which characterized the earlier one. Consequently, this questionnaire requires much more effort to complete than the other, and should be used when there is a greater seriousness of intent to place business with a company, short of undertaking a formal audit assessment exercise. This document could be used to discriminate between two possible vendors, both with apparently mature quality management systems, as a preparation for a full audit visit to the favoured candidate.

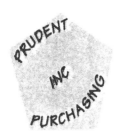

Software Procurement

QUALITY ASSURANCE AND
LIFE CYCLE METHODOLOGY ENQUIRIES

1. In what ways do you attempt to build quality into your software, rather than trying to test it in retrospectively?

2. Do you have a written quality management system to control the development process, and, if so, what procedures does it contain?

3. Do you use a life cycle methodology to develop software, and, if so, which model is followed and what documents does it deliver?

4. How do you handle complaints, and how do you prioritize defect repairs and enhancement requests?

5. Do you have a set standard layout in-house for your standard operating procedures in connection with software development? Can you send us some examples of procedures?

6. Do your programmers have a coding manual or style guide to work from when writing code? If so, which of the following categories does it cover:

    •   Header information (program name, description, when developed, by whom, input/output, use of library calls, interfaces, revision control, etc.)

    •   How variables are named

    •   How the code is structured (use of indentation to indicate loops & subs; use of labels; use of matching *if . . . then . . . else* or equivalent, chronological, process order, option menu or alternative logical sequencing; separation into modules; well-controlled integration of standardized or third party code)

- Secure error entrapment strategies (internal syntax error detection; internal audit trail procedure; internal logical error detection; avoidance of program termination in undefined states; noncritical error correction procedure through revisions & updates; critical error correction through immediate user notification)

- How function keys are assigned uniformly

- How menus, screen masks, and reports are structured

- How HELP text is structured

- Which program libraries are to be used

7. How do you ensure projects deliver software of the expected quality on time and within budget? What sort of project management disciplines do you use?

8. How do you ensure traceability from requirements, through design, through code, to test plans?

9. Do you have a procedure for reviewing designs against the requirements for suitability, traceability and testability?

10. How do you control changes to designs after they have been initially approved?

11. Do you draw up structured test plans, and, if so, what do they contain?

12. Are your test plans reviewed by a second person before being put to use?

13. How is testing carried out, and by whom (e.g., are the testers *independent* of the developers?)

14. Do you test error message routines? Do you use any automated test tools?

15. Do you have a written quality assurance policy (describing what your company's approach to quality is and how quality is to be achieved)?

16. Do you have a document change control system (e.g., describing who is authorized to make changes to which documents, who is in charge of technical control of such changes, who checks the quality, who implements the changes, who coordinates document changes and software changes)?

17. Do you have a written change control policy (how you police changes to your products)?

18. How do you control access to your source code?

19. Do you have a formal procedure for backing up your systems? If so, is it *documented*? If so, is it *actually followed*? How do you *know* this?

20. Do you have a written disaster recovery plan for your company (e.g., will you still be in business tomorrow if your premises burn down tonight . . .)? Is it up-to-date?

21. How secure are your premises and key business resources from theft?

22. What measures do you adopt to make sure your company procedures and standards are being followed (e.g., internal audits, etc.)?

Appendix 11

Sample Job
Description Template

Job Title:

Division: **Department:**

Present Holder: **Reports to:**

_____

Main Purpose of the Job: (One or two short paragraphs summarising the main purpose of the job)

Regular Duties: (Bullet points/numbers identifying specific tasks assigned to this position)

Responsibility: (Equipment, staff, and budgets. Special mention must be made where there is a responsibility for initiating and/or implementing staff training)

Personal Responsibility: (Specifically those aspects of the job which the job holder must perform personally)

Special Relationships: (Specify those to whom the job holder will have special contact)

Authority: (State what authority is delegated and what limits are imposed)

Education and Prior Work Experience Required:

Essential:

Ideal:

Departmental and Other Relationships:
(draw an organization chart showing job titles of superior, colleague, and subordinate positions, with numbers in the latter case)

_____	_____	_____
Job Holder	Manager	Department Head/Director
_____	_____	_____
Date	Date	Date

Appendix 12

The BuyIT Guidelines—
A Summary[1]

1. Planning business benefits

- Focus on business benefits, not technology.

- Plan to achieve measurable improvements.

- Don't leave it to professionals; the body responsible for delivering the business benefits should control the project.

- Plan sufficient resources for training.

- Review projects to confirm that expected benefits are being realized.

2. Identifying business requirement

- Insist on clear definitions of needs and benefits.

- Ensure end users are involved, committed and trained.

- Look beyond incremental changes; consider new ways of working.

3. Evaluate sourcing options

- The packaged solution should normally be the preferred option.

- If bespoke, ensure the system meets a need that is worth the risk.

4. Identifying skills

- Use a dedicated team with the correct skills.

- Each project should have a board sponsor, business manager and experienced project manager.

5. Managing supplier relationship

- Consider involving supplier in defining requirements.

- Create culture of cooperation rather than confrontation.

- Consider setting up a cross-functional IT procurement team.

6. Selecting the supplier

- Allow time and resources to make the right choice.

- Do no place too much reliance on lowest price; usability, functionality and supplier capability are critical to delivering business benefits.

- Insist on proof of performance from suppliers.

7. Writing and negotiating the contract

- Specify your own requirements for important clauses in the contract.

- Use the contract to manage risks, by specifying in more detail those aspects of the system that the supplier has not adequately demonstrated.

8. Managing simpler IT projects

- Take management of simpler projects seriously; they can still go wrong.

- Peoples' reactions to changes in working patterns probably constitute the greatest area of risk.

9. Managing complex IT projects

- Ensure appropriate risk management processes are in place and rigorously used.

- Once project management methods have been agreed on; do not take shortcuts.

- Split large projects into components that can be implemented separately, generating a constant stream of business benefits.

10. Ensuring delivery of business benefits

- Delivery of benefits must remain a board priority throughout the project.

- Focus attention on measuring the business improvements.

- Allow for other benefits to emerge as the system's capabilities are understood more widely.

- Do not expect the supplier to deliver the business benefits.

- At the end of each project, conduct an independent review of the extent to which the benefits were realized and record the (painful) lessons learnt!

Notes

1. Based extensively on a news item in *Computer Weekly,* 13 June 1996.

Appendix 13

The Health Implications of Intercontinental Travel

In contrast to the reassuring advertisements of the airlines and tour operators, frequent international travel is by no means free of risk. Its effects, both physical and psychological, have received scant attention, and I am indebted to the excellent article by Lucas (1987) for some of the insights shared here.

Most travellers suffer from nothing worse than swollen feet and jet lag. It is seldom realized that 0.01 percent of air passengers suffer illness to some extent during flight, a figure that rises to 2 percent after landing. The cabin of a modern airliner is pressurized to allow passengers to breathe normally, but this pressure is considerably less than that on the ground. It usually corresponds to that at the peak of a 7000-foot mountain, meaning 25 percent less ambient oxygen and a consequential 10 percent fall in blood oxygen level. While the healthy tolerate this unscathed, those predisposed to angina or asthma assume considerable risk. Flying can precipitate latent disorders, such as heart attacks, pulmonary embolism, and breathlessness.

Airlines face the continual temptation to reduce the cabin pressure still further in the interests of fuel economy, which exacerbates the situation. In this connection, airborne infection is another hazard; cabin air is recycled for about 10 minutes prior to being refreshed, a rate that can be further reduced by the crew, giving rise to a fetid atmosphere. A robust state of health (measured perhaps by the ability to climb stairs without strain and to take a brisk walk without discomfort) is, therefore, a key requirement for the international auditor.

The hazards from the temptations of free alcohol for business class flyers present another potential threat to safety. Lucas points out that alcohol aggravates all of the physiological, physical and mental stresses of flying, from Eustachian catarrh to mental confusion and irritability. Potentiated at altitudes due to its more rapid absorption, it impairs oxygen utilization and accentuates the thirst implicit in an environment of only 2–3 percent humidity. This potentiation persists after landing, making driving even more risky. Alcohol consumption should be tempered with water or fruit juices and accompanied by food. Since trans-time zone flight also interferes with the normal rhythms of digestion, food should not be consumed merely because it is available.

Well-being in the air is promoted by observing some simple precautions:

- Get a good night's sleep before flying.

- Take a brisk walk before check-in to stimulate the circulation.

- Choose an aisle seat, then walk around the cabin once every hour, and follow some simple exercises, such as those recommended by British Airways in their in-flight magazine.

- Exercise moderation with alcohol, but in any case drink plenty of aqueous fluids.

- Wear loose, comfortable clothing, since gas in body cavities expands in the lower ambient cabin pressure. Wear comfortable shoes, or use slip-ons if they are available (some airlines provide these free of charge for business class passengers).

- Rest the feet on hand baggage to avoid constriction of circulation at the thighs.

- Take another brisk walk after landing.

- Loneliness is stressful. Call home to strengthen the sense of identity with family and loved ones, and do not be unduly taciturn in conversation because of the perceived cost; it is worth every penny both to the traveller and to the firm paying the bill.

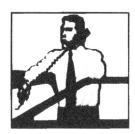

With prudence and wise preplanning, the auditor should arrive at his destination fit, unimpaired by the flight and ready to give the best to the audit assessment the next day.

Index

Printed and bound by CPI Group (UK) Ltd, Croydon, CR0 4YY

23/10/2024

01777686-0001